"A very complete compilation tha ....mmend to anyone interested in going to the Big Sur area."

—Ada Babine

Chair of the Sierra Club's Santa Barbara group
& veteran Big Sur hiker

HIKING&BACKPACKING

HIKING&BACKPACKING

BIG SUR

2ND EDITION

*Your complete guide to the trails of Big Sur,
Ventana Wilderness, and Silver Peak Wilderness*

Analise Elliot Heid

 WILDERNESS PRESS ... *on the trail since 1967*

Hiking & Backpacking Big Sur
Your complete guide to the trails of Big Sur, Ventana Wilderness, & Silver Peak Wilderness

2nd EDITION 2013
  3rd printing 2022

Copyright © 2013 by Analise Elliot Heid
The poem "Hands," by Robinson Jeffers, page 225, is copyrighted by Jeffers Literary Properties.

Front and back cover photos copyright © 2013 by Analise Elliot Heid
Interior photos by Analise Elliot Heid
Maps: Bart Wright, Fineline Maps
Cover design: Scott McGrew
Book design: Adapted by Annie Long
Book editor: Holly Cross

ISBN 978-0-89997-727-0 (pbk.); ISBN 978-0-89997-726-3 (ebook)

CATALOGING-IN-PUBLICATION DATA IS AVAILABLE FROM THE LIBRARY OF CONGRESS.

Manufactured in the United States of America

Published by: **Wilderness Press**
                  An imprint of AdventureKEEN
                  2204 First Avenue South, Suite 102
                  Birmingham, AL 35233
                  (800) 678-7006; FAX (877) 374-9016
                  www.wildernesspress.com

Visit our website for a complete listing of our books and for ordering information.

Distributed by Publishers Group West

ACKNOWLEDGMENTS

■ ■ ■ ■ ■ ■ ■ ■ ■ ■ ■ ■ ■

Foremost, I would like to thank Jeff Schaffer, author of Wilderness Press's *Hiking the Big Sur Country,* which this book replaces. I drew upon his incredibly accurate mapping and trail descriptions in writing this book.

My parents are at the head of the list of acknowledgments. Their love and support has given me the confidence to live passionately and follow my dreams. To Craig, for making my first experiences in the backcountry filled with adventure and fun. To Heid, for countless hours spent listening and encouraging. To Matt, for guidance and inspiration to go for it. To Jannie, for your willingness to stand up for what you believe in. To Laurie and Chris, for your incredible generosity. To Briezer and Wickland, whom I can always count on for an adventure. To E, for many words of advice. To Trevor, for your friendship and flexibility. To my community of friends and avid adventurers: Heart & Lissin, Hammer, Aaron, Pogen, Thomas, Isabel, Bill, and Joanne for accompanying me on unknown and overgrown trails. To Michelle and Leah, for taking the path less traveled. To Jan and Sid, for opening your home and hearts.

I wish to thank Thomas and Caroline Winnett at Wilderness Press for the opportunity to pursue professionally what I love. Thank you to David Lauterborn, who read the manuscript, contributing his knowledge and art of good writing, and to Roslyn, for picking up the pieces and guiding me through the process to completion.

A special thank-you goes to the hundreds of volunteers who built, maintained, and continue to work on the trails of the Santa Lucia Mountains. Unfortunately, the USFS has said that budgetary constraints preclude them from restoring most of the trails in the wilderness in the foreseeable future. Without the grassroots volunteer efforts of the folks at the Ventana Chapter of the Sierra Club and the Ventana Wilderness Alliance, many of the remote trails that traverse the heart of Ventana would be lost. The dedication of these volunteers to protecting and restoring the wildlands of the Big Sur coast is vital to the preservation of the rugged wilderness and biodiversity of the Northern Santa Lucia Mountains for generations to come. Without their efforts, this book would not have been possible.

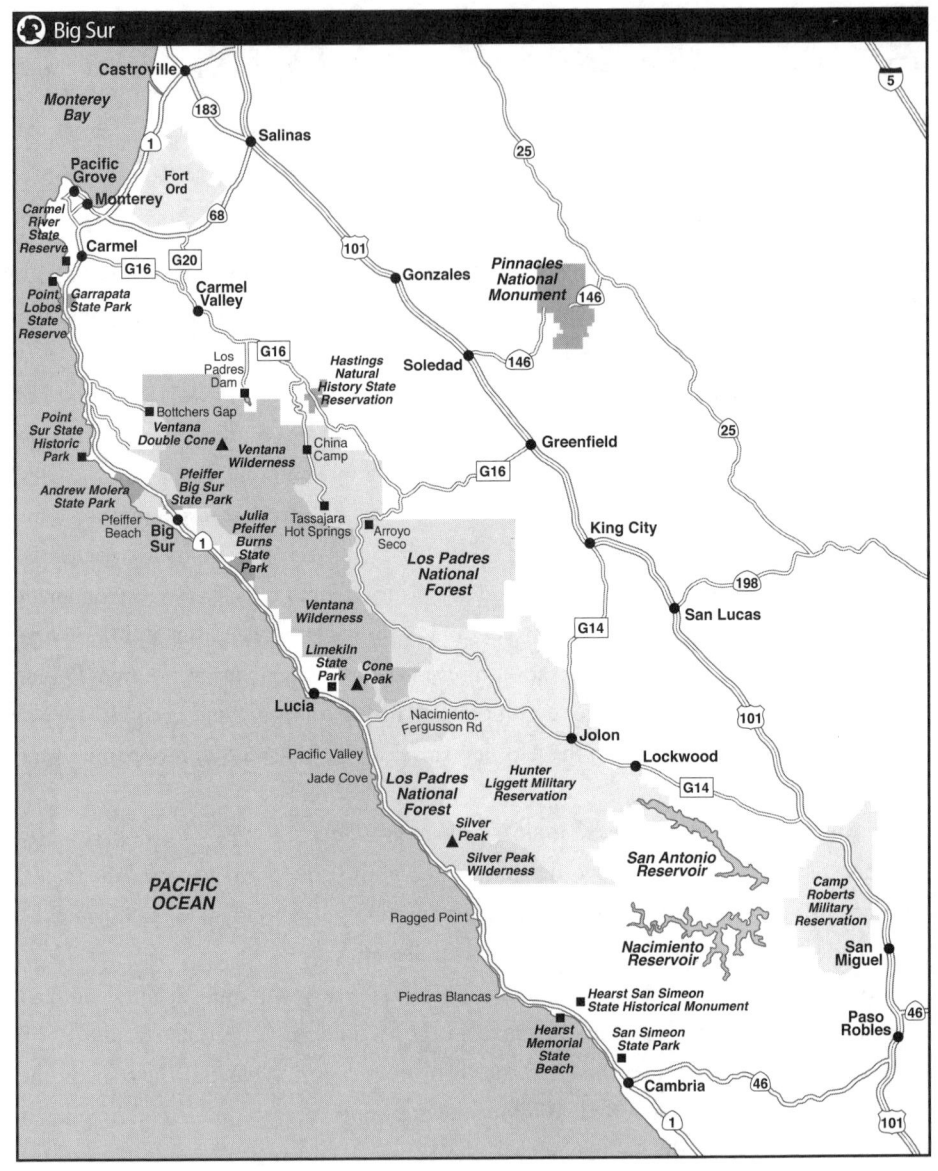

C O N T E N T S

■ ■ ■ ■ ■ ■ ■ ■ ■ ■ ■ ■ ■

PART I: State & Federal Lands of the Big Sur Coast

PART II Ventana & Silver Peak Wildernesses

Solitude overlooking a vast ocean at the edge of our continent

CHAPTER one

Introducing Big Sur

■ ■ ■ ■ ■ ■ ■ ■ ■ ■ ■ ■ ■

B IG SUR. THE NAME EVOKES IMAGES of a wild and rugged coast. In the mid-1800s, a handful of independent and adventurous homesteaders, fur traders, ranchers, and entrepreneurs settled the area along steep, narrow wagon roads. But Big Sur would remain remote until Highway 1 was completed in 1938. Modern-day visitors are struck by the drama of this two-lane roller coaster, which twists and winds through blankets of fog along sheer cliffs hundreds of feet above the Pacific.

Just where Big Sur begins and ends has long been a matter of debate. Historically, early Spanish explorers named the vague unexplored wilderness south of Monterey *El Sur Grande* ("The Big South"). Today, the region encompasses a 90-mile coastal stretch between Carmel to the north and San Simeon to the south, flanked on one side by the high peaks of the Santa Lucia Range and on the other by the jagged coast and broad Pacific Ocean.

While Big Sur is widely renowned for its exceptional beauty, few people venture beyond Highway 1. In addition, few roads cross the Santa Lucia Range, making it one of the largest roadless areas along the continental US coast. The result? A vast, remote wilderness waits to be explored.

About This Book

IN THIS BOOK, trips in Big Sur country are described in two parts: Part I, State & Federal Lands of the Big Sur Coast, and Part II, Ventana & Silver Peak Wildernesses.

Trips in Part I list day hikes only, as state and federal lands are limited to day use. While some state parks offer campgrounds, backcountry camping is forbidden. In contrast, the wilderness areas described in Part II offer more than 300 miles of trails and restricted roads to explore on either day hikes or extended backpacking treks. Each part is subdivided into chapters that list trips in geographic order from north to south.

Each trip includes summary information and the hike description itself.

Summary

Summary information for each trip includes:

TITLE The highlighted destination(s) along the route.

LENGTH AND TYPE The overall length of the hike and whether the route is out-and-back, point-to-point, or a loop. Distances to specific waypoints are listed in each hike description.

RATING This book rates each trip according to physical effort and ease of access. Ratings are as follows:

> *Easy:* Typically a short hike on level terrain with less than 500 feet of total elevation gain.
>
> *Moderate:* Hikes with a consistent medium grade with roughly 500–1000 feet of total elevation gain.
>
> *Strenuous:* Typically longer hikes with approximately 1000–2000 feet of elevation gain.
>
> *Challenging:* A very strenuous hike with roughly 2000–3000 feet of total elevation gain over many miles of steep, rugged trails in often remote regions. Wilderness experience and ethics required.

TRAIL CONDITION Many routes within the wilderness areas are ill maintained, suffering from landslides, encroaching brush, and vanishing tread. The five-level rating system described below summarizes the general navigability of the trail. This section also advises whether the trail is good for kids, and whether you're likely to encounter poison oak.

> *Well maintained:* Typically heavily used and regularly maintained.
>
> *Clear:* A well-defined trail with no major obstructions.
>
> *Passable:* The trail is evident with some encroaching brush and/or downed debris. Lightly traveled and not regularly maintained.
>
> *Difficult:* The trail is faint with waist-high or above brush and/or fallen debris.
>
> *Impassable:* The trail is unrecognizable with major trail obstructions, including encroaching brush, landslides, and/or much fallen debris.

HIGHLIGHTS The natural feature(s) that distinguish each hike.

TO REACH THE TRAILHEAD Concise directions to the start of the trail. Where necessary, information is provided regarding facilities, water, entrance fees, and parking fees.

TRIP SUMMARY A basic description of the route, including any day hike or extended overnight options. Includes information on potential difficulties/hazards, as well as advice on the best time of year to visit.

Maps

Each trip is shown on a map, which is placed adjacent to the trip itself or adjacent to a nearby trip. Please see the map legend for details about the maps.

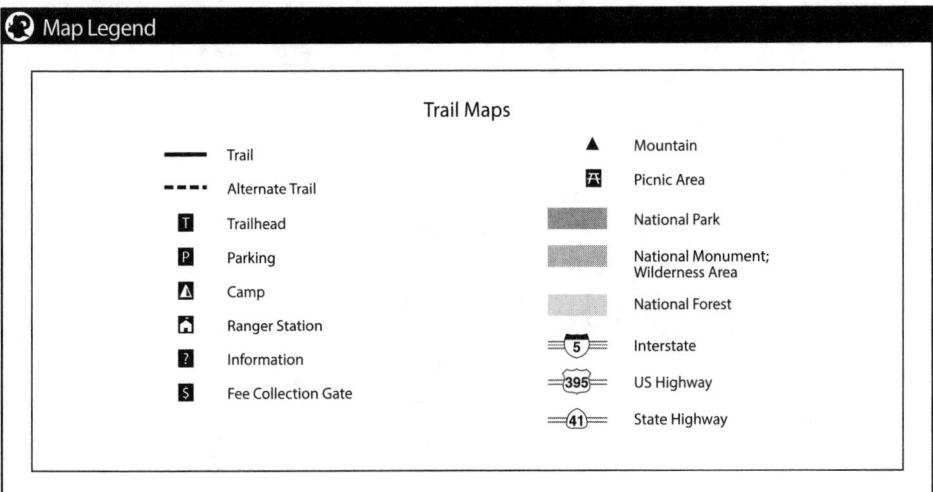

Map Legend

Trail Maps

—— Trail		▲	Mountain
- - - - Alternate Trail		🅰	Picnic Area
T Trailhead			National Park
P Parking			National Monument; Wilderness Area
Ⓐ Camp			National Forest
Ⓡ Ranger Station		(5)	Interstate
? Information		(395)	US Highway
S Fee Collection Gate		(41)	State Highway

Trip Description

Each trip description offers a thorough breakdown of the route, including trail conditions, seasonal considerations, water sources, historical notes, geology, plant and animal life, etc. Directions include all trail and spur junctions, camps, natural landmarks, and other notable features. Camps, junctions, and certain key features are listed in bold type followed by a parenthetical notation of the distance from the trailhead in miles and elevation in feet—for example, **Hiding Canyon Camp** (5.5 miles, 2500').

In certain instances, trail descriptions may overlap from one trip to the next. In such cases, the reader might be directed to a previous description for the route up to a certain point—for example, "See TRIP 49 Pine Valley (page 199) for the first 5.3 miles of this route to **Pine Valley.**"

If a spur leads to a notable feature (e.g., a camp, swimming hole, etc.), the trip description may include a Side Trip that elaborates on that feature. You'll also find sidebars throughout the text that offer more detail about natural features, historical anecdotes, and the like.

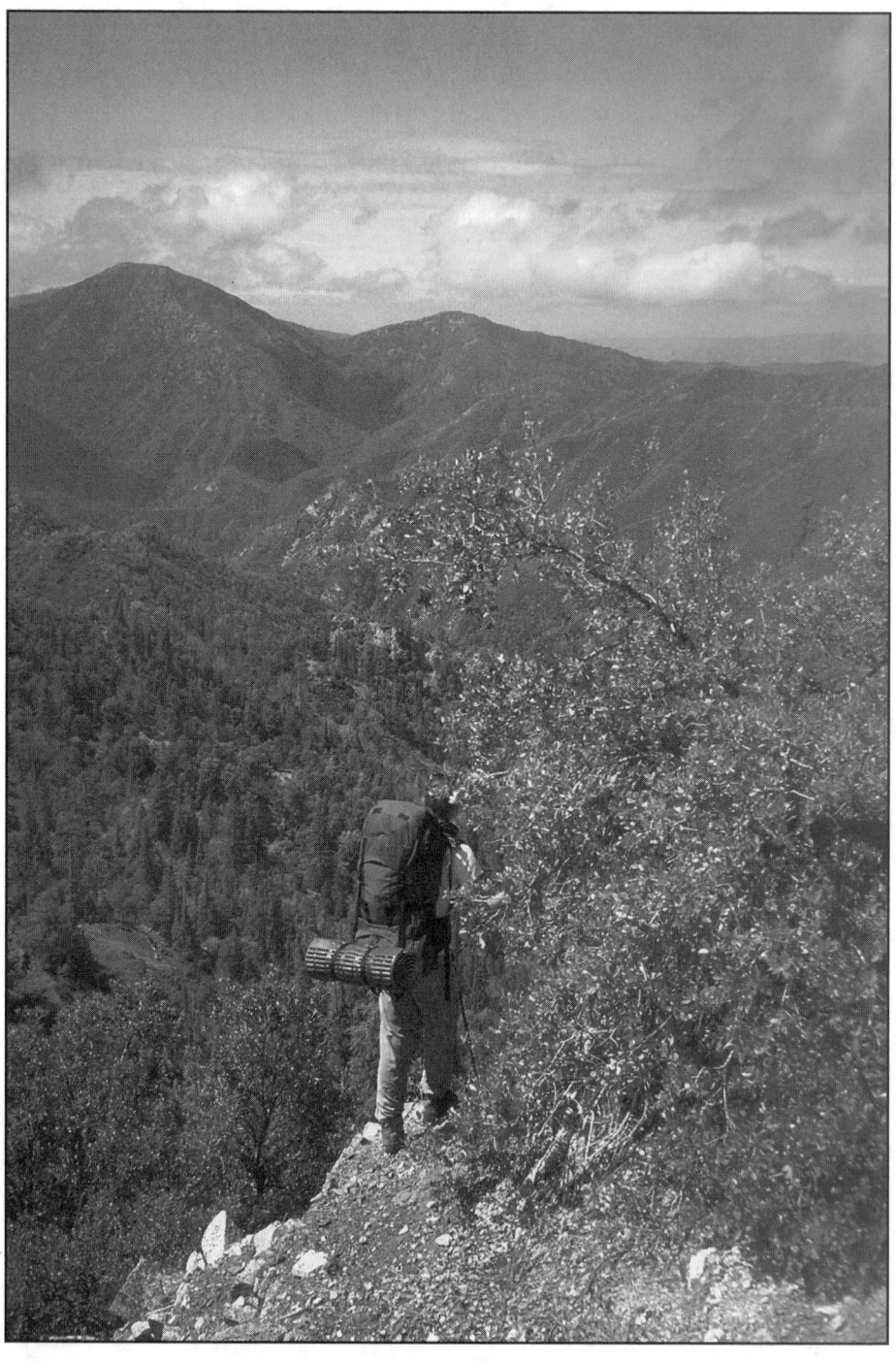

Tectonic activity created the prominent peaks and ridges of the Santa Lucia Range.

CHAPTER two

Natural History

■ ■ ■ ■ ■ ■ ■ ■ ■ ■ ■ ■ ■

Geology

BIG SUR'S RUGGED LANDSCAPE speaks to a tumultuous past, when ocean and rock collided in a dramatic convergence. It is a geologically youthful region. In just 5 million years, Big Sur has been smashed between colliding tectonic plates, compressed by massive faults, and rammed upward to form the jagged peaks, steep ridges, and deep gorges of the Santa Lucia Range.

While the mountains themselves may be relative toddlers, many of the rocks bear ancient origins, tens of millions of years old. The convoluted topography means that rock types formed under radically different conditions lie confusingly side by side. Ancient mountain ranges, seafloors, stream sediments, and molten rock form a jumbled matrix that continues to baffle geologists.

The story for most of these rocks begins 130 million years ago, amid sediments from an ancient mountain range 1800 miles southeast in present-day Mexico. In that era, North America's western shoreline lay about where the Sierra Nevada stands today, everything west was submerged beneath the ocean, and the Santa Lucia Range did not exist. In the following millennia, westbound rivers deposited the sediments along the coast, where these layers eventually solidified into sandstone, siltstone, and limestone.

Over subsequent millions of years, a massive oceanic plate slid slowly beneath the continental plate. The increasing depth and pressure melted the sandstone, siltstone, and limestone, which slowly cooled and solidified underground as various types of granite, marble, schist, and gneiss. The cooling process formed large crystals that lend these rocks a salt-and-pepper appearance in the sunlight. Geologists believe that rock types along the Big Sur coast and Santa Lucia Range share traits with granites of the Sierra Nevada, comprising a group called the Salinian block.

The hard, crystalline rocks of the Salinian block comprise many of the prominent high peaks of the range, such as Ventana Double Cone and Pico Blanco, as well as many of the rugged coves, cliffs, and promontories along the Big Sur coastline, particularly at Garrapata, Julia Pfeiffer, and Partington Cove. These durable, erosion-resistant granitic rocks hold up well in the pounding surf, producing little sediment to cloud the waters. Any sediment is coarse-grained and quickly sinks to the bottom, unlike finer sediments that cloud coastal waters elsewhere in California.

These rocks are readily identified when exposed. Limestone and marble outcrops are vivid white with a sugary texture. Granitic rocks in the surf zone appear coarse with reflective faces, while rocks higher on the bluffs weather a rusty orange. Collectively, the Salinian block rocks form the basement layers in the north half of the Santa Lucia Range.

As the denser oceanic plate dove under the lighter continental plate, mas-

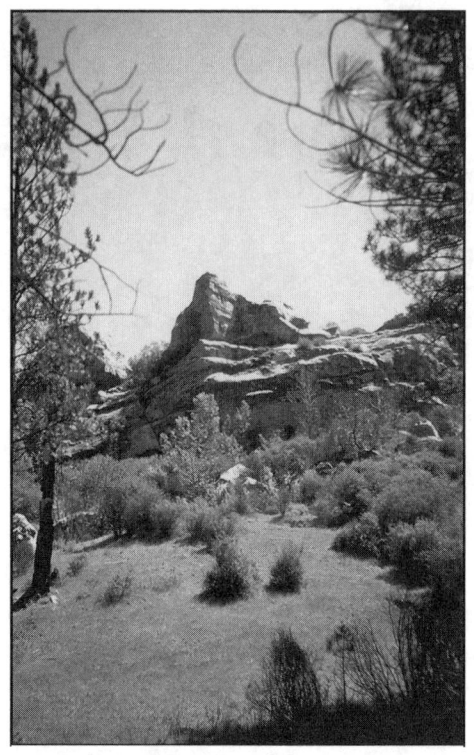

Sandstone cliffs tower above the open grasslands and pine-studded meadows of Ventana Wilderness.

sive accumulations of sand, mud, and the skeletons of microscopic sea creatures scraped off and slipped into a deep undersea trench. The resulting jumble appears along the Big Sur coast in the Franciscan formation, part of the Nacimiento block, which forms the underlying rock in the south half of the Santa Lucia Range.

The exposed cliffs at Andrew Molera State Park include excellent examples of Franciscan rocks. Formed from silica-rich sea creature skeletons, chert features jagged layering and an erosion-resistant glasslike texture. Sandstone is characterized by its tan color, rough surfaces, and fine sand grains. Comprising hardened, compressed mud, shale is gray-black in color with microscopic grains.

Serpentine, California's state rock, forms in layers that solidify above molten rock. These layers are scraped off and jumbled near the surface, where they react with groundwater to form this slippery green stone. You'll find dramatic serpentine outcrops in the Silver Peak Wilderness amid the Salmon Creek and San Carpoforo drainages.

Other younger rocks formed in the vicinity of the Santa Lucia Range before a single peak rose above the surface. A few million years ago, this area was a drainage basin that collected sediments in the form of sand, silt, and boulders. In time these solidified into sandstone, siltstone, and conglomerate. Conglomerate is least common, although at Point Lobos it is the dominant sedimentary rock and forms dramatic outcrops and cobblestone promontories.

While these theories may explain how the rocks formed, they don't explain how the rocks traveled hundreds of miles and rose to form the Santa Lucia Range. That story begins along the San Andreas Fault system some 30 million years ago. Once again, tectonic forces brought oceanic and continental plates together. This time, the North American plate and the Pacific plate met and began to grind past one another, marking the San Andreas Fault boundary.

Two massive chunks of Earth's crust, the Nacimiento and Salinian blocks, were ripped from their moorings along the North American plate and pushed northward along the numerous major faults associated with the San Andreas system. These faults generally run northwest-southeast, paralleling the coastline and general trend of the coastal mountains. A prime example is the Sur-Nacimiento Fault, which separates the Salinian and Nacimiento blocks, relieving pressure along the San Andreas Fault. As the tectonic plates collided, compressed, and fractured along these major fault lines, the land buckled in on itself like folds in a loose carpet, giving rise to the peaks, ridges, and gorges of the Santa Lucia Range.

Stream courses mark many of these otherwise indiscernible faults. The lower Big Sur River from the gorge to Andrew Molera State Park offers startling proof of how fault movement can alter a watercourse. Along this section, the river flows straight down the Sur Thrust Fault until it is forced into a conspicuous 90-degree turn out to Molera Beach.

Coastal bluffs, or marine terraces, offer evidence that the Santa Lucia Range continues its abrupt rise above sea level. These bluffs form as waves carve into the bedrock and deposit coarse sand and sediments. As land west of the San Andreas Fault buckles, these platforms rise above sea level, exposing the layered sand and cobblestones. Prominent marine terraces stretch from Point Sur to Andrew Molera State Park, while broader terraces form the flat terrain at Pacific Valley.

Erosion serves as a counteracting force to the recent uplifted Santa Lucia Range. As mountain flanks rise ever steeper, streams cut deep, fast channels through the rock, carrying away thousands of tons of sediment. A clear creek in summer can become a muddy torrent during heavy winter rains or after wildfires remove anchoring vegetation. Landslides are a common phenomenon in Big Sur. Of course, the Pacific Ocean also accounts for its fair share of erosion.

Geologists believe the recent uplift has thus far outstripped these erosive forces. If the uplift slows or stops, however, the tables will turn and gradually return the region to a rumpled landscape of low, rolling hills and plains.

Climate

CLIMATOLOGISTS HAVE LONG COMPARED California's climate to that of the Mediterranean coastline, with dry summers, wet winters, and moderate year-round temperatures. Big Sur's climate differs markedly, however, due primarily to consistent summer fog and the sheer topography of the Santa Lucia Range. Temperatures and humidity run the extremes along the fog-shrouded coast, atop 5000-foot mountain peaks, amid deep river canyons, and across the sun-drenched south-facing slopes.

An air circulation pattern known as the North Pacific High dominates regional weather patterns. From May through September, the sun most directly strikes the Northern Hemisphere. Surface air warms and rises into the upper atmosphere toward the North Pole. This heated air mass cools quickly in the upper atmosphere, subsequently sinking toward the surface as a large high-pressure cell. This massive high-pressure cell drives Big Sur's westerly winds and summer drought, as well as its summer fog, a very stable phenomenon off the California coast that is absent in the Mediterranean basin.

Thick fog forms when westerly winds brought by the North Pacific High push cold ocean water inland, forcing warmer surface water offshore. Rich in nutrients from nearshore submarine canyons, the cold water wells to the surface, sustaining abundant marine life along the Big Sur coast. With temperatures in the low 50s Fahrenheit, it also makes a swim here

In the wake of winter rains, fog retreats and grasslands and forests burst with new growth.

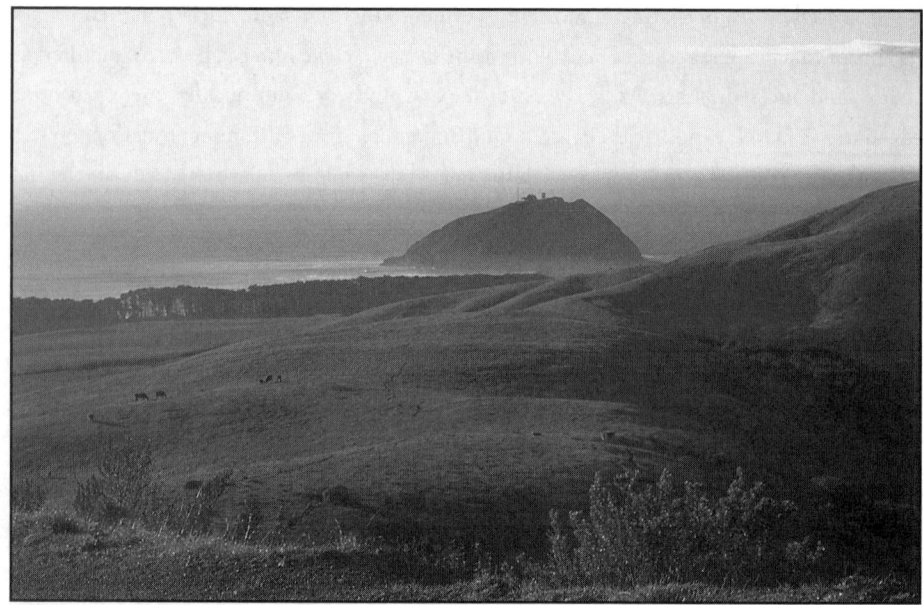

brisk at best, even in summer. The cold water chills the air directly above it. When this cold water comes in contact with warm, moist air along the coast, water vapor condenses into fog.

This pattern continues until late fall, when the sun strikes Earth farther south and the North Pacific High dissipates. No longer deflected by the high-pressure cell, the jet stream flows over California and brings with it strong winter storms. From November through April, California's wet season, these storms batter the coastal ranges until the sun's path again swings north to rebuild the North Pacific High.

Plant & Animal Communities

BIG SUR IS HOME TO A DIVERSE ARRAY of plant communities and associated wildlife. Botanists have long been fascinated by the proximity of northern and southern species living beside one another along the region's steep-sided ridges, narrow valleys, deep canyons, sun-drenched grasslands, and chaparral. Here, moisture-dependent redwoods may tower alongside drought-tolerant yuccas.

The story begins 5 million years ago, when the Santa Lucia Range was more of a low, rolling plain blessed with a moderate climate. Winters were warmer and summers wetter than today's more Mediterranean climate. The climate was likely too damp for chaparral species and too warm for redwoods and their shade-loving companions. Given the relatively uniform landscape and climate, botanists suggest the area supported fewer species than today's diverse topography permits.

Squeezed by tectonic plates and compressed by massive faults, the region rose and folded in on itself, creating the Santa Lucias' jagged peaks, steep ridges, and deep gorges. This topographic shift occurred in concert with climatic changes from the most recent Ice Age some 2.5 million years ago. These profound changes disrupted the uniform vegetation, paving the way for a major plant invasion.

The cool, damp climate allowed redwoods to take root in narrow, deep canyons along the coast. Fog encroached inland in dry months, supplying much-needed moisture to northern species. Thunderstorms became commonplace, as moist air rose abruptly to form thick cumulonimbus clouds, or thunderheads. These clouds arrived in summer, when temperatures were at a maximum and moisture at a minimum. Lightning sparked regular wildfires, and fire-adapted plant species thrived.

Drought-tolerant species also had an advantage. As the range continued to rise, coastal lands received the lion's share of precipitation, depriving eastern slopes of moisture. The steep topography also meant accelerated erosion, preventing mature soils from developing. The resulting shallow, primitive soils held considerably less ground water. But the hardy vegetation that populated these slopes shrugged at the arid conditions.

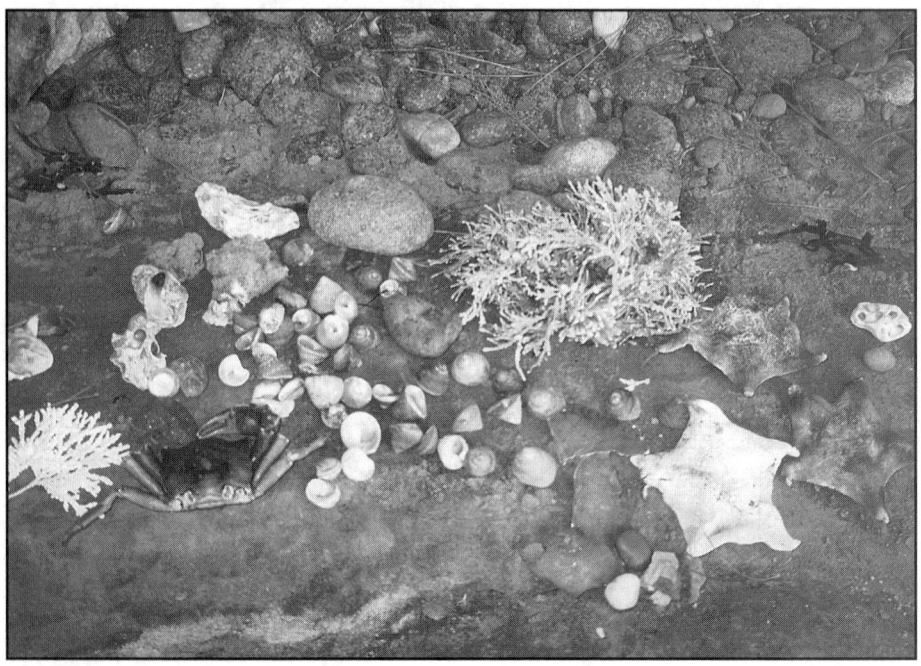

Low tide reveals diverse inter-tidal life.

Today, drought-tolerant plants still thrive on arid slopes, moisture-loving species grow along creeks and rivers, and shade-seeking plants retreat to the deep canyons and ravines. To categorize these patterns, botanists devised the concept of plant communities. A plant community is a group of species that grow together in a particular environment. Although it's possible to break these down into more detailed divisions, following is a basic breakdown of Big Sur's primary plant communities and their resident animals:

Coastal Scrub

Coastal scrub communities extend along the entire California coast and are divided into two major types: northern coastal scrub and southern coastal scrub. Although Point Sur is considered the loose boundary between the two types, northern and southern species intermingle along the Big Sur coast.

Common coastal shrubs include coyote brush (*Baccharis pilularis*), California lilac (*Ceanothus thyrsiflorus*), California coffeeberry (*Rhamnus californica*), and poison oak (*Toxicodendron diversilobum*). Headlands and bluffs feature such fragrant shrubs and herbs as California sagebrush (*Artemisia californica*), black sage (*Salvia mellifera*), hedge nettle (*Stachys bullata*), California mugwort (*Artemisia douglasiana*), and yerba buena (*Satureia douglasii*). Spring welcomes colorful purple, orange, and yellow blossoms from species such as silver and yellow bush lupine (*Lupinus albifrons* and *arboreus*), sticky monkeyflower (*Mimulus aurantiacus*), seaside daisy (*Erigeron glaucus*), and seaside wooly sunflower (*Eriophyllum staechadifolium*). Trees in this community are shrub-like, and few exceed 10 feet in height. California bay (*Umbellularia californica*) and coast live oak (*Quercus agrifolia*) nestle in ravines, while dense clusters of willows (mostly *Salix coulteri*) huddle near water.

The coastal bluffs and low rolling hillsides endure the constant assault of wind and salt spray, which sculpt and prune the plants to grow low and rounded. These species favor areas of heavy fog, average precipitation, abundant sunlight, and mild year-round temperatures. In Big Sur, northern plants thrive in moist locations, while southern species are more abundant in arid locations. When fire burns mature stands of coastal scrub, lush herbs and nutritious new growth thrive, providing prime foraging and nesting habitat to a greater number of animals.

Seeds, berries, roots, flowers, and young seedlings provide excellent food sources for herbivores, while woody plants provide nesting material. Omnivores and predators use the abundant scrub as cover from which to hunt, while prey species such as rodents, snakes, and small birds use it to hide from the former. Resident species include:

MAMMALS Mule deer, coyote, bobcat, gray fox, brush rabbit, black-tailed hare, California ground squirrel, Botta's pocket gopher, California meadow mouse, brush mouse, pinyon mouse, Merriam's chipmunk, long-tailed weasel, striped skunk, and dusky-footed woodrat.

BIRDS California condor, red-tailed hawk, white-tailed kite, California quail, western scrub jay, wrentit, California thrasher, song sparrow, white-crowned sparrow, bushtits, rufous-sided and California towhees, Anna's hummingbird, and western meadowlark.

REPTILES Western fence lizard, alligator lizard, western skink, gopher snake, California mountain king snake, western terrestrial garter snake, and western rattlesnake.

New growth of this native pine appears purple as new cones form the next generation of Monterey pines.

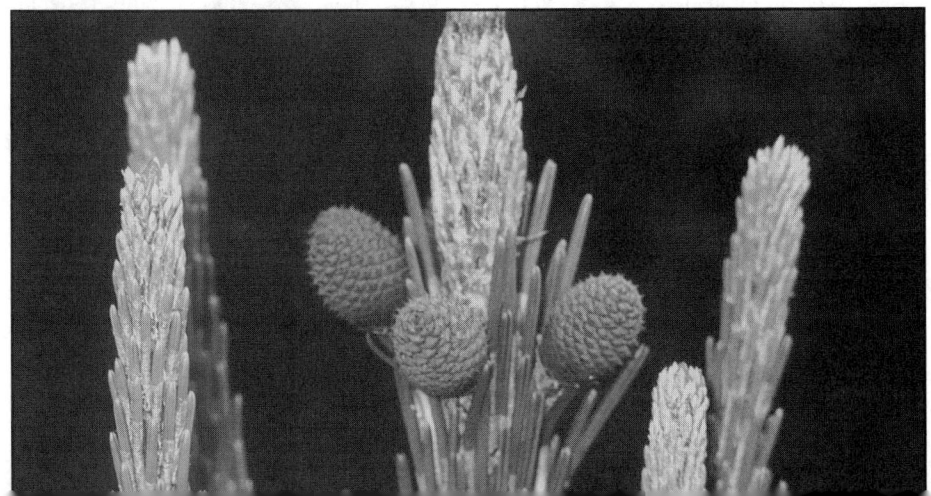

Chaparral

Comprising dense thickets of hardwood shrubs with stiff evergreen leaves, chaparral is unquestionably the dominant plant community in Big Sur, particularly in the Ventana and Silver Peak Wildernesses.

The predominant species of this fire-loving vegetation type is chamise, or greasewood (*Adenostoma fasciculatum*). This member of the rose family features a tough, woody stem, wiry branches, and bundles of needlelike evergreen leaves. It is named for its oily wood, which emits a pungent odor when brushed against. This brush species is a favorite perch for ticks, which wait to hitchhike on unsuspecting passersby.

The majority of chaparral in the Santa Lucias can be divided into two types: chamise chaparral and mixed chaparral. Chamise can grow in pure stands, while other plants grow in association with chamise to form mixed chaparral, where species such as ceanothus and manzanita dominate. The community includes manzanita species (*Arctostaphylos spp.*), buck brush (*Ceanothus cuneatus*), wartleaf (*Ceanothus papillosus*), California coffeeberry (*Rhamnus californica*), monkeyflower (*Mimulus bifidus*), California yerba santa (*Eriodictyon californicum*), poison oak (*Toxicodendron diversilobum*), and Our Lord's candle (*Yucca whipplei*).

Chaparral carpets the hottest, driest slopes, where summer temperatures can soar above 100°F. When lightning strikes, fire spreads quickly through mature chaparral stands. The volatile oils in some chaparral shrubs make this one of the most fire-adapted plant communities in the world. Historically, in the Santa Lucia Range, fire ravages chaparral slopes once every 10 to 40 years. The community provides critical stabilizing cover on steep, rocky slopes. When fire rips through, the slopes are left barren and unstable, resulting in massive floods and landslides when heavy winter storms strike.

Resident animal species include:

MAMMALS Mountain lion, coyote, gray fox, bobcat, mule deer, spotted skunk, ringtail, brush rabbit, California ground squirrel, Santa Cruz kangaroo rat, desert woodrat, California mice, deer mice, brush mice, Merriam's chipmunk, pallid bat, and Brazilian free-tailed bat.

BIRDS Turkey vulture, golden eagle, red-tailed hawk, Cooper's hawk, sharp-shinned hawk, California quail, mountain quail, Anna's hummingbird, wrentit, California thrasher, rufous-sided and California towhee, blue-gray gnatcatcher, Bewick's wren, bushtit, black swifts, white-throated swifts, and barn, violet-green, and cliff swallows.

REPTILES Western fence lizard, sagebrush lizard, western whiptail, coast horned lizard, garter snake, gopher snake, striped racer, western rattlesnake, and common kingsnake.

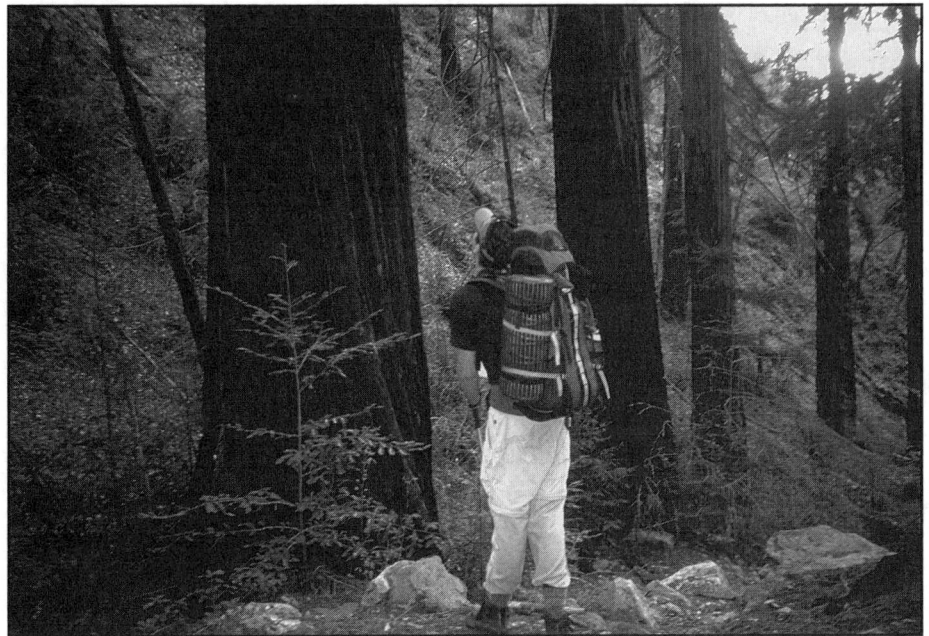

Coast redwoods show signs of vigorous regrowth after the 1999 Kirk Complex Fires in the narrow ravines of Hare Creek Canyon.

Redwood Forests

California is blessed with Earth's largest, oldest, and tallest living organisms. The largest tree in volume, the giant sequoia (*Sequoiadendron giganteum*), lords over the western slopes of the Sierra Nevada. The world's oldest tree, the bristlecone pine (*Pinus aristata*), perches along the flanks of the White Mountains. The tallest living organism, the coast redwood (*Sequoia sempervirens*), grows along the California coast, making its southern home in the Santa Lucia Range.

Redwood forests form a narrow belt along the coast from central California to southern Oregon. They are prized for their longevity (1000 years or more) and height (stretching some 250 to 300 feet above the forest floor). The tallest trees and healthiest groves rise farther north at Redwood National Park. Big Sur represents the redwood's southern stronghold, which peters out near Salmon Creek in southern Big Sur, close to the coastal California fog belt. As redwoods approach their southern limit, the trees are noticeably diminished in size.

In its warmer, drier southern range, this moisture-loving species is restricted to cool, damp valleys, canyons, ravines, and gullies. The fossil record proves that 50 million years ago redwoods were widespread throughout the Northern Hemisphere, including Greenland, Asia, and Europe. As the climate changed, so did the species' range.

Although redwoods can live for thousands of years, the desire for lumber makes the fast-growing, massive trees commercially valuable. At the turn of the century, the Big Sur region sustained massive logging operations that cleared much of the ancient stands. Remaining old-growth redwood forests are confined to a few coastal drainages, including the Little Sur, Big Sur, Partington, McWay, Big Creek, and Palo Colorado Canyons.

A number of other moisture-loving trees, shrubs, and herbs grow in association with redwoods. Common neighboring trees include tanoak (*Lithocarpus densiflorus*), California bay (*Umbellularia californica*), western sycamore (*Platanus racemosa*), white alder (*Alnus rhombifolia*), and bigleaf maple (*Acer macrophyllum*). Although redwood canopies all but blot out the sun, a surprisingly dense understory of ferns, herbs, and shrubs obtain enough sunlight to carpet stream corridors and steep slopes along the forest floor. Understory plants include western sword fern (*Polystichum munitum*), bracken fern (*Pteridium aqulinum*), giant chain fern (*Woodwardia fimbriata*), American maidenhair fern (*Adiantum pedatum*), California maidenhair fern (*Adiantum jordani*), coastal wood fern (*Dryopteris arguta*), fairy lantern (*Calochortus alkus*), western hound's-tongue (*Cynoglossum grande*), fairy bells (*Disporum hookeri*), western starflower (*Trientalis latifolia*), poison oak (*Toxicodendron diversilobum*), evergreen huckleberry (*Vaccinium ovatum*), and redwood sorrel (*Oxalis oregana*).

The lush forest seems surprisingly void of wildlife. The understory supports few seed-bearing plants to attract herbivores and their predators. One of the most common plants, redwood sorrel, is even toxic to herbivores. Regardless, a few animals do thrive here. One notable and highly visible resident is the banana slug, a bright yellow gastropod that grazes on understory plants and fungi. Its bright coloration is a defense mechanism, signaling predators that the slug is extremely distasteful. Other common species include:

MAMMALS Trowbridge shrew and broad-handed mole.

BIRDS Steller's jay, winter wren, brown creeper, Pacific slope flycatcher, dark-eyed junco, hermit thrush, varied thrush, American robins, chestnut-backed chickadee, common flickers, great horned owl, northern pygmy owl, and golden-crowned kinglet.

REPTILES & AMPHIBIANS Coast Range newt, red salamander, slender salamander, alligator lizard, western fence lizard, and sharp-tailed snake.

The ubiquitous banana slug

Riparian Woodland

By definition, riparian (riverside) woodlands follow clear water in Big Sur country. Characterized by moisture-loving trees, this community nestles alongside creeks, streams, and rivers in the heart of the wilderness. The most common trees are the deciduous western sycamore (*Platanus racemosa*), bigleaf maple (*Acer macrophyllum*), red alder (*Alnus rubra*), white alder (*Alnus rhombifolia*), and several species of willow (*Salix spp.*). In fall the major drainages of the Santa Lucia Range, notably the Carmel and Big Sur Rivers and Arroyo Seco, boast vibrant hues as autumn leaves catch the slightest canyon breezes. In spring the forest flaunts such delicate moisture-loving flowers as leopard lily (*Lilium pardalinum*), giant stream orchid (*Epipactus gigantean*), scarlet monkeyflower (*Mimulus cardinalis*), red columbine (*Aquilegia formosa*), and thimbleberry (*Rubus parviflorus*).

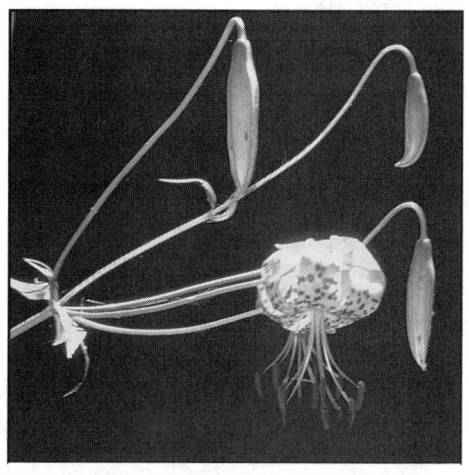

During spring tiger lilies adorn the banks of riparian corridors.

This is one of the best areas to view wildlife. Butterflies, dragonflies, amphibians, reptiles, fish, birds, and mammals all gather here to drink, hunt, forage, and mate. Resident species include:

MAMMALS Mule deer, mountain lion, bobcat, coyote, raccoon, gray fox, striped skunk, opossum, Pacific shrew, ornate shrew, western harvest mouse, deer mouse, dusky-footed woodrat, big brown bat, silver-haired bat, red bat, and hoary bat.

BIRDS American dipper, belted kingfisher, red-shouldered hawk, Cooper's hawk, western screech owl, long-eared owl, downy woodpecker, white-headed woodpecker, black phoebe, willow flycatcher, violet-green swallow, tree swallow, plain titmouse, white-breasted nuthatch, Bewick's wren, Swainson's thrush, warbling vireo, yellow warbler, Wilson's warbler, American goldfinch, lesser goldfinch, and song sparrow.

REPTILES Western pond turtle, western terrestrial garter snake, sharp-tailed snake, ringneck snake, rubber boa, California mountain kingsnake, western rattlesnake, western fence lizard, and alligator lizard.

FISH & AMPHIBIANS Pacific tree frog, steelhead trout, brown trout, rainbow trout, lamprey, arboreal salamander, red salamander, slender salamander, Coast Range newt, tiger salamander, bullfrog, and crayfish.

Grassland

Grasslands usually mix with coastal scrub along the slopes of the Santa Lucia Range. In the drier interior, they grow alongside arid thickets of chaparral on oak- and pine-studded hillsides. Grasslands also thrive along marine terraces and coastal bluffs, including El Sur Ranch north of Andrew Molera State Park, where cattle continually graze.

Those who believe the central coast to be void of seasonal changes have not taken a stroll through the grasslands of Big Sur. Following winter rains, vibrant green grasses sprout from the damp earth. This annual growth cycle may end before summer if little rain falls in spring. By late May, the rolling hills turn golden as the grasslands fade and lay dormant until the following winter's rains.

Most grasses responsible for these seasonal bursts of color are exotic species to the California landscape. In the mid 19th century, settlers brought in invasive annual grasses to feed livestock. These species quickly outcompeted native perennial grasses and thrived in areas ravaged by grazing, fire, or landslides.

Though grasses are the dominant species, forbs and herbs also thrive here, weaving colorful tapestries along the open slopes of the Coast Range. Among the most recognized are the blue, purple, and orange hues of sky lupines (*Lupinus nanus*) and California poppies (*Eschscholzia californica*). Other fragile, ornate flowers include the padres shooting star

Seasonal changes are most dramatic within the grassland ecosystem, where vibrant new growth carpets the landscape.

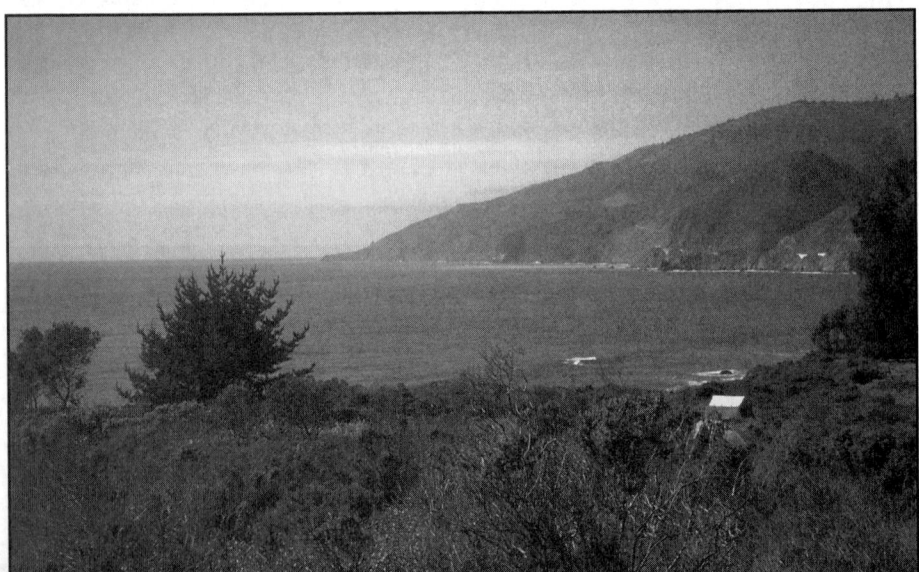

(*Dodecatheon clevelandii*), California buttercup (*Ranunculus californicus*), Johnny-jump-up (*Viola pedunculata*), and blue dicks (*Dichelostemma pulchella*).

Many animals forage and hunt in the grasslands, though few find safe refuge to nest and breed. Common species include:

MAMMALS Coyote, mule deer, bobcat, gray fox, pocket gopher, California ground squirrel, and long-tail weasel.

BIRDS Western meadowlark, grasshopper sparrow, savannah sparrow, lark sparrow, burrowing owl, horned lark, white-tailed kite, red-tailed hawk, red-shouldered hawk, American kestrel, golden eagle, barn owl, great horned owl, California quail, mourning dove, swallows, swifts, and finches.

REPTILES Gopher snake, western rattlesnake, yellow-bellied racer, ringneck snake, alligator lizard, and western fence lizard.

Oak Woodland

Majestic oak woodlands form some of Big Sur's most picturesque, enchanting forests. The southern region shelters centuries-old blue and valley oaks, while coastal slopes are studded with sprawling coast live oaks draped with lacy lichens. The most common trees are coast live oak (*Quercus agrifolia*), blue oak (*Quercus douglasii*), California black oak (*Quercus kelloggii*), valley oak (*Quercus lobata*), and canyon live oak (*Quercus chrysolepis*). Oak woodlands vary from dense forests to grassy savannas, and plants from neighboring communities often occupy the understory.

Unfortunately, tens of thousands of tanoaks, coast live oaks, and black oaks between Big Sur and the Oregon border are dying from sudden oak death. Researchers have isolated a previously unknown fungal species they believe causes the disease. This pathogen is a member of the genus *Phytophthora* (Latin for plant destroyer) and is related to species blamed for such agricultural plagues as the Irish potato famine. Scientists are conducting far-ranging research to determine how the fungus spreads and how it can be stopped. It's critical to slow the spread of the fungus by preventing the movement of infected leaves, wood, and soil. Visitors to Big Sur's oak woodlands should clean their tires, shoes, and animals' feet thoroughly before leaving the area.

Acorns are the most important food item for animals living in or around oak woodlands. In fall, as acorns ripen and fall, the forest chatters with excitement as birds and mammals flock to harvest the nutritious nuts. Resident species include:

MAMMALS Mule deer, bobcat, mountain lion, gray fox, coyote, striped skunk, wild boar (introduced from Europe), California mouse, western gray squirrel, pocket gopher, Audubon cottontail, lump-nosed bat, big brown bat, silver-haired bat, red bat, and hoary bat.

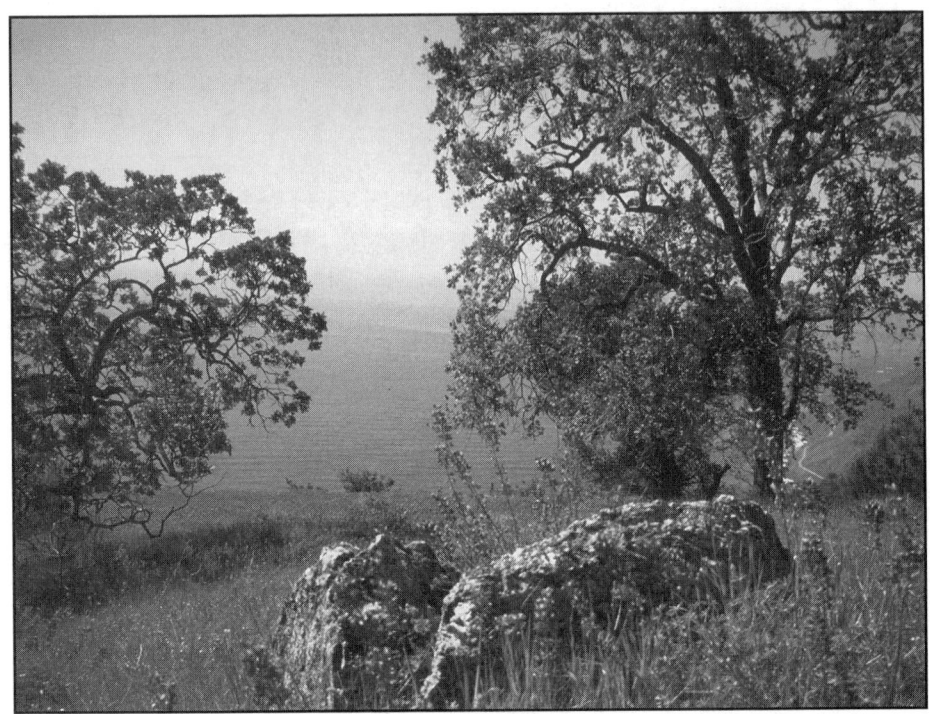

Sprawling black oaks filter views northwest toward the ocean along the Buckeye Trail.

BIRDS   Western bluebird; chestnut-backed chickadee; northern flicker; acorn, Lewis', and Nuttall's woodpeckers; violet-green and tree swallows; scrub jay; common raven; plain titmouse; bushtit; white-breasted nuthatch; orange-crowned and Townsend's warblers; Hutton's vireo; black-headed grosbeak; band-tailed pigeon; mourning dove; western screech and great horned owls; Cooper's, red-tailed, and red-shouldered hawks; and American kestrel.

REPTILES   Western fence lizard, alligator lizard, western skink, gopher snake, common kingsnake, and western rattlesnake.

AMPHIBIANS   Arboreal salamander, California newt, and western toad.

Mixed Evergreen Forest

The mixed evergreen forest is an extremely varied community, in which endemic, rare, isolated, or disjunct coniferous species grow amid a diverse array of hardwood trees. Member species include the Santa Lucia fir, Coulter pine, ponderosa pine, sugar pine, gray pine, Monterey pine, Douglas fir, and incense cedar.

Nestled along deep, dark canyon floors and atop the Santa Lucias' dry, rocky slopes and summits lives the rarest, most distinct, and narrowly distributed of all fir species, the endemic Santa Lucia fir. They are easily identified by droopy, densely foliated crowns that extend from the base of the tree with lower branches that nearly touch the ground. The tree's differing habitats share one characteristic: each is relatively fire resistant. Although the range is subject to periodic wildfires, the Santa Lucia fir is not fire adapted and cannot survive in areas susceptible to burning.

Fossil evidence from the Miocene period (22 million to 6 million years ago) proves the Santa Lucia fir was once widely distributed throughout western North America. During the Miocene, the climate was much warmer and wetter than today, including regular summer rainfall. During the Pliocene period (5.2 to 1.6 million years ago), the climate cooled, leading to the ice ages of the Pleistocene (1.6 million to 11,000 years ago). The Santa Lucia fir could not withstand these colder, drier conditions and thus retreated to milder coastal climates.

Botanist Thomas Coulter first described the Coulter pine in 1832 near Cone Peak. Its enormous, sharp-spurred cones are the heaviest of any pine species. The tree grows in association with canyon live oaks, tanoaks, California bays, and madrones. On the flanks of Junipero Serra Peak, Coulter pines grow alongside stately sugar pines.

A Scottish botanist first described sugar pines in 1831 while climbing Cone Peak. These largest of all pines boast enormous cones that are longer and more slender than the Coulter pine's cones. Distinct from their Sierra Nevada and Southern California cousins, Big

Climate change millions of years ago isolated this stand of Santa Lucia fir to the milder coastal climate of Big Sur.

Sur's sugar pines are restricted to isolated peaks and higher elevation slopes atop Cone and Junipero Serra Peaks.

The incense cedar is another disjunct tree removed from its Sierra Nevada population. When crushed, its flat, scaled foliage emits a pungent aroma. Botanists speculate that this tree was also once widespread, but as the climate warmed over the past 10,000 years and wildfires became more commonplace, its range shrank drastically.

The mixed evergreen plant community shares many of the plant and animal species commonly seen in Big Sur's oak woodlands. Consult that wildlife list for representative species.

BIG SUR SEASONS

Big Sur's steep, rugged topography and proximity to the ocean lead to a diverse array of regional microclimates. Deep, narrow canyons remain shady and cool even in sweltering summer heat. High, barren peaks regularly freeze and receive snow in winter. Cool onshore breezes sweep coastal terraces, while the sun beats down on arid south-facing slopes. Though visitors may complain about a lack of defined seasons along the coast, locals know Big Sur is markedly different and beautiful each season.

Summer

In summer, inland temperatures along the Santa Lucia Range often soar into the 90s Fahrenheit during the day and drop to the 40s Fahrenheit by night both in the valleys and at high elevation. This contrasts dramatically with stable, cool temperatures along the coast, which generally range from the low 50s to mid 60s Fahrenheit.

Separated from the ocean by 2000-foot Pfeiffer Ridge, the Big Sur River gorge is much warmer than the fog-shrouded beaches to the west. Campers and hikers flock to deep swimming holes within the gorge for bracing dips. Occasionally, the fog encroaches inland and is drawn up-canyon, bringing gray and overcast conditions even to high ridges.

Although rain is unlikely in summer, tropical low-pressure systems occasionally approach the coast in the form of puffy cumulus clouds. As this warm, humid air moves in, thunderheads may develop, spawning lightning and rain. During periodic summer droughts, wildfires are a real threat, so residents are watchful for any signs of lightning or smoke. Lightning sparked the 180,000-acre Marble–Cone Fire (1977), the 60,000-acre Rat Creek Fire (1985), the 90,000-acre Kirk Complex Fires (1999), and the 160,000-acre Basin Complex Fire (2008).

Fall

Indian summer brings warmer temperatures to the coast in fall. As the North Pacific High dissipates, nearshore cold-water upwelling stops, lowering humidity and driving fog well offshore. Views from high mountain peaks are outstanding in the crisp, clear air. Northwesterly winds diminish, and coastal waters become flat, calm, and warm (upper 50s instead of low 50s Fahrenheit). Deep within the riparian woodlands, deciduous trees change color and shed their kaleidoscopic leaves on the canyon floors.

Winter

Winter storms generally approach the central California coast from the northwest or southwest. Forming in the cold regions of the North Pacific and Bering Sea, northern fronts bring cold air masses and moderate rainfall. Forming over warm water in the South Pacific, southern storms typically bring extensive rainfall.

Arriving on the Big Sur coast, the moisture-laden air lashes the steep terrain and is forced upward. As the air rises, it cools and condenses, releasing moisture as rain or snow. When the North Pacific High lingers into winter, it prevents storms from reaching the coast and often leads to severe winter droughts.

Precipitation varies dramatically from year to year. Rainfall along the coast averages about 40 inches annually, while some 90 inches fall near the crests and ridges. In winter the high peaks are dusted in snow, which may remain on the ground for weeks or even months above 3500 feet.

A rain shadow effect occurs along eastern slopes, similar to that seen along the eastern slopes of the Sierra. Moisture-laden air deposits its precipitation along the rising western slopes and ridges, leaving eastern slopes drier on average, as the air warms and descends into the Salinas Valley. King City averages only about 11 inches annually.

Spring

Spring is glorious along the Big Sur coast. Plants and animals awake from dormancy, and the sights and sounds of life abound. In the wake of winter rains, grasslands and forests burst forth with new growth. Colorful, fragrant wildflowers carpet the grasslands and ridges, while oak and riparian woodlands bud in vibrant green hues. Views are spectacular on cold, crisp days.

The arrival of spring varies with the timing of winter rains. If rains continue until May, expect incredible wildflower displays through summer, while an end to rains in March turns the hillsides gold as dry season descends on Big Sur. Expect encroaching fog by late spring as the North Pacific High returns offshore, spawning cold-water upwelling.

CHAPTER three

Big Sur Cultural History & Lore

■ ■ ■ ■ ■ ■ ■ ■ ■ ■ ■ ■ ■

I MAGINE A LAND OF STUNNING BEAUTY with a wealth of resources, where thousands of steelhead swim upstream along crystal clear creeks and rivers. Grizzly bears, wolves, and mountain lions roam sheer mountains that jut toward the heavens. Sea otters, seals, and whales forage in nearshore waters. Condors, falcons, and eagles soar overhead. Acorns, wild berries, nutritious herbs, and medicinal plants flourish amid valleys and hillsides. This vision is perhaps what early Europeans saw as they explored the vast wilderness inhabited by the American Indians of Big Sur.

American Indians

ARCHAEOLOGICAL EVIDENCE PROVES that people have lived along the rugged Big Sur coast for some 8000 years. When Spanish explorers of the 16th and 17th centuries arrived in Big Sur, the native population numbered nearly 5000 people among three separate coastal tribes: the Ohlone (from Point Sur north to San Francisco), the Esselen (from Point Sur south to Big Creek and inland to the upper Carmel River and Arroyo Seco watersheds), and the Salinian (from Big Creek south to San Carpoforo Creek and inland from Junipero Serra Peak north up the Salinas River valley). These groups differed dramatically from one another, adopting different languages, religious beliefs, customs, and dress.

The American Indians were hunter-gatherers, harvesting a variety of food sources throughout the year rather than farming. In fall they moved inland to bountiful oak woodlands to collect acorns, in spring to the valleys and grasslands to harvest nutritious herbs, and in winter to the Pacific to fish and hunt along the rich coastal waters.

Ancient middens speak to this variety in their diet. Lying amid former Indian villages and encampments, middens are essentially trash heaps, offering a stratified record of animal bones, shellfish remains, stone tools, weapons, and ornamental artifacts. Coastal middens largely contain the remains of mussels, abalone, chitons, barnacles, seabirds, marine mammals, and fish, while inland middens feature the bones of deer, skunks, raccoons, coyotes, foxes, rabbits, squirrels, mice, and gophers.

Aside from the middens and written records from Spanish explorers, missionaries, and anthropologists, we know little about these people and how they lived. Tragically, their culture vanished soon after contact with the Europeans. Within a few decades, thousands succumbed to European diseases for which they had no immunity. Many of those who survived such diseases as whooping cough and measles were driven from their lands, converted to Christianity, and put to work raising cattle within the mission system.

Spanish Exploration & the Mission Period

IN 1542, Spain hired Portuguese navigator Juan Rodríguez Cabrillo to sail the California coast in search of riches and a water route between the Pacific and Atlantic Oceans. The first European to see Big Sur and the Santa Lucia Range, Cabrillo remarked, "There are mountains which seem to reach the heavens, and the sea beats on them; sailing along close to land, it appears as though they would fall on the ships." He also encountered Monterey Bay, naming it Bahia de los Pinos (Bay of Pines).

In 1602, 60 years after Cabrillo's expedition and nearly 20 years before pilgrims landed at Plymouth Rock, Spanish explorer Sebastian Vizcaíno sailed coastal California. His expedition spent two weeks surveying Monterey and Carmel Bays, proclaiming both to be excellent safe harbors. Vizcaíno named the coast Monte-Rey after Spain's new viceroy, the count of

In 1542, Cabrillo described the California coastline aptly: "There are mountains which seem to reach the heavens and the sea beats on them."

Monte-Rey. Vizcaíno's glowing reports and fears that Russian explorers were encroaching south along the coast from Alaska prompted Spain to claim Monterey Bay as its own.

In 1769, Gaspar de Portolá led an inland expedition north from Baja California near present-day San Diego. When the expedition reached the daunting coastal cliffs near Ragged Point, it turned inland. Protected by its sheer topography, Big Sur was left unexplored. After Portolá reached the San Francisco Bay, the expedition returned south, bypassing entirely Monterey, Carmel, and environs. Although disheartened, Portolá persevered and planned another trip.

In 1770, Portolá departed on another land expedition accompanied by Father Junipero Serra, who sailed north with the intent to establish Catholic outposts in the unknown territory. Serra established Mission San Carlos at present-day Carmel River State Beach and two other missions east of the Santa Lucia Range in the San Antonio River Valley and at Soledad in the Salinas Valley. Again, Big Sur was left unexplored.

The missionaries' arrival drastically altered native life in the Big Sur region. The newcomers claimed the land and brought Ohlone, Esselen, and Salinian natives into the missions. Some welcomed the priests, while others were lured by exotic gifts of glass beads, colored fabric, metal tools, and livestock. Forced conversion and de facto enslavement was not mission policy prior to 1800, but when natives resisted, more coercive methods were used. Missionaries justified their enslavement of "heathens" as acceptable if the natives ultimately converted to Christianity and found salvation.

In 1821, Mexico declared independence from Spanish rule, and in 1834 the vast mission lands were secularized and divided into livestock "ranchos." Any law-abiding Mexican Catholic was now eligible to receive land grants. California's ranching era had begun.

VISITING THE SAN CARLOS BORROMEO DE CARMELO MISSION ■ ■ ■

Step back in time and enter Father Junipero Serra's chosen home and final resting place, founded near the mouth of the Carmel River on August 24, 1771. Serra wished to build a permanent stone house of worship that required skilled masons to cut and dress the stones in the style of missions that Serra had erected in Mexico. With no skilled masons available in California, many of the missions never progressed past the humble adobe style, and the Carmel Mission we see today was delayed until years after Serra's death.

The construction of the stone church began in 1795 and was basically complete by 1797, when it was dedicated for worship on Christmas Day of that year. When the church was originally constructed, the sandstone walls were quarried from the Santa Lucia Mountains, but most of the exterior is different today. Inside, the statue of the

Virgin Mary in the side chapel of Our Lady Bethlehem is the same one that Father Serra carried back from Mexico in 1769.

Carmel Mission served both as headquarters for the mission's agricultural holdings in the Carmel Valley and as command center for the statewide California mission system. Today, the mission serves as a parish church, school, and basilica. Its distinction as a basilica is the highest honorary rank for a church and implies great historical and artistic importance. Pope John XXIII honored Carmel Mission's church with the rank of basilica in 1961 in recognition of Serra's work in the establishment of Christianity on the western coast of the United States, as well as the unique architectural features of the structure such as the Moorish dome and the parabolic ceiling. Since that designation, Carmel Mission Basilica was honored with a visit by Pope John Paul II, who visited the church to lay a wreath at the foot of the grave of Father Serra, who is buried beneath the floor of the sanctuary (near the altar).

Carmel Mission is open to the public Monday–Saturday 9:30 a.m.–5 p.m. and Sunday 10:30 a.m.–5 p.m. The admission fee to visit the mission grounds, basilica, and museums is $6.50 for adults, $4 for seniors (age 65 and up), and $2 for children age 7 and up (children under 6 are admitted free). These funds are used to support the continued maintenance and restoration of Carmel Mission. To get there, turn west from Highway 1 onto Rio Road and drive 0.7 mile to the corner of Lausen Drive. For more information, call (831) 624-1271 or visit **carmelmission.org**.

Ranching & Homesteading

As MEXICO REDISTRIBUTED the vast mission holdings as land grants, homesteaders claimed several outlying areas of Big Sur. Monterey soon developed into an important Pacific trading port, and the United States began to set its sights on California. Tensions arose between land-owning *Californios*, as they called themselves, and American pioneers immigrating through the treacherous passes of the Sierra Nevada. Conflict erupted at the outset of the Mexican War in 1846. In 1848, Mexico ceded California to the United States. The following year, gold was discovered in the foothills of the Sierra, and statehood was declared in 1850.

Pioneers and prospectors headed to California in droves. By this time, many outlying areas, including the Carmel, Nacimiento, and San Antonio River Valleys, were already privately owned. Two land grants spanned Big Sur: the 8984-acre Rancho El Sur, owned by Juan Bautista Alvarado, covering most of Point Sur, and the 8876-acre Rancho San Jose y Sur Chiquito, from the Carmel River to Palo Colorado Canyon.

Would-be homesteaders found the remaining steep, rocky terrain ill suited for farming, difficult to cross, and isolated from the world. Nonetheless, by the late 1800s a small community of determined pioneers had settled in Big Sur. These strong-willed folks survived by hunting, fishing, foraging, raising livestock, planting orchards, and tending gardens amid the lush canyons and steep ridges. Today, much of the land is named for these early pioneer families, including the Pfeiffers, Posts, Plasketts, Prewitts, and Partingtons.

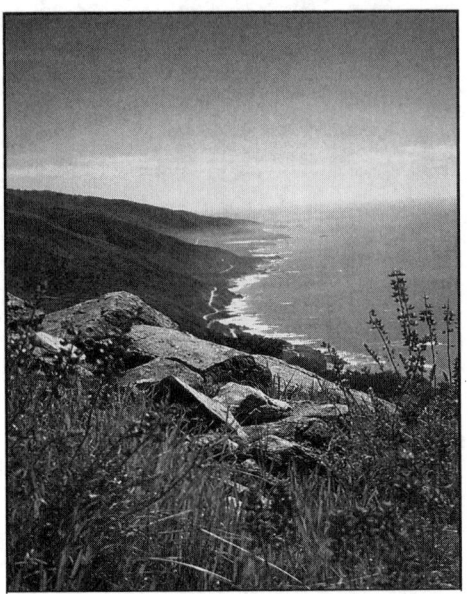

The sheer coastal topography has kept the Big Sur coastline rugged and largely uninhabited even to the present day.

Highway 1 Construction & Recent Settlement

UNTIL 1938, early settlers could only dream of a safe, fast route down the coast from Monterey to Big Sur. Even a simple supply trip to Monterey required a three-day trek up steep ridges and across creeks and deep canyons. In 1919, after lobbying pressure from a local politician, the federal government began construction of a road along the central California coast. The construction project pitted settlers who wanted to preserve their privacy against those who sought to profit from California's growing tourist trade.

Built by convicts and local labor, Highway 1 would become one of America's most popular roadways, revealing a gorgeous natural landscape. Artists and writers, social activists, scientists, philosophers, and other visionaries flocked to the area for inspiration, forming small artists' colonies and Bohemian sanctuaries. In the 1940s and '50s, playwright Henry Miller lived and worked in Big Sur. Other famous people who spent time here include Robert Louis Stevenson, Ansel Adams, Jack Kerouac, Mary Austin, Jack London, Sinclair Lewis, John Steinbeck, Robinson Jeffers, Lillian Ross, and Edward Weston.

Today, millions of annual visitors drive the Big Sur coast in appreciation of its unparalleled natural beauty. While the road literally paved the way for so many of us to access this wild, remote coast, it has also spurred government agencies, conservation groups, and local activists to preserve its exquisite beauty.

Big Sur Lore

WITHIN THE JAGGED cliffs and narrow valleys live generations of mysteries: tales of buried treasures, haunted beings, and supernatural speculation. The awe-inducing beauty and eerie isolation experienced by many who venture to Big Sur, whether to call it home or a place of refuge, gave birth to many interesting and irksome stories. In my countless days in the backcountry, I have yet to experience any evidence that these tales shed light on life within the Santa Lucia Mountains, yet they still remain an alluring part of Big Sur's cultural heritage, and I do not intend to endorse or debunk them.

The Dark Watchers

The sighting of the Dark Watchers originates from the Chumash Indians. They first spoke of these dark humanlike beings inhabiting the forests and high country of Big Sur in legends and their cave paintings. More recently, legendary author John Steinbeck described them in his story, "Flight":

"Pepe looked up to the top of the next dry withered ridge. He saw a dark form against the sky, a man's figure standing on top of a rock, and he glanced away quickly not to appear curious. When a moment later he looked up again, the figure was gone."

In 1937, the poet Robinson Jeffers mentioned them in his poem "Such Counsels You Gave to Me" as "forms that look human . . . but certainly are not human." If Jeffers or Steinbeck ever actually saw one of the Dark Watchers is unknown, but the local legend has been around since long before they wrote about it. Longtime Big Sur resident Rosalind Sharpe Wall claims to have seen the Dark Watchers near Bixby Bridge. If you happen to come across a Dark Watcher, the prevailing wisdom warns against looking at them.

The Ventana

The Ventana Wilderness is named for a unique notch called "The Window" on a granite ridge between Ventana Double Cone and Peak. According to local legend, this notch was once a natural stone arch that created a natural "window," which is supposedly what inspired the Spanish explorers gazing up toward the peaks to call it Ventana. The Ventana, or "The Slot" as local rock climbers call it, is the 200-foot-deep gap in the ridge. Geologists have yet to find rubble of a collapsed arch to support the legend, but nonetheless there are many arches and small complete "windows" in rock formations in the Santa Lucias. You can view the notch by looking west from Ventana Double Cone or along Coast Ridge Road with views north and looking northeast from Post Ranch Inn.

Supernatural Stories of Point Lobos

During the mission period, the Ohlone Indian neophytes at Carmel Mission would go out on foggy evenings to "cheer up" their lonely and forlorn fog spirits. The mission fathers strictly forbade any such pagan activity, and one night they followed them out into the fog and performed an exorcism. The fog spirits flew off angry and offended, departing with howls and causing sadness among the Indians. Some believe poetic justice prevailed, when the priest who performed the exorcism went mad, jumped off a cliff into the sea at Point Lobos, and was drowned.

A Goddess and a Hidden Gold Mine on Pico Blanco

With the discovery of gold and silver in Big Sur in the late 19th century, miners began searching for the precious metals along the flanks and valleys of the Santa Lucias. Today, the Pico Blanco area is littered with the rusting remnants of mining operations.

More than tales of fortunes found, historians have uncovered a curious tale that was circulated in response to the miners' arrival. According to local legend, an American Indian goddess zealously protected Pico Blanco. Historians recorded these accounts by miners claiming to have encountered the goddess, who cursed them with madness for pursuing gold.

During this same gold exploration period in Big Sur, a seemingly illiterate prospector named Al Clark became Pico Blanco's best-known resident. For decades he wandered the area around the mountain and told local ranchers stories of the goddess and a vast subterranean cavern filled with ancient pictographs that matched the descriptions of saber-toothed tigers and mastodons. In an effort to hide the cave, Clark said he used dynamite to destroy its entrance. Clark was an eccentric Columbia University graduate who posed as an illiterate. Rumors swarmed that he also found a hidden gold mine, but since he had no use for money, he left it alone and concealed the mine's location. Clark's hoard of gold still remains a mystery.

CHAPTER four

Driving & Destinations Along Highway 1

■ ■ ■ ■ ■ ■ ■ ■ ■ ■ ■ ■ ■ ■

M ORE THAN 3 MILLION VISITORS a year travel Highway 1, so it's no surprise that sightseers and vacationers have a myriad of services and attractions from which to choose— from resorts, spas, hotels, campgrounds, and retreats to galleries, hot springs, and coastal coffeehouses. The following attractions and businesses are listed in order from north to south under specific categories. While not comprehensive, the listings include many of the Hotels & Motels, Campgrounds & RV Parks, Restaurants & Cafés, Art Galleries, Automotive Services, and Events along Highway 1 between Carmel and San Simeon.

Hotels & Motels

LAMP LIGHTER INN SE corner of Ocean Avenue at Camino Real, Carmel-by-the-Sea, (831) 624-7372, carmellamplighter.com ($185–450/night). Just west of Highway 1, this is one of the most photographed inns in the country, offering rooms and cottages a short stroll from the beach and village.

CARMEL RIVER INN At Carmel River Bridge, (831) 624-1575 or (800) 882-8142, carmel riverinn.com ($165–450/night). Just past Carmel River State Beach, this inn is widely considered the best lodging bargain in Carmel.

PARK HYATT CARMEL, HIGHLANDS INN 120 Highlands Drive, Carmel, (831) 624-3801 or (800) 682-4811, highlandsinn.hyatt.com ($440–675/night). Ocean-view rooms with fireplaces and spa baths, as well as wine tasting and a fantastic restaurant.

RIVERSIDE CAMPGROUND & CABINS 22 miles south of Carmel, (831) 667-2414, river sidecampground.com ($90–200/night). Cabins on the Big Sur River.

BIG SUR RIVER INN 24 miles south of Carmel, (831) 667-2700 or (800) 548-3610, bigsur riverinn.com ($125–225/night). Balconies overlook the Big Sur River. Includes heated pool, restaurant, general store, and live entertainment in the bar on weekends.

GLEN OAKS BIG SUR 25 miles south of Carmel, (831) 667-2105 ($195–450/night). Standard rooms, as well as four separate cottages for rent in the redwoods, offering both river and forest views.

BIG SUR CAMPGROUND & CABINS 26 miles south of Carmel, (831) 667-2322 ($95–450/night). Tent cabins and A-frame cabins with kitchens, fireplaces, and redwood decks overlooking the river.

FERNWOOD RESORT 26 miles south of Carmel, (831) 667-2422 ($45–195/night). One of the least expensive spots above the Big Sur River, offering 66 campsites, 10 cabins, and 13 motel-style units.

BIG SUR LODGE 26 miles south of Carmel, (831) 667-3100, bigsurlodge.com ($159–364/night). Within Pfeiffer Big Sur State Park, this lodge offers simple cottages, a restaurant, gift shop, grocery, laundry, and a heated pool in summer.

RIPPLEWOOD RESORT 27 miles south of Carmel, (831) 667-2242, ripplewoodresort.com ($105–225/night). Another affordable option above the Big Sur River, with a convenience store, gas station, and café.

VENTANA INN 28 miles south of Carmel, (831) 667-2331 or (800) 628-6500, ventanainn .com ($440–1,500/night). Nestled on a hillside, this inn offers elegant cottages and luxury suites with ocean or mountain views, as well as a restaurant and spa services.

POST RANCH 28 miles south of Carmel, (831) 667-2200 or (800) 527-2200, postranchinn .com ($675–2,485/night). This cliffside ranch offers rustic yet elegant rooms with awe-inspiring ocean views. Voted one of the best hotels in North America. Award-winning Sierra Mar Restaurant serves world-class cuisine.

DEETJEN'S BIG SUR INN 28 miles south of Carmel, (831) 667-2377, deetjens.com ($105–260/night). Rustic, funky rooms offer an offbeat hideaway in a shady redwood canyon.

ESALEN INSTITUTE 8 miles south of Big Sur, (831) 667-3005, esalen.org ($140–220/night). Offering natural hot springs and workshops that emphasize the potentialities of human existence.

LUCIA LODGE 22 miles south of Big Sur and 38 miles north of San Simeon, (831) 667-2391, lucialodge.com ($150–275/night). These cabins are set along a 300-foot cliff above the Pacific, offering ocean views from the dining deck.

TREEBONES RESORT 37 miles south of Big Sur and 23 miles north of San Simeon, (877) 424-4787, treebonesresort.com (campsite: $90/night; yurt: $215–400/night). There are 16 canvas-covered yurts, along with ocean-view campsites and the Wild Coast Restaurant and Sushi Bar, which focuses on sustainably harvested local food. No children under age 6 allowed.

GORDA SPRINGS COTTAGES 42 miles south of Big Sur and 25 miles north of San Simeon, (805) 927-4600 or (805) 927-3918, gordaspringsresort.com ($150–300/night). Cottages feature a private patio overlooking the ocean; some have hot tubs, fireplaces, and ocean views. General store, restaurant, gift shop, and excellent whale-watching. Pet the resident llamas.

RAGGED POINT INN 50 miles south of Big Sur and 15 miles north of San Simeon, (805) 927-4502, raggedpointinn.net ($159–309/night). You'll find 21 rooms with coastal views, as well as a conference/wedding pavilion, restaurant, snack bar, gallery and gift shop, espresso stand, convenience store, gas station, and gardens.

Campgrounds & RV Parks

ANDREW MOLERA STATE PARK 21 miles south of Carmel and 70 miles north of San Simeon, (831) 667-2315 (24 sites, $25/night). A walk-in campground about 0.3 mile from the parking area. No dogs allowed. Sites are granted on a first-come, first-serve basis.

RIVERSIDE CAMPGROUND & CABINS 22 miles south of Carmel, (831) 667-2414, riversidecampground.com (45 sites, $40/night for tent site and $50/night for RV site). Perched along the Big Sur River in the shade of redwoods, this campground offers swimming and fishing in season.

BIG SUR CAMPGROUND & CABINS 24 miles south of Carmel, (831) 667-2322 (tent: $45–60/night for 2 people; $5 for each additional person up to 5; cabin: $180–535/night). Offers full-hookup campsites along the Big Sur River, as well as tent cabins and A-frame cabins.

FERNWOOD RESORT CAMPGROUND 25 miles south of Carmel, (831) 667-2422 (tent: $30–50/night for 2 people; $5 for each additional person up to 6; RV: $35–50/night). This campground offers 60 sites, showers, a restaurant, bar, and general store.

PFEIFFER BIG SUR STATE PARK 26 miles south of Carmel, (800) 444-7275, parks.ca.gov (218 sites, $35/standard site, $45/river site, $150/group site; reservations recommended). Along the Big Sur River, this 1006-acre park offers showers, Wi-Fi, and swimming.

VENTANA CAMPGROUND 30 miles south of Carmel, (831) 667-2712, ventanacampground.com (80 sites, $27–55/night prior to closure in 2008; will reopen summer 2013). Nestled in a redwood grove in Post Canyon, this rustic campground provides electricity and showers.

JULIA PFEIFFER BURNS STATE PARK 37 miles south of Carmel, (800) 444-7275, parks.ca.gov (2 tent-only sites, $30/night; reservations highly recommended). Near the trail to 100-foot McWay Falls, these primitive hike-in campsites are in high demand. Restrooms and water at the parking lot.

KIRK CREEK CAMPGROUND 54 miles south of Carmel and 40 miles north of San Simeon, (805) 434-1996, campone.com/campsites/kirk-creek (34 sites, $22/night; reservations recommended). This campground offers magnificent views of the Big Sur coast and a short trail to the beach.

LIMEKILN STATE PARK 56 miles south of Carmel, (831) 667-2403, parks.ca.gov (33 sites, $35/night; reservations recommended in summer and on holidays). At the mouth of Limekiln Creek, this campground amid the redwoods offers developed sites with picnic tables and fire rings. Some sites accommodate RVs and trailers. There are showers, picnic areas, and flush toilets.

PLASKETT CREEK CAMPGROUND 59 miles south of Carmel and 35 miles north of San Simeon, (805) 434-1996, recreation.gov (41 sites, $22/night; 3 group sites, $80/night; reservations recommended spring–fall and on holidays). This campground offers a parklike setting under the canopy of large pines and cypress a short walk from Sand Dollar Beach and Jade Cove.

TREEBONES RESORT 37 miles south of Big Sur and 23 miles north of San Simeon, (877) 424-4787, treebonesresort.com (campsite: $90/night; yurt: $215–400/night). There are 16 canvas-covered yurts, along with ocean-view campsites and the Wild Coast Restaurant and Sushi Bar, which focuses on sustainably harvested local food. No children under age 6 allowed.

SAN SIMEON CREEK CAMPGROUND Within San Simeon State Park, 5 miles south of San Simeon, (800) 444-7275, parks.ca.gov (134 sites, $35/night; reservations recommended in summer; first come, first served October 1–March 14). On a plateau overlooking the Pacific, this campground includes showers and RV sites (no hookups).

WASHBURN CAMPGROUND Within San Simeon State Park, 5 miles south of San Simeon, (800) 444-7275, parks.ca.gov (68 sites, $22/night; reservations recommended in summer; no showers). This campground lies a mile inland on a plateau overlooking the Santa Lucia Range.

Restaurants & Cafés

ROCKY POINT RESTAURANT 10 miles south of Carmel, (831) 624-2933, rockypoint restaurant.com. Promises spectacular coastal views from all tables.

BIG SUR RIVER INN 24 miles south of Carmel, (831) 667-2700 or (800) 548-3610, bigsur riverinn.com. Offers patio and indoor dining on the banks of the Big Sur River. Live entertainment on Sunday afternoons.

BIG SUR VILLAGE PUB 24 miles south of Carmel, (831) 667-2355. In the Village Shops, the pub features specialty beers and a pub-style menu.

REDWOOD GRILL 25 miles south of Carmel, (831) 667-2129, fernwoodbigsur.com. Serving buffalo burgers, salmon burgers, hamburgers, and veggie burgers in the shade of redwoods.

BIG SUR LODGE RESTAURANT & ESPRESSO HOUSE 26 miles south of Carmel, (831) 667-3100, bigsurlodge.com. Indoor and patio dining beneath the redwoods along the Big Sur River.

BIG SUR DELI 27 miles south of Carmel, (831) 667-2225, bigsurdeli.com. Known for reasonable prices, Big Sur Deli offers sandwiches, tacos, salads, and desserts at the deli, as well as groceries, camping supplies, and a gift shop.

BIG SUR BAKERY & RESTAURANT 28 miles south of Carmel, (831) 667-0520, bigsurbakery .com. Fresh pastries, breads, and pizza baked daily in a wood-fire oven, with sweeping views of the Big Sur River gorge.

CIELO 28 miles south of Carmel, (831) 667-2331 or (800) 628-6500, ventanainn.com. At Ventana Inn, this restaurant offers elegant dining, seasonal ingredients, and 50-mile vistas from the outdoor terrace.

SIERRA MAR RESTAURANT 28 miles south of Carmel, (831) 667-2800, postranchinn.com. At Post Ranch, this restaurant offers gourmet and eclectic California cuisine with a spectacular ocean view. Reservations required.

NEPENTHE 29 miles south of Carmel, (831) 667-2345, nepenthebigsur.com. Elegant dining in a rustic setting that overlooks 40 miles of incredibly scenic coastline.

CAFÉ KEVAH 29 miles south of Carmel, (831) 667-2344, nepenthebigsur.com. Just below Nepenthe, this café offers brunch and lunch on an outdoor terrace.

WILD COAST RESTAURANT AND SUSHI BAR At Treebones Resort, 37 miles south of Big Sur and 23 miles north of San Simeon, (831) 877) 424-4787, treebonesresort.com. Along with yurts and campsites, Treebones Resort features the Wild Coast Restaurant and Sushi Bar, which focuses on sustainably harvested local food.

WHALE WATCHER CAFE 25 miles north of Hearst Castle and 69 miles south of Carmel, (805) 927-1590, gordaspringsresort.com. At Gorda Springs Resort, this restaurant offers California cuisine and delicious homemade desserts, with spectacular ocean views.

RAGGED POINT RESTAURANT 14 miles north of Hearst Castle and 80 miles south of Carmel, (805) 927-5708, raggedpointinn.net. California cuisine, with ocean and mountain views.

Art Galleries

HEARTBEAT GIFT GALLERY 24 miles south of Carmel, (831) 667-2557, heartbeatbigsur .com. Adjacent to the Big Sur River Inn, this gallery offers art, jewelry, and collectibles from local artists and from around the world.

LOCAL COLOR 24 miles south of Carmel, (831) 667-0481, bigsurlocalcolor.com. Home to the Central Coast Artisan Gallery, where talented local artists display handmade goods.

STUDIO ONE 24 miles south of Carmel, (831) 667-1530. Owned by the Big Sur Arts Initiative, a local nonprofit arts enrichment organization. In addition to the gallery, the initiative provides teaching space for art classes, workshops, and seminars.

THE GARDEN GALLERY 27 miles south of Carmel, (831) 667-2000. The gallery offers local art, crafts, jewelry, clothing, and herbal products.

HAWTHORNE GALLERY 28 miles south of Carmel, (831) 667-3200, hawthornegallery.com. Represents local artists, featuring painting and sculpture in granite, wood, steel, bronze, glass, and ceramics.

THE PHOENIX SHOP 29 miles south of Carmel, (831) 667-2347, nepenthebigsur.com. At Nepenthe, this shop offers a collection of gifts, books, jewelry, and clothing.

HENRY MILLER LIBRARY 30 miles south of Carmel, (831) 667-2574, henrymiller.org. A nonprofit organization dedicated to the works of the American author, artist, and Big Sur resident Henry Miller. The gallery offers a wide assortment of art and fine and rare books.

COAST GALLERY BIG SUR 33 miles south of Carmel, (831) 667-2301, coastgalleries.com. A historic showplace for local artists and coastal craftsmen, featuring an art gallery, candle studio, and boutique.

Automotive Services

CHEVRON 3645 Rio Road, Carmel, (831) 624-7764. Open 6 a.m.–midnight; gas only.

CHEVRON CARMEL TOWING & GARAGE 4th Avenue and Junipero Avenue, Carmel, (831) 624-3827, carmeltow@redshift.com. Offers 24-hour towing and full-service repairs. Open 8 a.m.– 6 p.m.

BIG SUR GARAGE & TOWING 24 miles south of Carmel, (831) 667-2181. Offers 24-hour services: towing, tires, auto repair, and lockouts.

GORDA SPRINGS RESORT, RESTAURANT, STORE & GAS STATION 25 miles north of Hearst Castle and 69 miles south of Carmel, (805) 927-3918, gordaspringsresort.com. Open 8 a.m.–8 p.m.

RAGGED POINT INN RESORT & GAS STATION 14 miles north of Hearst Castle and 80 miles south of Carmel, (805) 927-4502, raggedpointinn.com. Open 8 a.m.–9 p.m.; gas only.

CAMBRIA TOWING 4363 Bridge Street, Cambria, (805) 927-4357. Offers 24-hour services: lockouts and tires.

Events

BIG SUR INTERNATIONAL MARATHON (831) 625-6226, bsim.org. Last Sunday in April. Voted best marathon in North America.

BIG SUR JAZZFEST (831) 667-1530. Spring. Three days of jazz at various Big Sur venues.

BIG SUR RIVER RUN (831) 624-4112, bigsurriverrun.org. Late October. Referred to as "the most beautiful run in the world," through redwoods along the Big Sur River.

HENRY MILLER LIBRARY (831) 667-2574, henrymiller.org. Summer calendar of international music, circus events, family entertainment, and community open mic.

HIDDEN GARDENS TOUR (831) 667-1530. Late June. One-day tour of various private Big Sur gardens, featuring presenters, artists, and musicians.

JADE FESTIVAL (831) 394-8315, surcoast.com/jfest.html. Early October. Jade, gems, wood, stone, barbecue, and live music in Pacific Valley.

Highway 1 Mileage Log: From Carmel River or Cambria

DESTINATION	Miles from Carmel River (*heading south*)	Miles from Cambria (*heading north*)
Carmel River Bridge	0	97.5
Carmel Meadows (Ribera Road)	0.6	96.9
Missionary Beach	1	96.5
Point Lobos State Reserve	1.9	95.6
Carmel Highlands general store	2.7	94.8
Malpaso Creek Bridge	4.5	93
Garrapata State Park (GSP north boundary)	5.2	92.3
GSP: Soberanes Canyon Trailhead	6.6	90.9
GSP: Whaleback Peak Trailhead	6.9	90.6
California Department of Fish and Game	7.8	89.7
Granite Creek Bridge	8	89.5
Garrapata Creek Bridge	9.4	88.1
Rocky Point Restaurant (turnoff west)	10.4	87.1
Palo Colorado Road (turnoff east)	11	86.5
Rocky Creek Bridge	12.5	85
Old Coast Road (turnoff east)	13	84.5
Bixby Bridge	13.1	84.4
Hurricane Point (viewpoint)	14.4	83.2

DESTINATION	Miles from Carmel River (*heading south*)	Miles from Cambria (*heading north*)
Little Sur River	16.4	81.1
Point Sur Historical Park & Lighthouse (turnoff west)	18.5	79
Point Sur Naval Facility (west gate)	18.9	78.6
Old Coast Road (turnoff east)	21.5	76
Andrew Molera State Park (west entrance)	21.5	76
River Inn Resort	24	73.5
Big Sur Center Village Shops (west)	24	73.5
Big Sur Campground & Cabins (west)	24.3	73.2
Riverside Campground & Cabins (west)	24.4	73.1
Ripplewood Resort, Gas Station, Store, Café	24.7	73.1
Glen Oaks (lodging & restaurant)	24.7	72.8
St. Francis of the Redwoods Catholic Church (west)	25.1	72.4
Fernwood Park Resort (west)	25.3	72.2
Pfeiffer Big Sur State Park (east)	26	71.5
Big Sur Lodge	26	71.5
Big Sur River Bridge	26.2	71.3
Big Sur Station (multi-agency facility; east)	26.4	71.1
Ripplewood Resort (west)	27	72.8
Sycamore Canyon Road (Pfeiffer Beach; turnoff west)	27.2	70.3
Big Sur Post Office & Store (east)	27.7	69.8
Big Sur Deli (gas station, store, bakery; turnoff west)	27.8	69.7
Ventana Inn turnoff (Old Post Ranch; east)	28.3	69.2
Post Ranch Inn & Cielo Restaurant (turnoff west)	28.3	69.2
Coastlands (residential neighborhood; turnoff west)	28.4	69.1
Nepenthe, Café Kevah, & the Phoenix Gift Shop (west)	29	68.5
Henry Miller Library (Graves Canyon; turnoff east)	29.3	68.2
Deetjen's (Castro Canyon; turnoff east)	29.7	67.8
Coast Gallery (turnoff east)	32.1	65.4
Torre Canyon Bridge	33.2	64.3
DeAngulo Trailhead (east)	34	63.5
Partington Ridge Road (residential; turnoff east)	34.3	63.1
Partington Cove & Tanbark Trailheads	35.1	62.4
Fire Road Trail to Tin House (turnoff east)	36	61.5
Large Vista Point (turnoff west)	36	61.5

DESTINATION	Miles from Carmel River (*heading south*)	Miles from Cambria (*heading north*)
Pfeiffer Burns State Park & McWay Creek Waterfall (turnoff east)	37.1	60.4
Anderson Creek Bridge	37.6	59.9
Burns Creek Bridge	38.7	58.8
Buck Creek Bridge	39.3	58.2
Esalen Institute (turnoff west)	40.3	57.2
Lime Creek Bridge	40.7	56.8
Dolan Creek Bridge	41.8	55.7
Rat Creek Bridge	42.9	54.6
Big Creek Bridge	45	52.5
Gamboa Point (west)	46.8	50.7
Vicente Creek Bridge	47.3	50.2
Lucia	50.1	47.4
New Camaldoli Monastery (east entrance)	50.6	46.9
Limekiln State Park	52.2	45.3
Vicente Flat Trailhead (east)	54.1	43.4
Kirk Creek Campground (turnoff west)	54.1	43.4
Nacimiento-Fergusson Road (turnoff east)	54.2	43.3
Mill Creek Bridge	54.5	43
Prewitt Loop Trailhead (north end turnoff east)	57.9	39.6
Pacific Valley Ranger Station & Prewitt Loop Trailhead (south end turnoff east)	58.5	39
Sand Dollar Beach parking & picnic area (turnoff west)	59.4	38.1
Plaskett Creek Campground; Pacific Valley School (turnoff east)	59.5	38
Plaskett Ridge Road (turnoff east)	59.6	37.9
Jade Cove turnout (west)	60	37.5
Willow Creek Bridge & Beach	61.5	36
Willow Creek Road & Treebones Resort (east turnoff)	62.1	35.4
Gorda (gas, lodging, store, restaurant)	63	34.5
Alder Creek Bridge	65.5	32
Villa Creek Bridge	66.2	31.3
Cruikshank Trailhead (east)	66.8	30.7
Soda Springs Trail (east)	69.5	28
Buckeye Trail (just past old ranger station on northeast side of highway)	71	26.5
Salmon Creek Bridge & Trailhead (east)	71.1	26.4

DESTINATION	Miles from Carmel River (*heading south*)	Miles from Cambria (*heading north*)
Monterey–San Luis Obispo county line	73.6	23.9
Ragged Point Inn (gas, lodging, restaurant; turnoff west)	75	22.5
San Carpoforo Creek Bridge	76.4	21.1
Arroyo de la Cruz Bridge	80.8	16.7
Piedras Blancas Lightstation (turnoff west)	84.1	13.4
Elephant Seal Vista Point (west)	85.1	12.4
Elephant Seal Vista Point (west)	85.4	12.1
Elephant Seal Vista Point (west)	86.4	11.1
Arroyo Laguna Bridge	87.5	10
W. R. Hearst Memorial Beach (turnoff west)	90.2	7.3
Hearst Castle entrance (turnoff east)	90.2	7.3
San Simeon Acres (lodging, restaurants; turnoff west)	93.3–93.7	4.2-3.8
San Simeon Creek Road to San Simeon State Park (turnoff east)	94.8	2.7
San Simeon Creek Bridge	95.1	2.4
Washburn Day Use Area & San Simeon State Beach	95.3	2.2
Moonstone Beach Road (north end; turnoff west)	95.7	1.8
Main Street, Cambria (turnoff east)	97.5	0

Driving & Destinations Along Big Sur Back Roads

■ ■ ■ ■ ■ ■ ■ ■ ■ ■ ■ ■ ■

I F Y O U A R E L O O K I N G T O E S C A P E the tourism and development of Highway 1, consider venturing east and turning along some of the back roads that gain access into the remote wildlands of Big Sur County.

With this remoteness comes ruggedness. Often county road departments and the US Forest Service close these back roads during storm events and keep them closed until the wet season dissipates in the spring. Maintenance is not high priority along these relatively unused roads, so expect to find ruts and debris (boulders, rocks, trees, and limbs) if you choose a more adventurous route.

Be prepared and note that most unpaved back roads are not suitable for low clearance vehicles, trailers, and RVs. Fortunately, there are a few paved roads that are suitable for your average two-wheel drive vehicle, but you should still expect a steep, windy, and, at times, single-lane ride. Regardless of the route you choose (paved or unpaved), inquire locally about road conditions before you head out, respect private property, fill up your tank, and make sure your vehicle is in good running condition with everything you might need to repair a spare or wait for some time for assistance.

If you plan to enter Fort Hunter Liggett, note the special rules at the three public-access points (Jolon Road, Nacimiento-Fergusson Road, and the northern end of Milpitas Road). All passengers will need to show photo identification to the sentry, and drivers will need to show car registration and proof of insurance. Entry may be denied due to security alerts or military training. Biking, hiking, camping, picnicking, and swimming are prohibited except to anglers and hunters who obtained the required permits from the Outdoor Recreation Office.

For information on road closures contact the following offices:

Fort Hunter Liggett: Call (831) 386-2503 or (831) 386-2310 for military road closures.

Los Padres National Forest: Call the King City office at (831) 385-5434 or visit www.fs.fed.us for seasonal or permanent closures of forest service roads.

Big Sur Station: Call (831) 667-2315 for information on state park and forest service roads.

Cal Trans: Call (888) 836-0866 for information about traffic and road conditions on Highway 1 from Carmel to Cambria.

Back Road Camping

IF YOU ARE TURNED OFF by the high price of camping along Highway 1, consider the primitive and remote camping that exists along Big Sur's back roads. The plus side is that many of these camps provide free camping (simply unheard of along the coast). With the exception of Arroyo Seco Campground and the developed sites at Nacimiento and San Antonio Reservoirs, these primitive, rarely maintained camps provide few to no amenities, so expect to bring in water and/or purifying systems and everything else you might need to be comfortable and safe.

Alder Creek Camp

DIRECTIONS: Located 8 miles from Highway 1 on Willow Creek Road (23S01).

CAMPSITES: 2 | **COST:** Free

WATER: On the creek; no potable water

COMMENTS: For more information contact the Los Padres National Forest Service at (831) 385-5434 or **www.fs.fed.us.**

Arroyo Seco Campground

DIRECTIONS: Coming from the south on Highway 101 to Greenfield, take the Arroyo Seco exit into town. Turn left on Elm Street. Go west to Arroyo Seco Road and turn left; campground is at the end of Arroyo Seco Road.

Coming from the north on Highway 101 just pass Soledad. Go west to Arroyo Seco Road and turn left; campground is at the end of Arroyo Seco Road.

CAMPSITES: 50 | **COST:** $15–30 (primitive sites), $20–40 (with showers and flush toilets), $75 (group site)

COMMENTS: For more information contact Rocky Mountain Recreation at (831) 674-5726.

Bottchers Gap Campground

DIRECTIONS: Located 8 miles inland, off Highway 1 on Palo Colorado Road (18S05), 15 miles north of Big Sur and 11 miles south of Carmel.

CAMPSITES: 11 | **COST:** $12/night, $5/day use

COMMENTS: For more information contact Parks Management Co. at (805) 434-1996, (805) 434-9199, or **campone.com.**

China Camp

DIRECTIONS: From Highway 101 north, exit at Arroyo Seco Road near the city of Greenfield. Proceed 16.2 miles to the junction of Carmel Valley Road and Arroyo Seco Road and bear right. Take Carmel Valley Road 17.2 miles to the junction with Tassajara Road and turn left. Go 11 miles to China Camp.

From Highway 101 south, exit at Arroyo Seco Road and make an immediate left at Elm Avenue. (If you get to the ENTERING GREENFIELD sign, you have passed the left turn.) Follow Elm Avenue for 6 miles and turn left at the T onto Arroyo Seco Road. Proceed 6.5 miles along Arroyo Seco Road to the junction with Carmel Valley Road and bear right. Take Carmel Valley Road 17.2 miles to the junction with Tassajara Road and turn left. Go 11 miles to China Camp.

CAMPSITES: 6 | COST: Free

COMMENTS: No water; vault toilets. For more information contact the Los Padres National Forest Service at (831) 385-5434 or **www.fs.fed.us**.

Escondido Campground

DIRECTIONS: Take Highway 101 to Jolon Road, turn onto Mission Road, to Del Venture Road. Travel 12 miles to the campground. Last 3 miles is unsurfaced.

CAMPSITES: 9 | COST: Free

COMMENTS: Closed during the winter and periodically during the wet season (November–March). No water, but the Arroyo Seco River is nearby (bring a water purification system); vault toilets. For more information contact the Los Padres National Forest Service at (831) 385-5434 or **www.fs.fed.us**.

Nacimiento Campground

DIRECTIONS: From the north, take Highway 101 south and take the Ft. Hunter Liggett exit. Then go 17.5 miles to the junction with Mission Road. From the south, take Highway 101 south to Exit 252. Drive 21.7 miles on County Road G18 to the junction at Mission Road. From the junction travel 3.2 miles on Mission Road to Nacimiento-Ferguson Road and turn left. It is 13 miles to Nacimiento CG from this point.

CAMPSITES: 8 | COST: $10/night

COMMENTS: No water; vault toilets. For more information contact Parks Management Co. at (805) 434-1996, (805) 434-9199, or **campone.com**.

Ponderosa Campground

DIRECTIONS: From Salinas take Highway 101 south and take the Ft. Hunter Liggett exit. Then go 17.5 miles to the junction with Mission Road. From Highway 101 south, take Exit 252. Drive 21.7 miles on County Road G18 to the junction at Mission Road. From the junction travel 3.2 miles on Mission Road to Nacimiento-Ferguson Road and turn left. It is 12 miles to Ponderosa CG from this point.

CAMPSITES: 23 | COST: $15/night

COMMENTS: No water (April–October); vault toilets. For more information contact Parks Management Co. at (805) 434-1996, (805) 434-9199, or **campone.com**.

Safety & Conservation

■ ■ ■ ■ ■ ■ ■ ■ ■ ■ ■ ■ ■

H UNDREDS OF MILES OF TRAILS AND ROADS crisscross Big Sur's state parks, the Ventana Wilderness, and the Silver Peak Wilderness. Plan carefully before you venture into the backcountry. This chapter describes potential hazards and offers gear suggestions to help you prepare for your hike.

The fact that a trail is described in this book does not mean it's safe for everyone. Trails vary greatly in difficulty and condition. Some sections are choked with poison oak, encroaching brush, fallen trees, and debris. The sheer landscape is also subject to floods and landslides. Conditions can change rapidly. A riverside trail that's safe on a dry day may be impassable during heavy rains, even for the fittest hiker.

It is essential that you tell someone where you're hiking and when you expect to return so rescue groups know where to look if you're overdue. Always respect your limits and avoid hiking alone. Stay on the trail, both to limit erosion and avoid injury.

Following the preparation tips is a partial list of regulations and advice on how to preserve this beautiful landscape for fellow hikers. If you'd like to volunteer your time, refer to the list of conservation organizations on page 50.

Wildlife Hazards

Ticks

Particularly in the Ventana and Silver Peak Wildernesses, trails are often overgrown with brush. This encroaching brush, in turn, harbors ticks. Tick numbers boom following winter's first major rains and don't drop again till early summer. They're most prevalent amid dense thickets of chamise, Big Sur's most widespread plant.

Once one of these blood-sucking arachnids latches on, it climbs till it reaches an exposed patch of skin. Deer ticks start out the size of a comma on a printed page, while wood ticks are only about twice that size. The tiny hitchhikers often go unnoticed until they swell with blood.

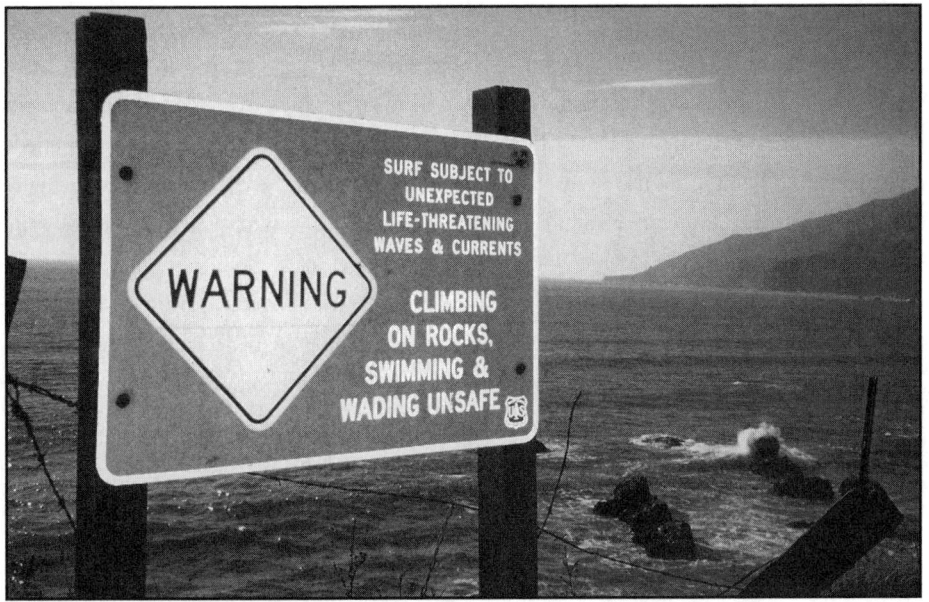

Along the coast, enjoy the coarse sand between your toes, but beware of cold water and dangerous currents.

Ticks usually take an hour or more to burrow into your skin, though in heavily infested areas you should check for them every few minutes. Wear long, light-colored clothing to make it easier to spot ticks. Consider wearing breathable rain gear, as the slow-moving insects have difficulty latching onto the synthetic material.

If you do find a tick burrowed into your skin, take a pair of tweezers, grip the tick as close to the skin as possible, and pull it straight out. Avoid squeezing the tick, as it may emit bacteria into the skin. While tick-borne Lyme disease remains rare in the northern Santa Lucia Range, that risk could change in the future. A tick must be attached for at least 24 hours to transmit the disease, which is very treatable if diagnosed early. If you develop a bull's-eye rash, pain, fever, headache, or muscle ache after a tick bite, see your doctor immediately.

Flies

How can such a small insect be so vexing? A number of fly species thrive when temperatures rise above 70°F. Though certain types can deliver a painful bite, these are typically slow and easy to swat. Much more of a nuisance are persistent nonbiting gnats, which continually buzz around your face. You may encounter flies on a warm winter day, but populations increase markedly between April and October. Dense oak woodlands are their favorite habitat in summer.

Rattlesnakes

Found throughout the Santa Lucia Range, these venomous snakes like to bask on warm rocks or sunny patches of dirt. They are most common in spring when their food supply (mostly rodents) also peaks. Rattlesnakes usually flee when startled and will only strike if threatened.

To avoid being bitten, stay on paths, always give snakes the right of way, wear high-sided hiking boots, and carry a walking stick. When climbing, watch where you place your hands and feet.

If someone is bitten, keep the person as calm and still as possible, gently wash the area with soap and water, apply a clean bandage, and seek immediate medical attention. Do not apply a tourniquet or pack the bite area in ice, as either method will only block circulation. Do not use your mouth to suck out venom, as that may lead to a complicating infection. Following treatment, most snakebite symptoms resolve within a few days.

Giardia lamblia

People often return from camping trips suffering from giardiasis, an infection of the small intestine that can cause nausea, diarrhea, loose or watery stool, and stomach cramps. A single-celled parasite, *Giardia lamblia* is passed in the stool of an infected person or animal or through contaminated food or water. Symptoms generally begin one to two weeks after being infected and may last two to six weeks.

Purify all water taken from springs, lakes, creeks, and rivers with a portable filter, chemical treatment, or by boiling it for one to three minutes.

Raccoons & Skunks

These night visitors are drawn by food left out by campers. Never leave your food unattended and always store it somewhere safe at night, preferably in a food canister hung from a tree. Avoid feeding wildlife. Raccoons and skunks are known carriers of rabies and are also infested with disease-carrying fleas, ticks, lice, and mites.

Mountain Lions

While mountain lions do roam throughout the Santa Lucia Range, they are extremely elusive and pose a minimal threat. Don't hike alone, and keep children within arm's length. If you encounter a lion, neither approach nor run from it. Do all you can to appear larger, and fight back if attacked.

Wild Boars

Hunters introduced these destructive, nonnative animals to the Santa Lucia Range as game in the 1920s, and their population has since exploded. Boar hunting is permitted within the

Ventana and Silver Peak Wildernesses, but regulations govern how far hunters must keep from trails and roads. For more information, contact the Los Padres National Forest Headquarters: (805) 968-6640 or www.fs.usda.gov/lpnf.

Plant Hazards

Poison Oak

Poison oak is a common trailside companion in Big Sur country. It grows as a low-lying bush, shrub, or vine along stream banks, rocky canyons, mountain flanks, and coastal bluffs from sea level to below 5000 feet (it's only absent on the highest rocky summits). Learning to identify this toxic plant is the first step toward avoiding a painful, annoying rash.

Poison oak leaves are clustered in threes. Shiny when young, the leaflets usually range from half an inch to 2 inches long. In fall the leaves turn a brilliant red, while branches are bare in winter. Unfortunately, all parts of the plant (the leaves, flowers, stem, roots, and fruit) are toxic year-round.

Since many trails are overgrown, particularly within the Ventana and Silver Peak Wildernesses, it's likely you'll brush up against poison oak at some point. It's best to wear long pants while hiking, regardless of temperature. If you're extremely susceptible, bring extra pants and long-sleeved shirts, and place each day's clothes in a plastic bag upon reaching camp. Wash your skin thoroughly with products designed to remove the plant's toxic oil, such as Tecnu.

Poison oak's oily resin contains the toxin urushiol. Contact can cause painful blistering, weeping soars, and maddening itching. The rash may appear in a few hours or days, depending on the extent of exposure and your degree of sensitivity. Most exposures are through direct contact with the plant. Other sources include smoke and secondary exposure from pets, soiled clothing, and gear. If your symptoms are severe, see a physician for treatment with strong corticosteroids.

Stinging Nettle

Another unpleasant plant you may encounter on the trail is the stinging nettle, which grows in clusters along the banks of creeks and rivers. Nettle leaves bear raised prickly hairs that stick in your skin, instantly delivering a painful sting and burning sensation. You'll know once you've walked through stinging nettles—the key is to recognize them in advance.

Growing in slender stalks up to 6 feet tall, nettles sport dense, drooping clusters of flowers where the leaves join the stalk. Leaves are heart-shaped, finely toothed, and grow on opposite sides of the stem. When you brush against the plant, the tiny hollow hairs break off and release an acid. Symptoms are usually gone within 24 hours.

You can neutralize the acid by mixing it with a base, such as baking soda. Bring a packet of baking soda with you, and apply it to your skin as soon as possible to soothe the burn. If baking soda is unavailable, try your own spit, which is somewhat basic and will help neutralize the acid.

Gear

Survival Essentials

You should always carry:

Water

Many wilderness trails are dry for several miles, and small seasonal creeks are not always reliable. Carry at least 1–2 liters of water and some means of purifying backcountry sources (filter or chemical treatment such as iodine).

Food

An energy bar, nuts, or trail mix may be critical if you're out longer than you planned to be.

First-Aid Kit

Accidents and injuries can happen to anyone. Properly preparing for these instances can save you from a backcountry disaster. Prepackaged first-aid kits are readily available at outdoor equipment stores. A basic kit should include at least the following:

- Ace bandages
- Advil or other anti-inflammatory medicine
- alcohol pads
- antibiotic ointment
- Band-Aids and moleskin
- cotton balls or swabs
- gauze pads and bandages
- hydrogen peroxide
- medical tape
- poison oak soap (Tecnu)
- space blanket
- tweezers (for removing ticks)
- Tylenol (fever and pain reduction)
- waterproof matches (for emergency fire)

Knife

Pocketknives and all-in-one tools can be invaluable in the event of a mishap.

Map & Compass

Some of the more remote trails are heavily overgrown with brush and easily lost to slides and fallen debris. A map and compass may help you find your way home.

Important Hiking Gear

Backpack

The ideal daypack should have enough room to carry survival essentials (see the previous page), ideally somewhere between 1000 and 2000 cubic inches of volume. Overnight packs should provide between 3000 and 4000 cubic inches.

Flashlight

Whenever possible, avoid hiking in the dark, as trails are steep, slippery, and lined with poison oak in places. However, if you're delayed or tire unexpectedly, you may end up hiking in the dark. Be prepared and always carry a flashlight. Hands-free headlamps are preferred over handheld flashlights.

Essential Overnight Gear

Sleeping Bag

Temperatures can drop dramatically at higher elevations along the Santa Lucia Range. Choose a sleeping bag with a temperature rating of 20°F or lower to ensure a warm and restful night's sleep. Be prepared for temperatures to occasionally drop below freezing from late fall through early spring.

Sleeping Pad

Inflatable and foam sleeping pads keep you off the cold, hard ground. They also provide spots to sit and lounge at camp.

Tent

Too often hikers leave tents at home, particularly in summer when rainfall is unlikely. However, fog creeps inland and can saturate a sleeping bag with condensation by morning.

The Kitchen Sink

Be sure to pack plenty of food, spices, cooking supplies, and utensils. There's nothing like eating gourmet in the backcountry. Don't forget the chocolate and warm drinks.

Camp Wear

Backcountry hiking can be a sweaty slog. When you arrive at camp, it's wonderful to hang out beneath the stars in a set of comfortable camp clothes (e.g., long underwear, comfortable fleece pants, and slip-on shoes). Again, those extremely sensitive to poison oak should store the previous day's clothes in a plastic bag.

Other Necessities

Don't forget a wide-brimmed hat, polarizing sunglasses, sunscreen, a towel, toiletries, a warm knit cap, waterproof backpack cover, duct tape, and trowel.

If there's still room in your pack, bring a camera, binoculars, a Frisbee, cards, and small travel games.

The Wilderness Ethic

TREATING BIG SUR'S PUBLIC LANDS as a precious resource will ensure they remain unspoiled for future generations. Please refer to the following commonsense guidelines:

Group Size

Visit in small groups. Although US Forest Service guidelines allow groups of up to 25 individuals at backcountry camps, most backcountry camps only have room for up to 10. You'll find designated group camping at Pfeiffer Big Sur State Park, Kirk Creek Campground, and Arroyo Seco Campground.

Camping

Camp at an established site. Keep your camp clean and never leave food out. Scout the area to be sure you leave nothing behind.

Fire Safety

Careless campfire use has sparked devastating blazes. Where fire use is authorized, please observe the following measures:

Campfires are permitted only in established fire rings and must be kept small, using as little wood as possible. Use only dead and downed wood. Always make sure your fire is completely extinguished before you break camp.

Regardless of the time of year, a fire permit is required for backcountry camping. The permits allow full campfires during the wet season (November through April) or the use of camp stoves the rest of the year. East side campers should contact the Los Padres National Forest Headquarters in Goleta at (805) 968-6640. West side campers can obtain a permit either at Big Sur Station, a half mile south of Pfeiffer Big Sur State Park, or at Pacific Valley Station, 5 miles north of Gorda.

Noise Pollution

Respect the natural peace, fellow hikers, and neighboring campers by keeping all trail and camp chatter down. Raucous behavior may also spook wildlife.

Camp at established sites to minimize your impact and "leave no trace."

Sanitation

Keep soap and detergent away from all natural water sources. If you're susceptible to poison oak and need to wash with medicated soap, do not bathe in the streams. Such products contain toxic chemicals that pollute water. Wash with water from a pot, and rinse at least 100 feet from any water source.

Also refrain from washing dishes or clothing in natural water sources. Wash using minimal water and dispose of wastewater at least 100 feet from any water source.

If a pit toilet is unavailable, dig a hole at least 6 inches deep, make your deposit, and cover it with the soil you removed. Do not bury toilet paper or trash, as an animal may dig it up.

Garbage

If you pack it in, you must pack it out. Before leaving camp, clean up and pack out any trash left by inconsiderate campers. Leave the site looking as lightly used as possible.

Pack Stock & Horses

Hikers must yield right-of-way to all pack and saddle animals. Forage is often scarce, so be sure to pack plenty of food for your animals. Such animals can severely damage trails and camps if not properly handled. Avoid tying animals to trees, as they may dig up roots and strip bark.

Wildlife

Do not feed wild animals. They will associate humans with food and may become aggressive pests. Juvenile animals may never learn normal foraging behavior, instead becoming dependent on handouts that are not part of their natural diets. Wild animals may also congregate in unnaturally high numbers, which might increase chances of disease transmission.

Conservation

WITH LITTLE MONEY ALLOCATED for maintenance, the US Forest Service is unable to devote much attention to trails within the Ventana and Silver Peak Wildernesses. Fortunately, groups of dedicated volunteers have taken responsibility for rebuilding trail networks and caring for this backcountry that belongs to us all. Many of these volunteers work for the following listed conservation groups, grass-roots organizations dedicated to protecting, preserving, enhancing, and restoring public lands within the Santa Lucia Range.

> Let us leave a splendid legacy for our children . . . let us turn
> to them and say, "This you inherit: Guard it well, for it is far
> more precious than money . . . and once destroyed, nature's
> beauty cannot be repurchased at any price."

Ansel Adams, American photographer, 1902–1984

We owe a debt of gratitude to such volunteers. The trails would not be passable and this book would not be possible without them. Be sure to do your part to leave Big Sur's natural spaces as pristine as you found them.

Conservation Organizations

The Big Sur wilderness hangs in fragile balance between humans and nature. Were it not for the foresight and efforts of grass-roots conservationists, much of the region's untamed splendor might be lost to development. Please contact the following groups if you'd like to get involved:

Big Sur Land Trust
PO Box 221864
Carmel, CA 93922
(831) 625-5523; **bigsurlandtrust.org**

Ventana Wilderness Alliance
PO Box 506
Santa Cruz, CA 95061
(831) 423-3191; **ventanawild.org**

Sierra Club, Ventana Chapter
PO Box 5667
Carmel, CA 93921
(831) 624-8032; **ventana.sierraclub.org**

Ventana Wilderness Society
19045 Portola Dr., Suite F-1
Salinas, CA 93908
(831) 455-9514; **ventanaws.org**

PART ONE

■　■　■　■　■　■　■　■　■　■　■　■

State & Federal Lands of the Big Sur Coast

THIS SECTION COVERS the 90-mile stretch of coast from Carmel River State Beach south to San Simeon State Beach. All lands are accessible from Highway 1, which winds past golden hillsides, redwood-lined ravines, ancient oak forests, and sheer granite cliffs. Lying primarily west of the highway, the region comprises six state parks (Garrapata, Andrew Molera, Pfeiffer Big Sur, Julia Pfeiffer Burns, Limekiln, and San Simeon), seven beaches (Carmel River, Pfeiffer, San Simeon, Hearst Memorial, Piedras Blancas, Jade Cove, and Sand Dollar), one reserve (Point Lobos), and one historic park (Point Sur). These public spaces are relatively small, thus trails are short and for day use only.

Due to its proximity to the ocean, the region is fertile in both terrestrial and marine life. Northern and southern biogeographical regions converge here in a kind of suture zone that supports a wide range of vegetation. Fog shrouds the coast in summer, nurturing moisture-loving plants in deep ravines, while the sheer, exposed slopes host such drought-tolerant species as yuccas. Cold-water upwellings from deep marine canyons bring nutrient-rich waters to the surface, luring fish, seals, birds, whales, and sharks close to shore.

Recreational opportunities are equally diverse. Visitors can dive the waters off Point Lobos or Jade Cove, summit granite peaks, marvel at 5,000-pound male elephant seals, plunge into swimming holes along the Big Sur River, explore Hearst Castle, surf the rollers at Andrew Molera, learn about maritime history at Point Sur Lighthouse, or simply take a barefoot stroll on the beach. Whatever you choose, you're bound to return.

CHAPTER seven

Carmel River State Beach & Point Lobos State Reserve

■　■　■　■　■　■　■　■　■　■　■　■　■　■

Carmel River State Beach

THIS PARK ACTUALLY comprises two beaches: Carmel River State Beach at the river mouth and San Jose Creek Beach (aka Monastery Beach) farther south. Together they form a mile-long crescent of coarse sand backed by bluffs that offer spectacular views. Visitors can go for a stroll, build a sandcastle, picnic, or watch wildlife on the sheltered inland side of the beach at Carmel River Lagoon.

While the turquoise Pacific may look inviting, neither beach is safe for swimming or wading. A deep underwater canyon just offshore contributes to hazardous surf conditions. Even on calm days, unpredictable "sleeper waves" have risen up to surprise waders, sometimes dragging them in. Year-round strong currents and water temperatures that linger in the mid-50s Fahrenheit make submersion a real danger, though experienced, properly trained surfers and scuba divers do brave these waters.

> **DIRECTIONS:** From Carmel, drive south on Highway 1 and turn right at the Rio Road signal light. In a half mile you'll pass Carmel Mission (Mission San Carlos Borromeo de Carmelo) on the left. One block past the mission, turn left on Santa Lucia Avenue. Drive 0.4 mile west on Santa Lucia to Carmelo Street and turn left. Within a half mile Carmelo dead-ends at the beach's north parking lot.
>
> **VISITOR CENTER:** Point Lobos State Reserve, off Highway 1, 2.2 miles south of the Rio Road intersection. Open daily 9 a.m.–7 p.m. in summer, 9 a.m.–5 p.m. in winter.
>
> **NEAREST CAMPGROUND:** See Chapter 10: Pfeiffer Big Sur State Park (page 98) for coastal campgrounds or Chapter 14: Bottchers Gap (page 148) for inland options.
>
> **INFORMATION:** Open 7 a.m.–10 p.m. Dogs must be on a leash.
>
> **WEBSITE:** parks.ca.gov
>
> **PHONE:** (831) 649-2836

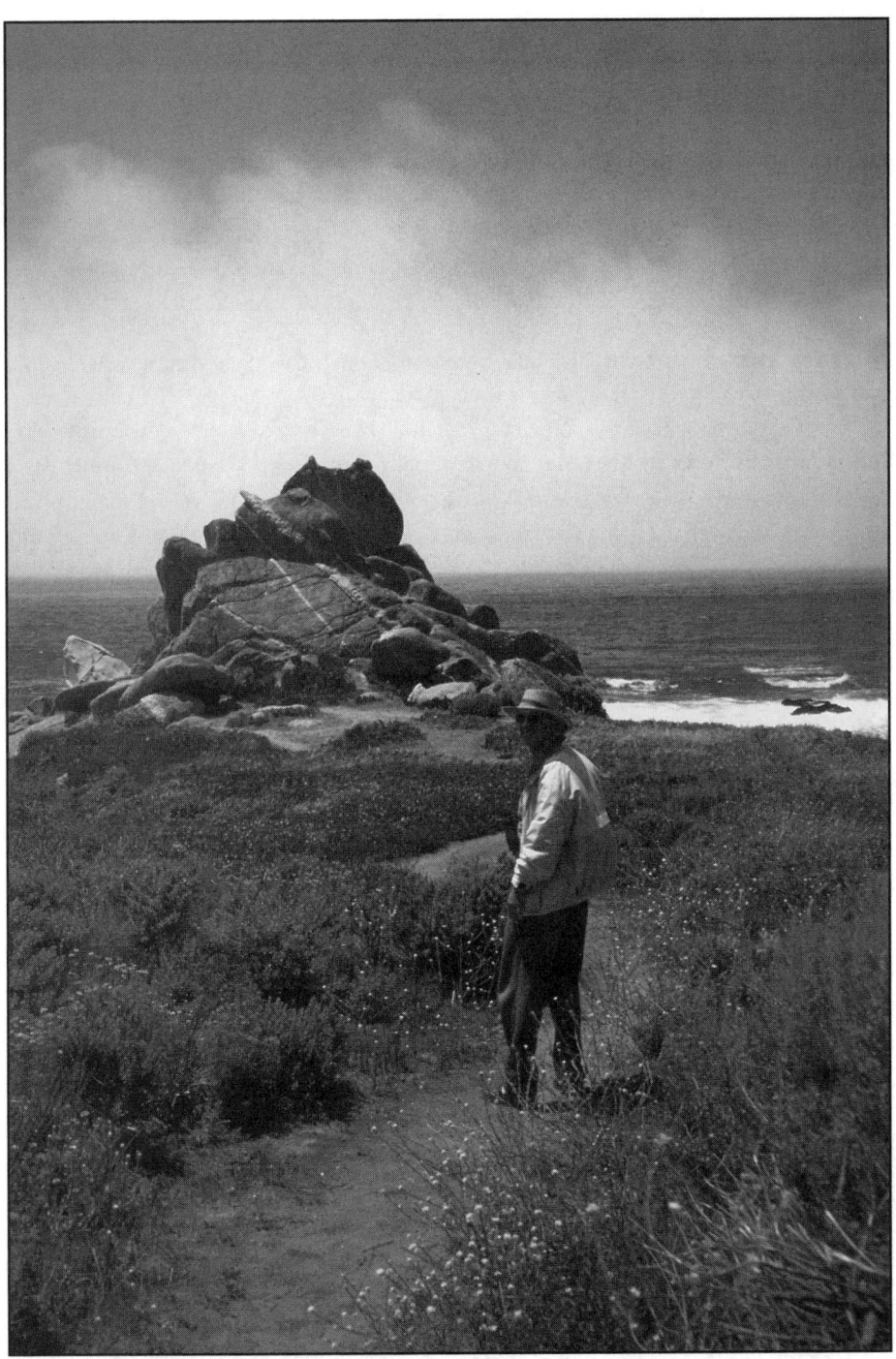

Short spur trails lead to stunning views from rocky granite outcrops along Carmel River State Beach.

Trip 1

CARMEL RIVER STATE BEACH

LENGTH AND TYPE: 2-mile out-and-back

RATING: Easy

TRAIL CONDITION: Well maintained, poison oak, good for kids

HIGHLIGHTS: A wildlife haven amid the Carmel River lagoon and estuary, featuring a mile-long crescent of coarse white sand and views of the open ocean

TO REACH THE TRAILHEAD: This hike begins at Carmel River State Beach, where you'll find a phone, restrooms, and water at the free parking lot.

TRIP SUMMARY: Carmel River State Beach actually comprises two beaches: Carmel River State Beach, at the river mouth, and Monastery Beach (aka San Jose Creek Beach), just south of the river. The trail saunters along these wave-washed beaches and atop the adjacent bluffs. The first 0.2 mile of the route crosses soft sands deposited by the Carmel River and pounded into fine powder by the often-heavy surf. The bluffs overlook granite pinnacles, wind-sculpted Monterey cypress, and a marsh and estuary that teem with life.

Trip Description

From the north end of **Carmel River State Beach,** the hike strikes out across sand and heads southwest toward the river mouth. Sand bridges the river mouth in summer, but expect a wet crossing after winter rains. If you prefer to keep your feet dry, park at Monastery Beach and hike north, following this trail description in reverse. Parking stretches for 0.2 mile along

Monastery Beach offers views inland that give rise to its name.

Highway 1 at Monastery. Just south of the lagoon you can either continue along the shoreline or climb atop the bluffs for sweeping views of Carmel Bay, the lagoon, and the marsh.

The bluff trail leads up a half dozen stairs to a fork (0.2 mile, 25'). The left spur traverses the east edge of the bluff for views of the marsh and lagoon. This spur then turns south through thickets of coyote brush, sagebrush, and lupine, ascending a small knoll capped by a large **wooden cross** (0.3 mile, 35'). A plaque explains its significance. In 1769 the Portolá-Crespi expedition traveled overland from Mexico. After waiting in vain for the long-overdue supply ship *San Jose*, they erected a cross here to signal their early return to San Diego. From here the spur veers west and rejoins the main bluff trail.

The direct route to the south end of the beach leads from atop the stairs along the west edge of the bluff, blanketed in fragrant coastal chaparral. A half mile south, the trail passes very large, striking homes in the **Carmel Meadows** subdivision. Farther along you'll encounter another short, narrow spur that leads down to prominent boulders pounded by surf. Beyond this spur, the main trail curls southeast to emerge at **Monastery Beach** (0.9 mile).

WHERE RIVER & SEA COLLIDE ■ ■ ■ ■ ■ ■ ■ ■ ■ ■ ■ ■ ■ ■ ■

The opposing forces of the Carmel River and Pacific Ocean form a unique ecosystem at Carmel River State Beach. Longshore currents deposit sand on the beach at the river mouth, forming sandbars that periodically dam its flow. The water that accumulates in the lagoon and surrounding marsh is a mix of freshwater and saltwater, creating a rare habitat. In the 160 miles between San Francisco Bay and Morro Bay, coastal salt marshes occur only at Elkhorn Slough, Pescadero Marsh, and here. It takes heavy rainfall to flood the river and once again break through the sandbars, allowing the lagoon to drain into the ocean.

Among Monterey County's prime birding locations, the lagoon and marsh shelter a wide variety of waterfowl and songbirds during their migration along the Pacific Flyway. Pelicans, seagulls, and several duck species bathe in the brackish water, while great blue herons, egrets, sandpipers, and plovers work the shallows for food. Red-winged blackbirds enact courtship displays atop tule reeds at the edge of the marsh. In the evenings, cliff swallows swoop down from nests south of the lagoon to nab flying insects. Also watch for the occasional northern harrier, black-shouldered kite, or red-tailed hawk, which soar over the wetlands in search of prey.

The river also hosts the southernmost major steelhead trout run in North America. Native steelhead return annually from the ocean to spawn. Strict rules protect this population, as the run dwindled to just a handful of fish in the early 1990s. As of 2002, the Carmel River averaged 123 juvenile steelhead per hundred feet of stream—numbers reflective of well-stocked streams, though this group and other California steelhead populations remain threatened species under the federal Endangered Species Act. Contact the California Department of Fish & Game for current fishing regulations: (831) 649-2870.

■ ■

Dramatically different rock formations anchor either end of the beach. On the north end, the trail passes large granitic outcrops laced with veins of blocky white crystals—excellent examples of Hobnail granite. Over the past 65 million years, the Pacific plate carried these ancient rocks hundreds of miles north from their origin in Mexico. In contrast, the south end features a narrow ridge of russet and tan conglomerate, composed of well-cemented stream sediments from a flood plain that was later supplanted by the Santa Lucia Range.

Monastery Beach is a popular launching spot for divers exploring the nearshore kelp forests. Cold upwelling in the Carmel Submarine Canyon brings nutrient-rich water to the surface, supplying food to abundant marine life. The canyon extends 3.5 miles west before deepening and turning northwest for 12 miles along an active fault to join the Monterey Submarine Canyon, the West Coast's largest submarine canyon.

Enjoy the coarse sand between your toes before returning the way you came.

Point Lobos State Reserve

THIS EXCEPTIONAL STRETCH of the Big Sur coast has been dubbed "the crown jewel of the California state park system." Seven hundred of the reserve's 1250 acres lie underwater, encompassing rocky coves, shallow tide pools, and broad kelp beds. The remaining 550 acres take in 14 trails that crisscross through wind-sculpted pines, across jagged rocky headlands, and along white sand beaches beside cobalt waters. Strolling this dynamic, diverse landscape, you'll find plenty of opportunities to sightsee, take photos, paint, picnic, and study nature, while water lovers can scuba dive or snorkel.

In addition to harboring incredibly diverse flora and fauna, unique geology, rare plant life, and spectacular scenery, Point Lobos is also rich in human history. At one time or another over the past 200 years, the point has been home to American Indians, Chinese fishermen, Japanese abalone harvesters, and Portuguese whalers. Throughout the park, historic relics and endangered archaeological sites offer visitors insight into the varied occupations that once thrived here.

Whether you walk the windswept coastline or head inland through Monterey pine groves and meadows, you'll hear the raucous barking of sea lions from their nearshore colonies—an enduring reminder of the earlier Spanish name for the reserve: *Punta de los Lobos Marinos* (Point of the Sea Wolves).

DIRECTIONS: The reserve entrance is off Highway 1, 2.2 miles south of the Rio Road intersection in Carmel and 1.2 miles north of the Highlands Inn entrance road (Highlands Drive) in Carmel Highlands.

VISITOR CENTER: An information kiosk at the entrance offers books, maps, and interpretive displays about the zoology, geology, and botany of Point Lobos.

NEAREST CAMPGROUNDS: See Chapter 10: Pfeiffer Big Sur State Park (page 98) for coastal campgrounds or Chapter 14: Bottchers Gap (page 148) for inland options.

INFORMATION: Open daily 9 a.m.–7 p.m. in summer, 9 a.m.–5 p.m. in winter. There's an $10-per-vehicle entrance fee (discounts offered to seniors and the disabled). Entry is limited to 450 visitors at any one time. Bicycles are restricted to paved

Point Lobos State Reserve

roads. Fires and the use of stoves are prohibited. Fishing, Frisbee, kite flying, and other games are prohibited. Pets are not allowed in the reserve, though guide dogs for the blind and certified service dogs are permitted. Diving is restricted to Bluefish and Whalers Coves with advance permits and proof of dive certification.

WEBSITE: pointlobos.org

PHONE: (831) 624-4909

Trip 2

CARMELO MEADOW, GRANITE POINT, & MOSS COVE TRAILS

LENGTH AND TYPE: 4.4-mile out-and-back

RATING: Easy

TRAIL CONDITION: Well maintained, good for kids

HIGHLIGHTS: Visit the Whaling Station Museum and adjacent Whalers Cabin Museum to learn about the area's cultural history.

TO REACH THE TRAILHEAD: Once at Point Lobos, park in the lot just past the entrance kiosk. If that lot is full (often the case on weekends), bear right at the first fork and head north 0.3 mile to Whalers Cove. Follow the trail description from Whalers Cove, bypassing the 0.2-mile Carmelo Meadow Trail description.

TRIP SUMMARY: This hike begins amid colorful coastal wildflowers in Carmelo Meadow and leads to Whalers Cove, the former site of a prosperous whaling station. A short stroll up the road leads to the Whalers Cabin Museum and Whaling Station Museum, each of which display historical artifacts, diagrams, and photographs. The **Granite Point Trail** leads through dense Monterey pines to Coal Chute Point, which overlooks the surging surf and thick floating kelp mats. Keep a close watch for harbor seals and sea otters amid the kelp.

Trails at Point Lobos lead to jagged, rocky headlands, turquoise waters, and wind-sculpted pine forests.

Trip Description

The **Carmelo Meadow Trail** leads from the entrance road north to Whalers Cove or south toward Gibson Beach and Bird Island. Head north through **Carmelo Meadow**. In spring, grasses and herbacious plants give way to a spectrum of wildflowers. At 0.2 mile the Carmelo Meadow Trail ends at **Whalers Cove** and a junction with the Granite Point Trail. Turn left onto the **Granite Point Trail** and stroll 0.1 mile to the **Whaling Station Museum** and **Whalers Cabin Museum** (0.3 mile, 30').

WHALE TALES ■

In the 1850s, Chinese fishermen sailed to California in 30-foot junks in order to harvest abalone along these rocky shores. Their settlement at Whalers Cove consisted of about a dozen structures, one of which now houses the Whalers Cabin Museum. Artifacts and memorabilia span several time periods in the cultural history of the cove.

Portuguese whalers arrived at Point Lobos in 1862 and established the Carmel Bay Whaling Company, one of 16 whaling stations on the California coast. The men hunted gray whales, which still roam these waters from mid-December through May during their migration from Baja to Alaska. The station closed in 1879, but the Whaling Station Museum offers a historical perspective of the industry alongside equipment, photographs, and drawings that depict the lives of whalers and their families. Docents are often on hand to answer questions.

After killing a whale, the whalers towed it into the cove and sliced its blubber into strips. They then cut the blubber into smaller pieces and melted it down in large iron cauldrons called try pots. The reduced blubber was used primarily as lamp oil. Two try pots are on display next to the museum alongside an enormous finback whale skeleton.

■ ■

Just past the museums, the trail leads to a small parking lot where an abalone cannery and a granite quarry once operated. At the height of abalone harvesting, the cannery supplied 75% of the abalone sold in California, while granite from the quarry was used to build the U.S. Mint in San Francisco. From here return to the junction with the Carmelo Meadow Trail.

Past this junction the Granite Point Trail leads through dense stands of Monterey pine and climbs toward **Coal Chute Point,** the first spur on your left (0.4 mile, 30'). At this site in the mid-1870s, coal was dumped from ore carts down a coal chute to the cove below, where deep water enabled coastal steamships close access to shore. The 200-foot spur loops back to Granite Point Trail.

The trail continues through dense, fragrant coastal scrub, descends to the edge of a former pasture, then reaches a junction with the spur toward **Granite Point**. Turn left and climb 0.1 mile to the point (1.6 miles, 30'), where spectacular views abound. Carmel Bay lies to the north, boasting wave-washed beaches and rocky promontories. Abundant life teems in the kelp forests, which rise and fall with the tides. Herons and egrets often "surf" atop these floating mats. The spur loops around to join the **Moss Cove Trail.**

This trail follows the road once used to transport coal from the hills above Point Lobos to Coal Chute Point. It also leads to the newest addition to the reserve, a pasture that once supported grazing cattle. Today small mammals such as mice, voles, and rabbits scurry in the underbrush, while hawks, kestrels, and kites soar overhead, taking advantage of the open hunting grounds. The trail emerges at the south end of **Monastery Beach** (2.2 miles, 20'). Return the way you came.

Trip 3

CYPRESS GROVE TRAIL

LENGTH AND TYPE: 0.8-mile loop

RATING: Easy

TRAIL CONDITION: Well maintained, good for kids

HIGHLIGHTS: Stroll past gnarled Monterey cypress trees in one of only two remaining native groves of this species.

TO REACH THE TRAILHEAD: From the entrance station of the park, drive 0.8 mile to the Sea Lion Point parking area. The trailhead is on the north side of the lot, just past the restrooms and information kiosk. Water is available at the trailhead.

TREES THAT INSPIRED A RESERVE ■ ■ ■ ■ ■ ■ ■ ■ ■ ■ ■ ■

Monterey cypress trees bear distinct twisted branches, shallow exposed roots, and dense flattened canopies. Their contorted appearance attests to the harsh environment of salt spray, rocky granite soil, and gale-force winds the trees must endure. Protection of the celebrated cypress prompted the acquisition of Point Lobos as a state reserve in 1933.

The Monterey cypress trees along North and South Point stand as a memorial to Mr. and Mrs. A.M. Allan, former owners of Point Lobos. In 1888 several land claimants banded together to develop a portion of the headland as residential lots. Fortunately, A.M. Allan, in conjunction with the Save-the-Redwoods League, had the foresight to buy back the residential lots, limit access, and seek public support to make Point Lobos part of the new state park system.

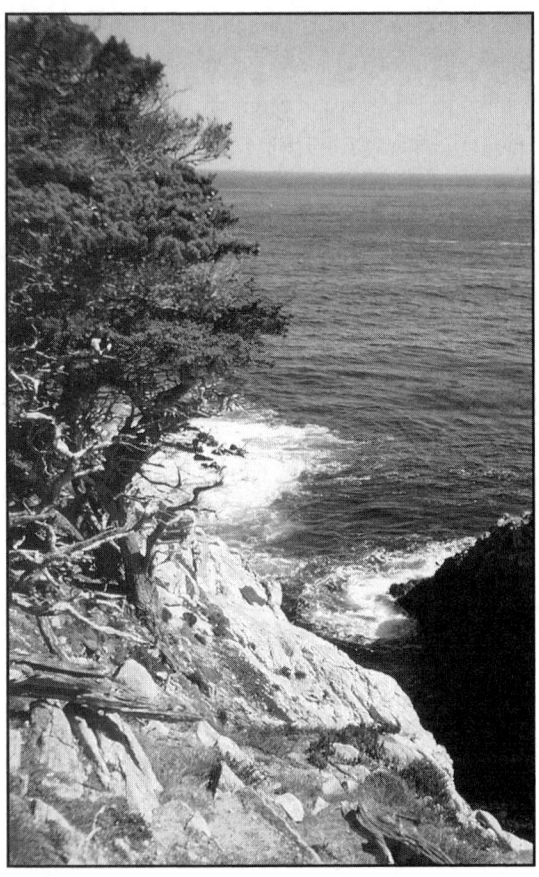

The Monterey cypress clings its bare roots to the sheer granite cliffs of Point Lobos.

TRIP SUMMARY: This short, easy trail leads to overlooks of near-shore islands and rocky coves, where sea otters, harbor seals, and sea lions frolic amid multicolored kelp beds.

Trip Description

From the information kiosk, the trail leads north and soon forks. The **North Shore Trail** heads off to the right, while the **Cypress Grove Trail** veers left 0.1 mile, then splits again into a loop trail through the **Allan Memorial Grove**. Taking the loop in either direction will lead you back to this junction.

Along the northwest fork, the trail offers views into **Headland Cove,** where with any luck you'll see all three species of resident marine mammals: California sea lions, sea otters, and harbor seals. If thick summer fog obscures your view, listen for the boisterous barking of sea lions from nearshore rocks.

Strolling past Headland Cove, you soon enter the grove, one of only two naturally growing stands of Monterey cypress in the world (the other grove is at Cypress Point on the north end of Carmel Bay). In the colder, wetter climate of the Pleistocene epoch some 15,000 years ago, these wind-sculpted trees extended over a much wider range. As the climate slowly turned hotter and drier, the cypress trees withdrew to the cool, fog-shrouded coast. Closely inspect the branches and buttressed trunks to spot a deep orange velvety encrustation. This plush substance is lichen that coexists with the tree, using its branches merely as a roost rather than obtaining nourishment at the tree's expense.

The trail soon veers right, offering dramatic views of secluded coves and granite pinnacles stretching north to Cypress Point. At **North Point** a spur climbs 50 feet to a rocky ledge. Clinging to crevices along the granite walls are such coastal plants as *Dudleya,* or bluff lettuce, featuring succulent silver leaves arranged in a spiral. In summer and fall especially, be sure to bring binoculars, as humpback and gray whales pass within sight of shore along their migratory route from Alaska to the Sea of Cortez, in Baja, Mexico.

Farther along the main trail, a long staircase leads down toward the blue-green waters of **Cypress Cove,** where you may distinguish the heads of several sea otters, resting on their backs atop an underwater forest of 70-foot giant bull kelp. Ascend the steps and continue along the main trail 0.1 mile to complete your loop around the peninsula. From here retrace your steps to the parking area.

Trip 4

SOUTH SHORE, BIRD ISLAND, SOUTH PLATEAU, & PINE RIDGE TRAILS

LENGTH AND TYPE: 2.6-mile loop

RATING: Easy

TRAIL CONDITION: Well maintained, good for kids

HIGHLIGHTS: Explore cliffside gardens, pebbly beaches, blue-green waters, wave-sculpted archways and coves, and forests of majestic Monterey pines.

TO REACH THE TRAILHEAD: From the entrance station of the park, drive 0.8 mile to the Sea Lion Point parking area, bear left, and follow the road another 0.3 mile toward Little Mound Meadow. A parking area on the right leads to the South Shore Trail. If this lot is full, turn left and drive 100 yards farther to the Piney Woods parking and picnic area. You'll find picnic tables, water, and restrooms at the trailhead.

TRIP SUMMARY: This scenic loop takes in an array of habitats, from cliffside gardens, coarse pebbly beaches, and wave-sculpted archways and coves to Monterey pine forests and golden grasslands. Watch egrets walk atop dense rafts of floating kelp, listen for barking sea lions, and smell the salt spray. You may spot the fluke of a passing gray whale or surprise grazing black-tailed deer in a wildflower-strewn meadow.

Trip Description

From the parking area, the **South Shore Trail** leads west toward the typically gentle surf along this rocky shoreline, protected by its southern orientation and wave-thwarting offshore rocks. Low tide exposes pools teeming with unfamiliar life. Pause a moment to peer into a pool. At first you may only notice a few rocks and plants, but the longer you wait, the more alive the pool becomes. Blue-handed hermit crabs scurry nervously along the bottom, while camouflaged sculpin fish dart across the pool to new hiding places. Do be careful where you step—the exposed rocks are covered with slippery seaweed, not to mention tiny tide pool creatures. Check at the information kiosk for daily tide charts.

EBB & FLOOD ■

Ocean tides have perplexed humans throughout history. One ancient theory stated that a water god swallowed seawater and a few hours later released it, thus creating the tides. Science has since explained the phenomenon. High (or flood) tide is when the water level is at its maximum and the beach is covered. During low (or ebb) tide, the water recedes and the beach is exposed.

The tides are generated when the combined gravitational forces of the moon and sun tug on the planet's surface against the force of gravity pulling inward toward Earth's core. Both the sun and moon draw ocean water to positions directly beneath them. High tides are actually bulges that form as water flows toward two regions on the surface—one facing the moon, where gravitational pull is strongest, and the other facing directly away, where gravitational pull is weakest. Low tides represent the corresponding withdrawal of water from regions midway between these bulges. The tides shift as Earth's daily rotation moves the surface closer or farther from these gravitational pulls.

■ ■

Onward, the trail turns southeast toward a junction with the **Mound Meadow Trail** (0.3 mile, 15'), on the left heading northwest. You could take this to the Pine Ridge Trail for a short half-mile loop back to **Piney Woods**. For a richer visit, continue on the South Shore Trail along the reserve's exquisite southern boundary, encompassing some of the state's most beautiful coves and inlets.

The trail meanders within sight of the shore and colorful kelp beds off **Weston Beach**. These rocky promontories are typical of the Carmelo formation, a mix of water-sculpted rocks, fine sediment, and debris deposited by ancient avalanches that occurred in a narrow underwater canyon. Wave action, erosion, and uplift over the past 39 million years have exposed the formation, leaving a complex pattern of graded beds and pebbly beaches.

Leaving Weston Beach, you may want to duck off the trail and descend a few feet to **Hidden Beach** (0.4 mile). Look amid the intertidal rocks for feeding shorebirds such as the black oystercatcher, which boasts a red bill and loud whistled yelps.

Past Hidden Beach the South Shore Trail emerges at the southern parking area, where the **Bird Island Trail** begins (0.6 mile, 25'). If you're short on time, you could park here and explore China Cove and Bird Island, favorite destinations in the reserve.

The short detour to **China Cove** leads up a set of stairs to the headland, where another long, steep set of stairs descends to the white sand beach and sparkling waters. This calm, protected cove is a safe place to wade or explore nearby arches. Year-round water temperatures hover in the 50s Fahrenheit, so you may only want to get your feet wet.

Bird Island Trail heads west to a 0.4-mile loop around **Pelican Point,** passing brittle granite cliffs that do battle with the pounding Pacific. Over time these cliffs crack and fault, forming caves and archways that eventually collapse, leaving spires like **Bird Island.** Bring your binoculars to scan the thousands of migratory and residential seabirds and shorebirds. In spring and summer the island is a nesting site for hundreds of cormorants, known for their sleek black torsos and snakelike necks. Also keep watch for sea otters floating atop the kelp forests and great blue herons surfing on the thick nearshore kelp rafts. Eventually retrace your steps to the junction with the **South Plateau Trail.**

As you turn inland along the South Plateau Trail, you'll soon pass a short spur to **Gibson Beach,** one of the few wide, protected sandy beaches at Point Lobos. The South Plateau Trail is a nature trail, where numbered markers correspond to a pamphlet in a box at the trailhead near the entrance kiosk. When the trail forks (1.9 miles, 50'), turn left onto the **Pine Ridge Trail.**

Farther from the sea breeze and salt spray, the Pine Ridge Trail winds through a tall shady grove of Monterey pines—one of only three remaining natural groves on Earth. Similar to the cypress, Monterey pines require heat or fire to release seeds from their cones. Hiking on a carpet of pine needles, you may notice charcoal or basal fire scars on the pines, evidence of controlled burns. In general, natural processes at the reserve are left undisturbed.

Pristine pocket beaches are nestled under stands of Monterey pine.

However, rangers do use fire to promote healthy pine regeneration and to limit wood debris and understory regrowth. Black-tailed deer, white-rumped northern flicker woodpeckers, and western gray squirrels may remind you of the Sierra Nevada. But the ever-present noisy barks of California sea lions carry deep into the grove, a reminder that you're but a short walk from the fresh, fragrant sea air, salty spray, and soothing waves.

As you begin a shady moderate climb, you'll cross several small plank bridges conveniently placed along the trail over seasonal wet areas. Half a mile later the trail gently descends 0.2 mile to a Y junction. Turn left toward Piney Woods on a level walk, catching ocean glimpses beyond the towering pines. You'll soon emerge at the parking area. Restrooms, water, and picnic tables are 50 feet farther on your left. If you're parked along the shore adjacent to the South Shore Trail, continue 100 feet along the paved road.

CHAPTER eight

Garrapata State Park & Point Sur State Historic Park

■ ■ ■ ■ ■ ■ ■ ■ ■ ■ ■ ■ ■ ■

Garrapata State Park

GARRAPATA STATE PARK offers a scenic slice of the beauty and ruggedness we associate with Big Sur, where redwoods burrow deep within the folds of steep mountains that abruptly rise above a rocky shoreline and wave-washed sandy beaches. On the northern edge of the Big Sur coast, the park features 4 miles of coastline and spans 2879 acres between Andrew Molera State Park to the south and Point Lobos to the north. Created in 1983, Garrapata is one of the more recent additions to the state park system along the central California coast. Coastal and inland access and miles of hiking trails promise numerous recreational opportunities.

Do heed tick warnings. In 1830, Spanish explorers were so exasperated by these blood-sucking arachnids, they named the canyon and creek *Garrapata* (Spanish for "tick"). Despite its unappealing name, the park shelters rich and diverse plant and animal life. The terrain encompasses five vegetation zones: coastal scrub, chaparral, redwood forest, riparian wood-land, and mixed evergreen forest. From late December through January and March through April, gray whales migrate along the coast—south for the winter to Baja, then back north to arctic waters in spring, marking the longest migratory route of any mammal in the world. Near the park's south end, Soberanes Point offers a good vantage point for whale sightings.

As with the other state lands along the Big Sur coast, Garrapata limits trail and road access to day use only, so if you're planning a visit, arrive early. There is no main entrance or entrance fee. Access is via Highway 1 turnouts, which are often crowded by midday in summer and on weekends. The climate is moderate year-round, with average temperatures between 50°F and 65°F. Weather varies from cool, damp fog to strong onshore winds and

Garrapata State Park

the occasional warm, glorious day. Wear layered clothing and be prepared for changing conditions. Fall promises more consistent, warm fogless days, while summer days are often cool, as fog shrouds the coast. After winter rains the bluffs and hillsides sprout verdant plant life that by spring blankets the headlands, valleys, and hillsides amid decadent orange, purple, yellow, and red wildflower blooms.

DIRECTIONS: Garrapata State Park lies 7 miles south of Carmel and 18 miles north of Big Sur. There is no official park entrance. Parking and trail access is via 19 turnouts along Highway 1, the first on the Monterey County line at Mile 67.2 and the last at Mile 65.3. The turnouts correspond to numbered gates. Gates 17, 17A, 18, and 19 lead to Garrapata State Beach, while gates 8, 9, and 10 lead to the Soberanes Point trails.

VISITOR CENTER: Big Sur Station: (831) 667-2315. The station is on Highway 1, 18 miles south of Garrapata State Park. Open daily 8 a.m.–6 p.m. Memorial Day through Labor Day, 8 a.m.–4:30 p.m. the rest of the year.

NEAREST CAMPGROUNDS: The nearest developed state campground is at Pfeiffer Big Sur State Park (see page 98 for details). The nearest walk-in campground is at Andrew Molera State Park (see page 82 for details).

INFORMATION: Park closes at sunset. Camping and fires are not permitted. Dogs are only allowed on Garrapata Beach (not on trails) and must be kept on a leash at all times (6-foot maximum). Bicycles are permitted only on Rocky Ridge Trail. Do not remove plants, minerals, or other natural features.

WEBSITE: parks.ca.gov

PHONE: (831) 624-4909

Enjoy the journey along the many short spur trails that lead to dramatic vistas and sheltered coves within Garrapata.

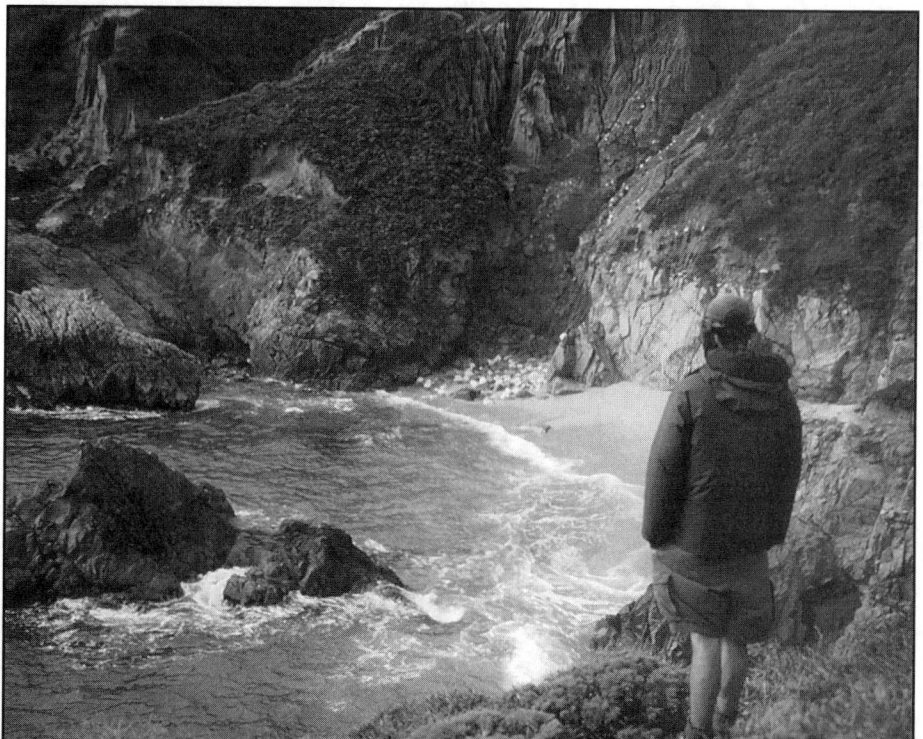

Trip 5

COASTAL ACCESS TRAILS

LENGTH AND TYPE: 2-mile out-and-back

RATING: Easy

TRAIL CONDITION: Well maintained, poison oak, good for kids

HIGHLIGHTS: Rugged rocky shores, wave-washed beaches, and isolated coves

TO REACH THE TRAILHEAD: This hike description begins from turnout 17 along Highway 1.

TRIP SUMMARY: The hike stretches about a mile to the south end of the park via the headlands or the beach.

EARLY BEACHCOMBERS ■ ■ ■ ■ ■ ■ ■ ■ ■ ■ ■ ■ ■ ■ ■

Between dense thickets of coastal brush, shellfish remains and the bones of seals, otters, and land mammals such as deer and rabbits poke up from the bare sand, marking ancient middens, or human garbage heaps. The middens in Garrapata State Park date to coastal tribes that roamed the coast centuries before Spanish missionaries arrived. One shell bead dated from 100 to 300 A.D., while archaeologists traced obsidian flakes to the Borax Lake region of the Coast Range, nearly 200 miles north of Big Sur.

Garrapata's natives were likely members of the Rumsen subgroup of Ohlone Indians. Through extensive trade, the Ohlone were able to obtain items from both neighboring and distant tribes. The tribe relied on hunting and gathering along the coast in mild summer months, moving inland for the winter. They ate primarily mussels and other shellfish.

Before the arrival of Spanish missionaries, an estimated 10,000 Ohlone lived in an area stretching from San Francisco Bay south to Big Sur and east to the Central Valley. By the late 1700s, the Spanish had claimed much of the land and missionaries' conversionary zeal had all but erased native culture. Within a few short decades, exposure to deadly European diseases reduced Ohlone's numbers to some 2500 people. Today, descendants of the Ohlone still live in the area and preserve their ancestors' native traditions.

■ ■

Trip Description

From 17, the northernmost turnout, a short spur leads a few yards west to a bench atop a scenic overlook, an ideal spot to watch migrating whales in winter and spring. April and

A natural symphony of seals barking, creeks gurgling, and waves pounding is common along the 4 miles of rocky shoreline and wave-washed sandy coves in Garrapata State Park.

May are the best months, as mothers steer their calves closer to shore for safety from such predators as great white sharks and orcas. Park naturalists often lead whale-watching hikes on spring weekends (call the park for specific dates).

The trail meanders south and then west past dramatic views of a rocky shoreline pounded continuously by foamy surf. You'll soon turn east past a small isolated cove and an overlook south to Garrapata Beach. A spur veers left to **turnout 17A** (0.3 mile, 40'), while the main trail continues south past another spur, this one to **turnout 18** (0.5 mile, 40'). From here you'll descend to a narrow canyon carved by **Doud Creek** (0.6 mile, 10'). Cross the creek and head south, either farther along the headlands or across **Garrapata State Beach.**

Beyond the creek, the bluff trail climbs and curls east a few paces to the spur for **turnout 19** (0.8 mile, 30'). Past this spur, the main trail descends west to emerge on the south end of Garrapata State Beach (1 mile). Pause to appreciate its timeless beauty before heading back the way you came.

Trip 6

ROCKY RIDGE TRAIL

LENGTH AND TYPE: 6-mile out-and-back or 4.6-mile loop

RATING: Strenuous

TRAIL CONDITION: Well maintained, poison oak

HIGHLIGHTS: Breathtaking views from mountains that rise dramatically beside a craggy coast

TO REACH THE TRAILHEAD: Both the Rocky Ridge and Soberanes Canyon Trails start from turnout 8, amid a strip of Monterey cypress on the east side of Highway 1, 7.1 miles south of Carmel Valley Road (County Road G16) and 14 miles north of Andrew Molera State Park. The trailheads lie beyond the numbered gate adjacent to a dilapidated barn. There are no facilities or water at the trailhead.

TRIP SUMMARY: You can approach this hike either as a 6-mile out-and-back along the Rocky Ridge Trail or as a 4.6-mile loop trip through Soberanes Canyon via the Soberanes Canyon Trail. Both routes are strenuous. The Rocky Ridge Trail drops abruptly from a 1435-foot ridge to 400-foot Soberanes Creek. Although the loop is 1.4 miles shorter, it's along a steeper, more strenuous grade, plunging 1000 feet to the canyon bottom in less than 0.7 mile.

The 3-mile Rocky Ridge Trail climbs past creekside willows and fragrant coastal scrub along a ridge of arid, boulder-strewn golden grasslands to a promontory more than 1600 feet above the sea. You'll enjoy 360-degree views, stretching from Point Sur to the Monterey Peninsula and the Santa Cruz Mountains to the Pacific. The topography is so sheer that despite a long climb, you'll still hear barking sea lions less than a mile away. Its difficulty keeps crowds at bay, though hikers, joggers, and bicyclists do flock here in summer. The best time to visit is in spring when coastal scrub is in bloom, migrating gray whales pass just offshore, and fog rarely encroaches inland.

Trip Description

From turnout 8, the trail begins a gentle climb up a closed road past the barn, soon crossing **Soberanes Creek.** Thirty yards beyond the creek, the trail meets the Soberanes Canyon Trail junction (0.1 mile, 120'), which branches right. Keep left and head north. Fifty yards farther, the trail passes a spur on the left, which descends some 130 yards to **turnout 12** (parking here would shave 0.2 mile off your hike). A minute farther north, the trail leaves the canyon and passes the first sign for the Rocky Ridge Trail (0.3 mile, 180').

Onward, the trail climbs 0.3 mile southeast up to a ridgetop (410') that boasts views of Garrapata's inland mountains and valleys. Pause for a breather, as your easy walk is over. The trail climbs more than 1200 feet in the next 1.5 miles, crests a knoll, then contours along a prominent saddle, nearly topping another ridge marked with a U.S. Geological Survey benchmark (1435'). Hints of even more spectacular views will draw you up the final 250 feet.

Farther up the main trail, look east for glimpses of the lush redwood groves that line Soberanes Creek, in stark contrast to the surrounding arid slopes of coastal scrub and grasslands. The trail heads northeast across a saddle, then north to its terminus atop a ridge (3 miles, 1680'), 1600 feet above Highway 1.

From this point, you have three options: (1) retrace your steps along the Rocky Ridge Trail, 3 miles to the trailhead, (2) hike a mile farther, climbing the **Peak Trail** up 1977-foot **Doud Peak,** or (3) descend into **Soberanes Canyon** along the upper Rocky Ridge Trail to the **Soberanes Canyon Trail.** The latter two routes continue east along a north-facing ridge 0.3 mile to a fork—the right branch descends into Soberanes Canyon, while the left branch leads to Doud Peak. The remaining 0.7 mile along the Peak Trail offers sweeping views of the untamed central coast as far north as **Fremont Peak,** at the north end of the **Gabilan Range.** On exceptionally clear days, you may even spot **Pacheco Peak,** about 50 miles northeast.

If you're taking the 4.6-mile loop, head southeast, where an extremely steep passage leads down the Rocky Ridge Trail to the upper end of the Soberanes Canyon Trail. In just under a mile the trail plunges 1200 feet down loose gravel and sand. You'll find steps in sections where the grade exceeds 30%, but be sure to pace yourself. The trail eventually emerges from the coastal scrub to enter the shady, damp redwood forest. A final few steep, short switchbacks lead you down to the gurgling creek and the junction with the westbound Soberanes Canyon Trail.

See TRIP 7 Soberanes Canyon Trail (on the following page) for that trail description.

Trip 7

SOBERANES CANYON TRAIL

LENGTH AND TYPE: 2.2-mile out-and-back or 4.6-mile loop

RATING: Easy to strenuous

TRAIL CONDITION: Well maintained, poison oak

HIGHLIGHTS: A canyon that shelters primeval groves of the world's tallest living organism, *Sequoia sempervirens*

TO REACH THE TRAILHEAD: Both the Soberanes Canyon and Rocky Ridge Trails start from turnout 8, on the east side of Highway 1, 7.1 miles south of Carmel Valley Road (County Road G16) and 14 miles north of Andrew Molera State Park. The trailhead lies beyond the numbered gate adjacent to a dilapidated barn. There are no facilities or water at the trailhead.

TRIP SUMMARY: Depending on your time and fitness level, you can approach this as either an easy 2.2-mile out-and-back hike or a strenuous 4.6-mile loop. In this direction the 4.6-mile loop features a particularly grueling climb—instead, consider beginning with the Rocky Ridge Trail and returning along the Soberanes Creek Trail (see TRIP 6 Rocky Ridge Trail, page 72, for details).

The trail meanders upstream along Soberanes Creek. Where the canyon narrows, a dense redwood canopy shelters a myriad of shade- and moisture-loving plants.

Trip Description

From turnout 8, the trail climbs a closed road past the barn, soon crossing **Soberanes Creek**. Thirty yards beyond the creek you'll reach the **Soberanes Canyon Trail junction** (0.1 mile, 120'), which branches to the right. The left branch heads north along the Rocky Ridge Trail (see page 72 for description).

Spanish missionaries introduced prickly pear cacti to the coast.

Head east along the creek past clusters of coastal prickly pear cacti. Though not a native species, the plant thrives here. Spanish missionaries likely brought the plant north from Mexico as early as 1769. Beyond, the trail bends northeast past stunted, wind-sculpted redwoods (0.4 mile, 50') that are continually battered by salty onshore winds. As you hike farther up the canyon away from the surf, you'll find much healthier redwoods nestled along the canyon bottom. Farther inland, the trail enters a forest of mature redwoods that harbor a lush understory of ferns, mosses, and other creekside plants.

At 0.8 mile, the trail again crosses Soberanes Creek, then crosses it three more times over the next 0.3 mile. Just past the final crossing, a conspicuous spur branches off along the south bank. The main trail continues briefly along the north bank, ascends and descends several small, steep slopes, then descends a series of short switchbacks to the creek, where it meets the **Rocky Ridge Trail junction.** Over the years, high winds and flash floods have knocked down several large redwoods, providing excellent creekside seating, an ideal spot to rest and picnic. When ready, head back the way you came to complete the 2.2-mile round-trip.

The Rocky Ridge Trail continues up a few short, steep switchbacks, climbing above the cool redwood forest to exposed slopes of coastal scrub (see TRIP 6 Rocky Ridge Trail, page 72, for details).

Trip 8

SOBERANES POINT TRAILS

LENGTH AND TYPE: 2-mile loop

RATING: Easy

TRAIL CONDITION: Clear, poison oak, good for kids

HIGHLIGHTS: Roam the bluffs along one of California's most dramatic coastlines.

TO REACH THE TRAILHEAD: The Soberanes Point Trails are accessible via Highway 1 turn-outs 7 through 11. The trail description that follows starts on the west side of the highway at turnout 7.

TRIP SUMMARY: From turnout 7, the trail meanders south past uninhabited coves toward Soberanes Point. Along the way, watch pelicans skim wave crests in formation, peer down as surf surges into narrow inlets and coves, and maybe spot migrating whales. Some spurs lead to spectacular overlooks, while others descend to the beach for a barefoot stroll.

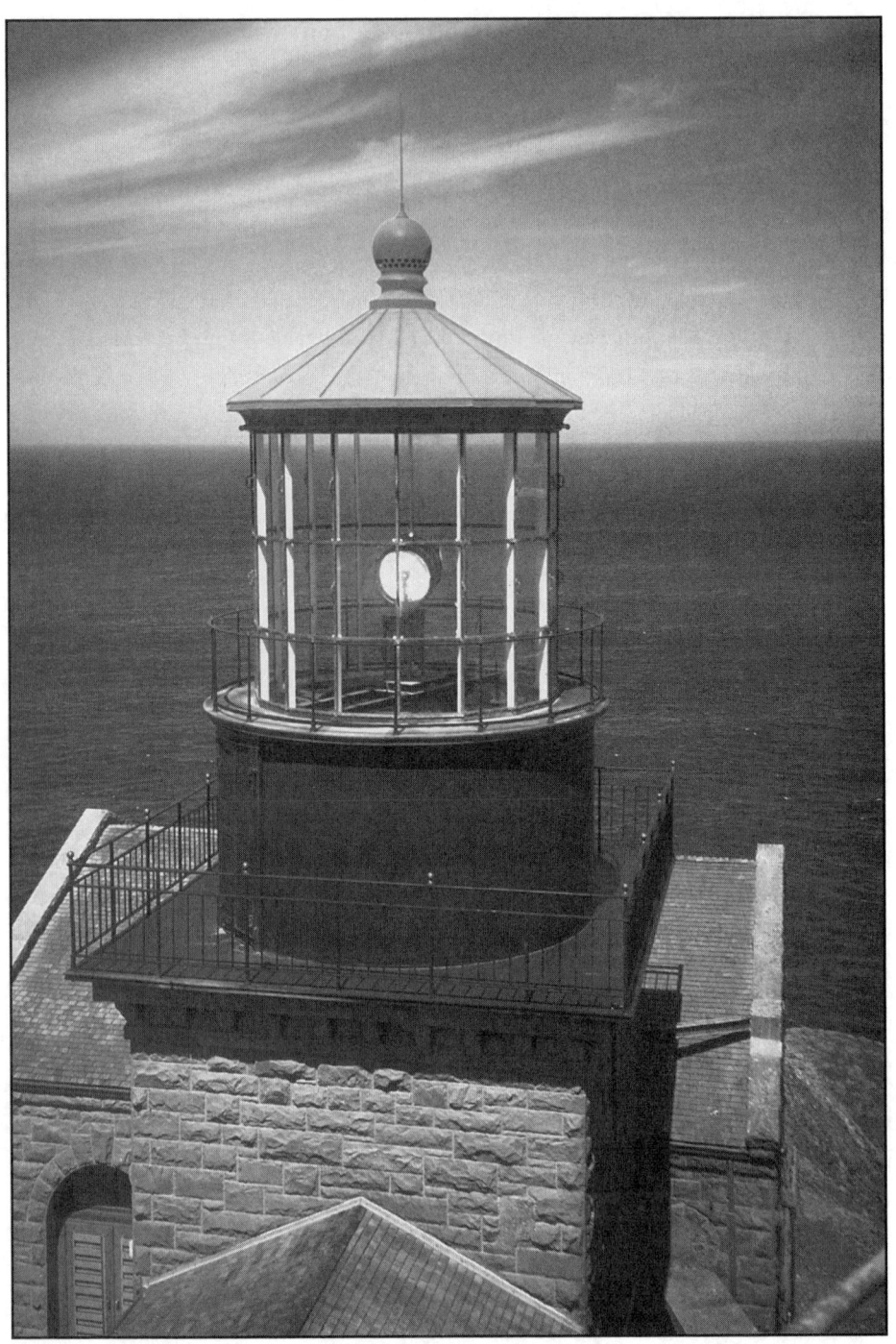

Point Sur Lighthouse stands as a sentinel of the bygone era of dangerous marine travel.

Trip Description

From turnout 7, the trail quickly reaches **Soberanes Creek** and a junction with a short spur down to the water's edge. Veer left across the creek through a dense stand of Monterey cypress between turnouts 8 and 9, where you'll find a portable toilet. If you parked at the Rocky Ridge and Soberanes Canyon Trailhead (turnout 8), your hike will begin here.

A few steps south of the cypress grove, you'll pass a junction with a trail to the left that skirts Highway 1. Those taking the 2-mile loop will return along this trail. Stay right and you'll soon reach a fork. Veer right to explore the dramatic shoreline that leads to rocky **Soberanes Point**. The route crosses bluffs covered with California sagebrush, bush lupine, coyote brush, coffeeberry, and other coastal scrub plants.

Beyond the point, the trail curls east and then north past the western flanks of **Whale Peak** to the junction between gates 8 and 9. If you parked at turnout 7, retrace your steps north across Soberanes Creek.

BIG SUR ROCKS ■

Big Sur's coastal topography is a stunning blend of clear, cobalt water and the rugged granitic rocks of the Santa Lucia Range. Geologists believe these rocks originated in the southern Sierra in present-day Mexico and moved northwest hundreds of miles along the San Andreas Fault. These hard, crystalline rocks of the Salinian block also comprise many of the prominent high peaks of the range, such as Ventana Double Cone and Pico Blanco.

Deep underground, the molten rock slowly cooled, forming large crystals that glisten in the sun, lending the stone a grayish, salt-and-pepper appearance in the surf zone and a weathered rusty orange farther up the bluffs. As they slowly erode in the pounding surf, these durable rocks produce coarse-grained particles that sink quickly to the bottom, leaving little sediment to cloud the water.

■ ■

Point Sur State Historic Park

THE CENTERPIECE OF THIS historic park is Point Sur Lighthouse, perched 270 feet atop an isolated volcanic rock at the mouth of the Little Sur River. Built in 1889, the light provided invaluable warning to thousands of ships that plied this treacherous coast. Life for keepers and their families was lonely and isolated until the completion of Highway 1 in 1937. Then, in the 1960s, the U.S. Coast Guard began automating lighthouses. The last keeper left Point Sur in 1974. Year-round guided walking tours feature the lighthouse and supporting structures.

DIRECTIONS: The park is on the west side of Highway 1, 19 miles south of Carmel and a quarter mile north of the Point Sur Naval Facility.

VISITOR CENTER: Big Sur Station: (831) 667-2315. The station is on Highway 1, 18 miles south of Garrapata State Park and just south of Pfeiffer Big Sur State Park. Open daily 8 a.m.–6 p.m. Memorial Day through Labor Day, 8 a.m.–4:30 p.m. the rest of the year.

NEAREST CAMPGROUND: The nearest developed state campground is at Pfeiffer Big Sur State Park (see page 98 for details). The nearest walk-in campground is at Andrew Molera State Park (see page 82 for details).

INFORMATION: Closed to public except by guided tour. Docents lead three-hour tours year-round: Saturdays and Sundays at 10 a.m., Wednesdays at 1 p.m. The summer schedule includes Wednesday tours at 10 a.m. and 2 p.m. (April through October) and Thursday tours at 10 a.m. (July and August). Moonlight tours vary. Arrive early, as tickets are first come, first served. Admission: adults $12; ages 6–17, $5; children age 5 and under, free. Groups of 10 or more must call in advance. Groups of up to 40 people may also arrange private tours (minimum $200 charge). Visitors with disabilities should contact the park in advance to discuss access. No pets (even if left in car), picnicking, RVs or campers, strollers or baby carriages, beach access, or smoking.

PHONE: (831) 625-4419 or (831) 667-0528 (disabled access)

WEBSITES: pointsur.org or parks.ca.gov

Trip 9

POINT SUR STATE HISTORIC PARK

LENGTH AND TYPE: 0.4-mile out-and-back

RATING: Easy

TRAIL CONDITION: Well maintained, good for kids

HIGHLIGHTS: Experience life at a remote lighthouse perched on the edge of the Pacific.

TO REACH THE TRAILHEAD: At the park, meet at the farm gate along the west side of Highway 1 at the scheduled tour time. Arrive early, as tours occasionally fill up and reservations are not accepted. A docent or state park ranger will open the gate and direct you where to park. You'll drive less than a mile along a narrow paved road to the base of massive Point Sur. From here the three-hour tour begins.

TRIP SUMMARY: Point Sur Lighthouse is a lonely sentinel perched atop a massive rock formation at the mouth of the Little Sur River. The beacon reminds visitors of a bygone era,

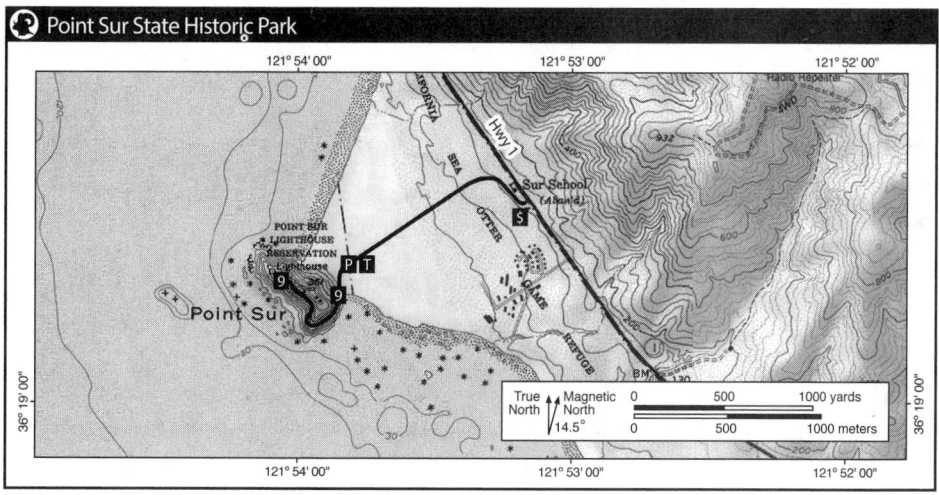

Point Sur State Historic Park

when mariners sailed blindly along the fogbound coast, often unaware of their proximity to the rocky shoreline. Swept by strong winds and big Pacific swells, the surroundings here remain largely unchanged.

Staffed from 1889 until 1974, Point Sur was home to families who stoically endured long months of isolation and solitude. Today, the lighthouse is automated and only traces of the keepers' stories remain in empty buildings, workshops, and barns.

Trip Description

From the parking area, you'll climb a steep paved road and two stairways to **Point Sur**. Count on plenty of rest stops along the way as your guide shares dramatic tales of life at this remote lighthouse.

Wildlife abounds on and around the point. Migrating gray whales pass within sight of shore. Pelicans fly by in formation, while cormorants vanish underwater and oystercatchers clamber across the rocks. Sea otters and seals swim beyond the surf line, feasting amid the kelp forests below. Also keep watch for golden eagles, peregrine falcons, and California condors, which soar overhead in search of prey or carrion.

Point Sur is a complete turn-of-the-century **lighthouse**. Your guide will lead you up the circular stairwell for a look at the lens and to stroll the catwalk. Weighing 4330 pounds, the first-order Fresnel lens is nearly 8 feet high and more than 6 feet in diameter. Its 16 panels of prisms bend light into a single focused beam visible for 23 nautical miles. Pause at this exposed point, taking in the fog, wind, sun, salt spray, and other raw elements.

CHAPTER nine

Andrew Molera State Park

THE LARGEST STATE PARK on the Big Sur coast, Andrew Molera is also one of the few places you can actually get your feet wet rather than just enjoying ocean viewpoints. This is an excellent place for beachcombers, surfers, and anglers, as well as hikers, joggers, bicyclists, and equestrians. Its 7.4 square miles boast more than 20 miles of trails, offering hikers passage across driftwood-strewn beaches, beside rivers lined with redwoods, and atop high ridges that overlook the Santa Lucia Range and broad Pacific. The wild and scenic Big Sur River winds amid the park's mountains, meadows, and a walk-in campground on its way down to the sea.

Diverse ecosystems shelter a broad range of plant and animal communities. Birders know the park well. In 1992 the nonprofit Ventana Wilderness Society established a research and education center and bird observatory here. The Big Sur Ornithology Lab has documented more than 380 migratory, resident, and transitory birds. Researchers point to multiple factors, including biotic diversity, the mild climate, a healthy lagoon and estuary, and a nearby lighthouse that may attract nocturnal migrants.

DISCOVERY CENTER

Don't miss the Discovery Center in Big Sur, located at Andrew Molera State Park. At the Discovery Center, you can see and interact with the exhibit Bringing the Condors Home and learn about the recovery efforts to bring the condors back to the wild. Enjoy a picnic or sign up for tours with on-site biologists and naturalists. Best of all, the Discovery Center is open to the public and free of charge.

But this park isn't just for the birds. Keep watch for sea otters, seals, and sea lions amid the kelp beds and migrating gray whales just offshore. At dusk and dawn, deer graze in the Creamery Meadow as steelhead rise to feed on insects in the Big Sur River. Catch-and-release steelhead fishing is permitted from mid-November through February, while surf casting for rockfish and surfperch is permitted year-round. Fishing regulations change from year to year, so contact the Department of Fish & Game at (831) 649-2870 for current information.

The day-use fee is $8/vehicle, or you can park on the highway and hike in for free. The free turnout is on the west side of the highway, 0.1 mile north of the park entrance. A trail

The mouth of the Big Sur River is a dynamic place that is subject to dramatic seasonal changes—be prepared to get your feet or more wet if planning to cross.

leads from the turnout to Cooper's Cabin, just west of Trail Camp. If that turnout is full, there's another 0.3 mile south of the park's entrance. Water and toilet facilities are available at the official park lot.

DIRECTIONS: The park lies at the junction of Highway 1 and Old Coast Road, 22 miles south of Carmel and 4.2 miles north of Pfeiffer Big Sur State Park. The entrance is on the west side of the highway.

VISITOR CENTER: Big Sur Station: (831) 667-2315. The station is on Highway 1, 4.2 miles south of Andrew Molera State Park and just south of Pfeiffer Big Sur State Park. Open daily 8 a.m.–6 p.m. Memorial Day through Labor Day, 8 a.m.–4:30 p.m. the rest of the year.

NEAREST CAMPGROUNDS: The park's Trail Camp walk-in campground (24 sites, $25/night; register at the entrance kiosk) is in a large meadow near the Big Sur River, an easy 0.3-mile walk from the parking lot. Sites are granted on a first-come, first-serve basis and fill up quickly in summer and on holidays. Another option is Pfeiffer Big Sur State Park (218 sites, $25/standard site, $35/river site; reservations recommended in summer and on holidays).

INFORMATION: The park is day use only unless you're camping. Dogs are not allowed on trails or at Trail Camp. Bikes are permitted only on Ridge, Beach, Trail Camp, and Creamery Meadow Trails. Horses are not allowed on the Hidden, Headlands, or Spring Trails, or in Trail Camp. To reserve a guided horseback tour, call Molera Horseback Tours at (831) 625-5486 or visit molerahorsebacktours.com.

WEBSITE: parks.ca.gov | **PHONE:** (831) 667-2315

Trip 10

TRAIL CAMP & HEADLANDS TRAILS

LENGTH AND TYPE: 2-mile out-and-back

RATING: Easy

TRAIL CONDITION: Well maintained, poison oak, good for kids

HIGHLIGHTS: An array of migratory and resident birds, seals, whales, and otters make their home amid the marsh, estuary, and ocean along Molera Beach.

TO REACH THE TRAILHEAD: At the park's entrance kiosk, turn right. The trailhead is at the north end of the parking lot.

TRIP SUMMARY: Among the region's easiest coastal bluff hikes, this hike offers gorgeous overlooks of the Big Sur River, distant peaks, sheer cliffs, and a driftwood-blanketed beach.

Tracing the final mile of the river's 15-mile journey to the Pacific, the trails lead through a walk-in campground nestled in an expansive meadow, past views of the Santa Lucia Range to the east, to emerge at the river mouth. Watch for migrating gray and humpback whales, foraging seals and sea otters amid the kelp, and hundreds of soaring, diving, and foraging seabirds aloft on coastal air currents.

Trip Description

Trail Camp Trail starts on the north end of the parking lot, then turns west along the north bank of the **Big Sur River,** skirting a lush riparian habitat. After 0.2 mile the trail broadens into a road and enters the spacious **walk-in campground.** You'll find 12 primitive sites scattered throughout the meadow. Campers are rewarded with a night's sleep under giant sycamores and a short walk to one of Big Sur's most scenic beaches. Bring a tent, especially in summer, when fog blankets the meadow with condensation.

Facilities include toilets, potable water, tables, and a fire ring. Purchase firewood at the entrance kiosk or at the Big Sur Village store, less than 5 miles south on Highway 1. California State Parks reduced the number of sites from 50 to 12, conforming to state health codes and protecting park resources.

A hundred feet beyond the campground, the trail forks. A short spur on the right leads to historic **Cooper Cabin,** then continues east 0.2 mile to a Highway 1 turnout (a free place to park and still access the park). Continue along the riverbank 0.2 mile through a dense forest of twisted alders and willows. Less than 0.1 mile farther the path narrows and reaches the **Headlands Trail junction** (0.9 mile, 20').

COOPER & THE BUTTERFLIES ■ ■ ■ ■ ■ ■ ■ ■ ■ ■ ■ ■ ■ ■ ■ ■

In 1834 this area was part of a Mexican land grant known as Rancho El Sur, owned by Juan Bautista Alvarado. Six years later Alvarado sold the land to Juan Bautista Rogers Cooper, a Monterey sea captain and merchant. Built in 1861, Cooper Cabin remains the oldest standing structure in Big Sur. Cooper used the land to graze livestock and also launched the first large-scale production of Monterey Jack cheese.

In the late 1800s the narrow wagon road from Monterey went only part way down the coast, so settlers gathered annually near Cooper's riverside cabin to picnic, fish, and dance while awaiting the arrival of supply schooners. Andrew Molera was Cooper's grandson, and in 1965 his sister donated the land in his name.

Visitors still wonder at enormous bluegum eucalyptus trees, planted when the cabin was built. In 1986 state park officials, concerned that this introduced Australian species was crowding out native willows and alders and negatively affecting wildlife, began to remove eucalyptus saplings. Biologists opposed the cutting, as monarch butterflies roost here during their long migration. The biologists and butterflies ultimately prevailed, preserving the giant trees.

From October through January, monarchs return to Big Sur to roost amid the stands of eucalyptus. By day watch them glide from branch to branch in the spacious canopy of this exotic tree.

■ ■

Turn right and head north up the old wooden stairs. You'll find yourself 30 feet above the shoreline as you pass thick patches of poison oak, golden yarrow, and sagebrush. Continue the gentle climb for ever-expanding panoramic views of **Molera Point** and the rugged coastline to the north and south.

Look south to spot sculpted driftwood strewn across the white sand. Look below and see if you can discern where the sand is tinged purple. This purple sediment is eroded almandite, a rare mineral. Also notice the jagged rocks in the surf. These contorted rocks were heavily metamorphosed within the numerous faults that divide, break, and reshape the Big Sur coastline, most all of them associated with the San Andreas Fault.

Skirt the secluded coves and beaches till you reach a bench atop the bluff overlooking 2-mile **Molera Beach,** a great spot to watch for sea lions, seals, and sea otters as they feed and play among the giant kelp beds. California gray whales migrate south to Baja from December through January and return north to Alaska in March and April. Take a moment to enjoy the sweeping view before returning the way you came.

Back at the Trail Camp Trail junction, turn right and continue your route west. In less than a hundred feet, the path emerges on the beach at the mouth of the Big Sur River.

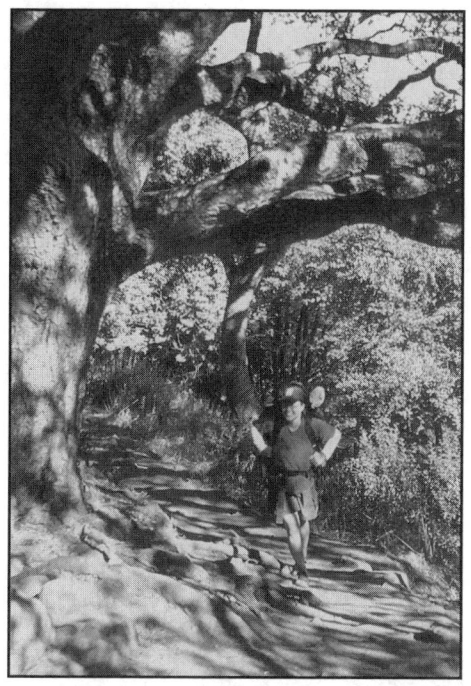

Trail Camp is a short jaunt through massive oaks and sycamores along the Big Sur River.

During the dry season (May through October), when less water flows into the ocean, sand builds up and blocks the river mouth, flooding the lagoon and inland marsh. This diverse ecosystem creates a unique habitat for shorebirds and water-fowl, including great blue herons, egrets, gulls, and pelicans.

Big Sur is also home to steelhead trout (a rainbow trout that spends part of its life in the sea), which migrate upstream to spawn and lay eggs. Each spring thousands of 6-inch steelhead smolt venture downstream into the ocean. For every 100 smolt that reach the sea, fewer than 5% will return as a spawning adult. At dawn and dusk in summer and fall, watch as dozens of young steelhead leap through the air to enjoy a banquet of aquatic insects.

When you're ready, return the way you came. In drier months you could cross the river and head back following the **Beach** or **Creamery Meadow Trails** (see following trip description).

Trip 11

BEACH & CREAMERY MEADOW TRAILS LOOP

LENGTH AND TYPE: 1.8-mile loop

RATING: Easy

TRAIL CONDITION: Well maintained, poison oak, good for kids

HIGHLIGHTS: A barefoot stroll across windswept, driftwood-strewn Molera Beach

TO REACH THE TRAILHEAD: From the park's entrance kiosk, continue straight to the picnic area. The route begins at the bridge across the Big Sur.

TRIP SUMMARY: Adjacent to the Big Sur River, Creamery Meadow is lined with dense riparian woodland. You'll stroll past twisted sycamores, head-high yellow bush lupines, and gnarled redwoods. Once a cattle pasture, today it boasts some of the best bird-watching in California.

Trip Description

From the picnic area, cross the **Big Sur River** on the narrow footbridge. In winter the bridge is removed so steelhead trout can migrate upstream—expect a knee- to waist-high wade. After heavy winter storms, the river may be too swift to cross. If you prefer to stay dry or cannot cross, take the **Trail Camp Trail** to the beach (see page 83).

Once across the Big Sur, turn right and head west on the **Beach Trail** alongside **Creamery Meadow,** a turn-of-the-century pasture for cows that produced Monterey Jack cheese. Park officials are replanting and slowly restoring the area to a beautiful open meadow dotted with willows, cot- tonwoods, red alders, sycamores, and a few scraggly, salt-stunted redwoods. Abundant wildlife includes coyotes, bobcats, and deer along the trails; lizards, mice, and rabbits in

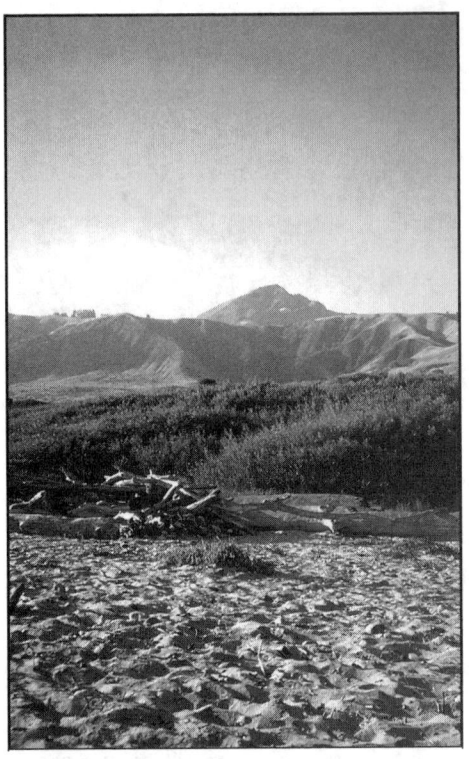

Views from Molera Beach lead toward the triangular marble-topped Pico Blanco.

the high grass; and white-tailed kites, kestrels, and red-shouldered hawks soaring overhead.

Closer to the beach, the wind and salt spray have taken a toll on vegetation. As you turn north toward the river, notice the contorted redwood to your left across the meadow. Farther down the trail you'll pass the rocky end of a bluff midway to the surf. During large swells, waves surge halfway up this stretch, stranding massive logs and driftwood. On your left, just before you reach the beach, you'll pass the **Bluffs Trail** (1.1 miles, 10'), which heads southeast along the edge of a marine terrace.

Before heading back toward the **Creamery Trail,** stroll windswept **Molera Beach.** You'll likely spot sea otters, sea lions, and harbor seals feeding in the nearshore kelp forests. Notice the low bluffs of deformed rocks, part of the Franciscan complex, a mix of sedimentary rocks and basalt slices from the seafloor. The San Andreas Fault and associated faults continually wrench this region and metamorphose the gray, tan, and brown sandstone, and shale. Look closely to spot almandite, a rare mineral that tints the sand purple and pink.

Stroll farther to escape the crowds and find an isolated cove all to yourself. Keep in mind, though, that your hike is tide-dependent—the beach can be impassable or even dangerous in places during high tides. Tide tables are posted on the information sign in the parking lot, or you can check at Big Sur Station, 4.2 miles south of the park entrance road on Highway 1.

PERFECT PEELING WAVES ▪ ▪ ▪ ▪ ▪ ▪ ▪ ▪ ▪ ▪ ▪ ▪ ▪ ▪ ▪

As you stroll Molera Beach, you may notice surfers paddling past marine mammals to greet perfect peeling waves on the north end of the beach. In fact, this stretch is one of Big Sur's most reliable surf spots. The beach is ringed in from all directions except west, in a semi-point setup. The water sculpts and sustains a gravelly sandbar, and prevailing northwest winds create fast right-hand lanes on days that are blown out elsewhere. Access the break by walking nearly a mile from the park entrance. Though the walk deters some surfers, expect a crowded lineup during big west or south swells.

Heading back up the Beach Trail, you'll pass thick patches of toxic poison oak amid colorful flowering plants. Many of the latter display vibrant yellow blossoms, including bush lupine, seaside wooly sunflower, sedum, *Dudleya*, and yellow sand verbena. A tenth of a mile from Molera Beach, you'll reach the **Creamery Trail junction**. Turn right on this wide trail to take in the opposite side of Creamery Meadow. In the meadow you'll spot coyote brush, poison hemlock, California poppies, and more lupines, while large coast live oaks, sycamores, and bay trees line the ridge to your right. The trail gradually bends northeast to rejoin the Beach Trail at the footbridge over the Big Sur (1.8 miles, 40').

Trip 12

EAST MOLERA TRAIL

LENGTH AND TYPE: 3.2-mile out-and-back

RATING: Strenuous

TRAIL CONDITION: Clear, poison oak

HIGHLIGHTS: Coastal vistas, sweeping panoramas of the Santa Lucia Range, and a secluded ridge capped with redwoods

TO REACH THE TRAILHEAD: Access the trailhead via either Highway 1 or from the park's official lot.

On Highway 1, the trailhead lies 0.3 mile south of the park entrance road and is marked by a small, worn wooden cattle chute on the east side of the road. Park at either of two turnouts, about 0.1 mile north and south of this chute.

If you're starting from the parking lot, plan to hike another 0.6 mile overall. From the lot, walk up the entrance road 75 feet past the kiosk and take the service road on your right, which heads southeast toward Molera Trail Rides. Follow this road past the barn, where you'll find a signed trailhead. The trail parallels the highway, then passes beneath it through a large culvert. You'll emerge on a dirt road on the east side of the highway. Follow this road a few yards until you reach the East Molera Trail, which rises from the highway turnout, crosses the dirt road, and continues uphill.

TRIP SUMMARY: This trail switchbacks up a sheer hillside to a secluded ridge capped with redwoods. The 1.6-mile trail reaches 1550 feet, offering sweeping views of the coast and Santa Lucia Range. Bring plenty of water and a wide-brimmed hat for the exposed stretch to the ridge, and pack a sweater or windbreaker for the return hike.

Trip Description

The **East Molera Trail** climbs gradually, first beneath the large twisted branches of coast live oaks and then across open grassland. From its junction with the dirt road (0.1 mile, 180'), the trail up to the redwood saddle is 1.5 miles long with nearly 1500 feet of elevation gain. Heading left uphill, the trail climbs less than 0.1 mile past a water-storage tank to rejoin the road. You could stay on the road for a gentler though longer ascent. Over the next 0.2 mile the trail parallels a narrow band of lush redwoods, bays, and oaks that shelter in a narrow gully. This gully hosts a small creek in wet months and channels a ribbon of thick fog in drier months.

Just before the main trail turns left up a steep rise, a narrow **spur** (0.4 mile, 360') branches right to enter the redwood-shaded gully. The spur traverses the gully past redwoods and fragrant bay trees to open oak woodlands. At trail's end, a majestic oak tops a grassy knoll, a peaceful spot to picnic, offering views south along the **Big Sur River,** north to **Point Sur Lighthouse,** and west to **Molera Beach.**

From the spur junction, continue up the road to your left, where the ascent quickly turns strenuous, climbing nearly 1000 feet in about a mile. The trail switchbacks and climbs directly up a ridge. After a steep climb east, the trail ascends another ridge. From here you can see the redwood saddle, less than 0.1 mile away. The views only improve, and hints of even better ones urge you on.

The final 0.1 mile gradually ascends grassy slopes that in spring are blanketed in the deep purple and orange hues of abundant lupines and poppies. The trail ends on a **ridge crest** (1.6 miles, 1550') amid towering redwoods, which seem blatantly out of place. The cool shade is a blessing, especially after strenuous hikes on hot summer days. In summer, fog may obscure the view, but in spring and fall you'll likely be rewarded with stunning views. Northeast is the narrow **South Fork Little Sur River** canyon and the massive marble **Pico Blanco,** southeast lies the **Big Sur River** watershed, and the park stretches south and southwest to the Pacific. When you're rested, head back down the trail.

NORTH MEETS SOUTH ▪ ▪ ▪ ▪ ▪ ▪ ▪ ▪ ▪ ▪ ▪ ▪ ▪ ▪ ▪ ▪ ▪ ▪

Northern and southern biogeographical regions converge in Andrew Molera State Park, forming a kind of suture zone with sharp differences in vegetation. Canyons filled with redwoods, lush ferns and mosses, slithering salamanders, and chatty winter wrens lie adjacent to semiarid grasslands dotted with yuccas, scurrying alligator lizards, and rufous-crowned sparrows. This blend of distinct zones, along with the park's mild climate, topographic diversity, and proximity to the ocean, supports a remarkable 17 distinct plant communities.

▪ ▪

If you'd like to hike farther, the trail continues up an overgrown **fire road**. Heading southeast, this road stretches 2 miles to the park boundary, marked by an old fence line, then climbs through Forest Service land another 1.25 miles to **Post Summit**. Be aware that the summit trail is steep, overgrown, and hard to follow. Diehards will be rewarded with spectacular views of the coast, the **Little Sur River** drainage basin, and the crags of **Ventana Double Cone**. The rocky gorge below shelters a pristine stand of Santa Lucia firs, endemic only to the Santa Lucia Range.

Trip 13

RIVER TRAIL LOOP

LENGTH AND TYPE: 4-mile loop

RATING: Easy

TRAIL CONDITION: Well maintained, poison oak

HIGHLIGHTS: This oasis within the Big Sur River canyon offers a chance for a refreshing dip in a natural swimming hole.

TO REACH THE TRAILHEAD: From the park's official parking lot, walk up the entrance road 75 feet past the kiosk and turn right on the road toward Molera Trail Rides and the Ventana Wilderness Society. Considered the start of the Bobcat Trail, this road leads 0.3 mile to a horse corral. From there the trail narrows and follows the river.

TRIP SUMMARY: Skirting crystal clear water amid a verdant canyon, these riverside trails promise a wonderful year-round stroll. In fall a radiant display of sycamore, maple, alder, and cottonwood leaves brightens the river's course. Following winter storms, the 15-mile Big Sur River provides critical habitat for steelhead trout and a variety of other wildlife. In spring new life abounds, as bare golden hills sprout carpets of blooming wildflowers. Summer welcomes perfect weather for a picnic and swim.

Trip Description

From the trailhead at the horse corral, the **Bobcat Trail** narrows and begins a gentle climb alongside the **Big Sur River,** passing dense thickets of blackberry and poison oak. These are often mistaken for one another due to their similar three-leaf arrangement (blackberries have thorny stems). At the first **junction** (0.1 mile, 150'), a spur leads right (south) to the river. If you prefer an easy 1-mile loop, this spur leads to the **River Trail,** then back to the parking lot. The spur heads upstream a few feet, crosses the river, climbs the south bank, and eventually joins the River Trail. From there walk downstream to the parking lot.

Back at the junction, another short spur climbs east to a Highway 1 parking turnout, 0.75 mile south of the park entrance road. For the next 0.1 mile the Bobcat Trail parallels Highway 1, which drowns out the river and birdsong. The trail soon leaves the highway and emerges at an open meadow (1 mile, 150'). Large yellow and purple lupine bushes dot the meadow amid a colorful tapestry of California poppies, shooting stars, Indian paintbrush, blue dicks, and wild oats. Deer often graze here at dawn and dusk.

The trail crosses the meadow and rejoins the river at a **junction** with two spurs (1.2 miles, 170'). Both spurs offer optional 2.5-mile loops back to the parking lot. The first spur crosses the river diagonally, meets the opposite bank beneath a small cliff, then leads 200 feet downstream to the River Trail. A few feet upstream, the second spur heads across a bend in the Big Sur and also joins the River Trail.

Past this junction, the Bobcat Trail briefly follows the east bank, heads north up a shallow seasonal creek, then branches at **Coyote Flat,** an expansive meadow. The left branch skirts the meadow and leads to turnouts along Highway 1 (2 miles south of the park entrance road) before rejoining the main trail. The more scenic main trail branches right along the meadow's southeast edge to another fork. At this **junction** (1.5 miles, 180'), a spur leads southwest, crossing a narrow stretch of the Big Sur. Here a large outcrop channels water into a deep emerald **swimming hole,** an ideal spot for a summer picnic and swim.

Back at the junction, continue along the Bobcat Trail across the river to the Cooper Loop (1.8 miles, 180'), a 0.3-mile circuit through a redwood grove carpeted in dense ferns, mosses, and redwood sorrel. Pfeiffer Ridge and Franciscan cliffs just west of the river flats shelter these trees from harsh ocean winds and salt spray.

Complete the loop, recross the river, and head to the swimming hole mentioned above (2.3 miles, 180'). You'll have to wade across here to hook up with the **River Trail**. After heavy winter storms, the water may rise dangerously high, in which case you'll have to retrace your steps to the parking lot via the Bobcat Trail.

Across this ford, the River Trail winds downstream beside cottonwoods, bigleaf maples, and western sycamores, heading northwest to a junction with the **Hidden Trail** (3.1 miles, 170'). Continue on the River Trail past live oaks and coyote brush for a gentle descent alongside **Creamery Meadow**. North of the meadow, a spur on your right leads across the river to the Bobcat Trailhead, sparing you 150 yards of extra walking. For more exercise, continue northwest 0.1 mile to a junction on the left with the **Creamery Meadow Trail**. A few yards past this junction, the route darts east across the Big Sur back to the parking lot.

Trip 14

CREAMERY MEADOW, RIVER, HIDDEN, & RIDGE TRAILS LOOP

LENGTH AND TYPE: 3.6-mile loop

RATING: Moderate to strenuous

TRAIL CONDITION: Well maintained, poison oak

HIGHLIGHTS: Panoramic views from Pfeiffer Ridge of marble-rimmed ridges carved by the meandering Big Sur River and broad marine terraces that slope down to Point Sur

TO REACH THE TRAILHEAD: From the park's entrance kiosk, continue straight to the picnic area. The route begins at the bridge across the Big Sur.

TRIP SUMMARY: The route crosses the Big Sur and follows the river past mature sycamores, cottonwoods, maples, and alders before climbing high above the coastal bluffs. The Hidden Trail ascends Pfeiffer Ridge for 360-degree views of the region's diverse topography and vegetation. The Ridge Trail gently descends to Molera Beach, offering sweeping ocean views. Bring your binoculars, as you may glimpse migrating gray whales in spring. Hundreds of bird species make this one of the state's best bird-watching spots.

Trip Description

From the picnic area, cross the **Big Sur River** on the narrow footbridge. In winter the bridge is removed so steelhead trout can migrate upstream—expect a knee- to waist-high wade. After heavy winter storms, the river may be too swift to cross. If you prefer to stay dry or cannot cross, take the **Trail Camp Trail** to the beach (see page 83).

A healthy and stable population of native mule deer can now be seen along Creamery Meadow, once grazed by cattle that supported the Monterey Jack cheese creameries.

Once across the river, head left on **Creamery Meadow Trail** about 100 yards southwest to a junction. The right fork follows the **Beach Trail**. Instead, veer left along the Creamery Meadow Trail, passing both the meadow and a junction with a dirt road (the continuation of the Creamery Meadow Trail).

Continue southeast on the **River Trail** along the south bank of the Big Sur. For its first 0.1 mile the trail follows a level dirt road south to the broad meadow at **Coyote Flat**. At dawn and dusk, coyotes stalk the shoulder-high bush lupine in search of scurrying rabbits, voles, and mice, while black-tailed deer (also known as mule deer for their large ears, which twitch and turn at any sound) feed on herbs and grasses. Past the meadow, the vegetation quickly changes to sprawling live oaks amid thickets of coyote brush. Pause to gaze across the river toward 3709-foot marble-topped Pico Blanco.

After 0.8 mile you'll reach the **Hidden Trail junction**. This 0.7-mile trail is steep and strenuous, with an average 15% grade. The first 0.1 mile is a moderate ascent beneath live oaks, followed by a steep stretch that climbs beyond the oaks to slopes covered in coyote brush. Stop to catch your breath and admire the rugged foothills and folds of the Santa Lucia Range.

Hidden Trail climbs the spine of **Pfeiffer Ridge** to the **Ridge Trail junction** (1.5 miles, 720'). On a clear day you'll see **Point Sur,** which rises from broad marine terraces 10 miles north. Turn right onto the Ridge Trail and head west toward **Molera Point**. The trail slopes gently 1.1 miles down Pfeiffer Ridge (aka **Molera Ridge**) toward **Molera Beach** and the Creamery Meadow Trail. Hit the beach to stroll barefoot in the sand and wonder at the sculpted driftwood before turning right (northeast) on the Creamery Meadow Trail.

The trail skirts a mile of **Creamery Meadow,** a former pasture that once supported cattle raised to produced Monterey Jack cheese. Recent restoration efforts have attracted abundant wildlife. Watch for grazing black-tailed deer, elusive coyotes and bobcats, hundreds of small songbirds, and soaring raptors overhead. Just past the meadow is the familiar River Trail junction. Head left to recross the Big Sur on the footbridge (or ford in the wet season).

Trip 15

BLUFFS, SPRING, PANORAMA, & RIDGE TRAILS

LENGTH AND TYPE: 8.4-mile loop

RATING: Moderate

TRAIL CONDITION: Well maintained, poison oak

HIGHLIGHTS: Spectacular views of marble mountains and secluded coves awash in foamy surf

TO REACH THE TRAILHEAD: From the park's entrance kiosk, continue straight to the picnic area. The route begins at the bridge across the Big Sur. You'll need to follow the first mile of the Beach Trail to reach the Bluffs Trail junction.

TRIP SUMMARY: This hike leads to an idyllic cove at the west end of the Spring Trail, where the sand is tinged with pink and purple hues. The return along the Panorama and Ridge Trails promises spectacular views as you cross golden grasslands and pass beneath robust redwoods, oaks, and bays. Seals and sea otters feed in the nearshore kelp forests, raptors soar overhead, rabbits and lizards scurry into the brush, and elusive bobcats slink past the trails.

Trip Description

From the picnic area, cross the **Big Sur River** on the narrow footbridge. In winter the bridge is removed so steelhead trout can migrate upstream—expect a knee- to waist-high wade. After heavy winter storms, the river may be too swift to cross. If you prefer to stay dry or cannot cross, take the **Trail Camp Trail** to the beach (see page 83).

Once across the Big Sur, turn right and head west on the **Beach Trail** alongside **Creamery Meadow.** About a mile down the trail on your left, just before you reach **Molera Beach,** you'll meet the **Bluffs Trail junction,** which heads southeast along the edge of a marine terrace.

The trail begins with a half dozen stairs and a steep 100-yard climb atop bluffs formed by uplifted marine terraces. Pause to watch stout waves slam into the boulder-strewn beach.

A spur on the right skirts the cliffs for daunting views, then loops back to the main trail. At this point (1.2 miles, 50') the trail widens into a road, leaving plenty of room for passing hikers, bicyclists, and equestrians.

The Bluffs Trail is a kaleidoscopic experience, a blend of glistening blue ocean, golden grasses, rich rust-colored earth, and coastal brush in varying hues of green, yellow, orange, and purple. The trail crosses two small gullies, dry in all but the wettest months of the year. Bicyclists are not allowed past the second gully, as posted on a sign. The trail narrows and then widens as it crosses a barren sandstone landscape, perhaps a beach during the Ice Age, when ocean levels were several feet higher. California poppies thrive here, among few plants capable of surviving such harsh conditions. The trail ends at the **Spring Trail junction** (2.8 miles, 50').

The Spring Trail leads 0.1 mile down a narrow, slightly overgrown trail, following a small gully to a dramatic beach, one of my favorites along the Big Sur coast. After heavy winter storms, a tangle of driftwood blankets the beach entrance, creating a beautiful obstacle course of water-sculpted roots, limbs, and trunks. Under high tide and large winter surf, much of the beach disappears, but most other times you can enjoy a barefoot stroll nearly half a mile in either direction (north toward **Molera Point** or south toward **Cooper Point**). Beyond that, the beach is too narrow and dangerous to traverse in all but the lowest tides. Check tide tables at the entrance kiosk before setting your sites on a long stroll. To reach the Bluffs and Panorama Trails, return to the Spring Trail junction.

At this junction, the 1.9-mile **Panorama Trail** begins. The trail crosses the previously mentioned gully, then gradually switchbacks inland, ascending to a ridge capped by a cluster of stunted redwoods that hardly resemble the species renowned as the world's tallest tree. This close to the ocean, the redwoods are exposed to salt spray and gale-force winds that warp the trees into their gnarled state.

The trail follows a minor depression, then ascends to one of the park's best viewpoints, allowing plenty of time to catch one's breath and enjoy the hike (4.3 miles, 930'). Following a 200-foot climb, you'll be rewarded with panoramic views of Point Sur to the northwest, Pico Blanco to the north, and Cone Peak lording over the southeastern horizon some 40 miles away.

Pressing on, you'll reach a junction with a 200-foot spur (4.4 miles, 950'), which leads south toward a cluster of homes nestled along a hillside beside the fence and road. The steep ascent continues 0.3 mile to the **Ridge Trail junction** (4.7 miles, 1050') and the park's highest viewpoint west of Highway 1. Find the well-placed bench in the shade of a Monterey cypress to rest and take it all in.

The 2.75-mile Ridge Trail gently descends a closed fire road through incredibly diverse plant communities of coyote brush, sagebrush, coffeeberry, and the ubiquitous poison oak,

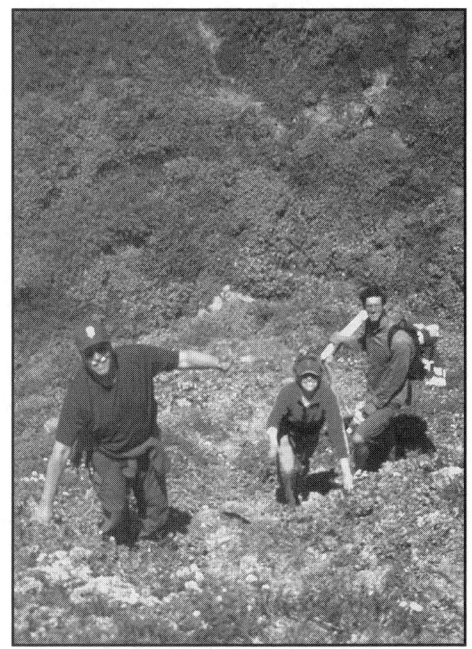

From Bluffs Trail, follow the spurs for dramatic vistas atop coastal bluffs.

then past clustered tanoaks and sprawling coast live oaks draped with lacy sage-colored lichen. Next come stately redwoods accompanied by redwood sorrel (a large four-leaf clover) and sword fern, easily identified by its large serrated fronds.

In half a mile the trail reaches the **South Boundary Trail junction** (5.2 miles, 900'). For a change of scenery and a chance to commune with nature, you could descend this lightly used 1.9-mile spur to the **Big Sur River** and Highway 1. Refrain from hiking the 2 miles along Highway 1 back to the parking lot, however, as narrow lanes leave little room between speeding cars and you.

Continuing along the Ridge Trail, you'll reach the **Hidden Trail junction** (6.3 miles, 730'). Pause to admire an awesome view that encompasses the lower Big Sur watershed, bordered by sprawling willows, alders, cottonwoods, and bigleaf maples against a backdrop of prominent peaks along the **Santa Lucia Range.** To the southeast, **Manuel Peak** (3379') rises amid a dark green patchwork of redwoods that border the Big Sur on its way through a narrow gorge. On a clear day you'll also see **Cone Peak** (5155'), which rises from the shoreline some 40 miles southeast. Less steep but perhaps more impressive, conical, marble-capped **Pico Blanco** (3709') towers over the nearby Santa Lucia foothills.

The return to your vehicle via the Hidden and River Trails, then across the Big Sur along the final stretch of the Creamery Meadow Trail (see TRIP 14 Creamery Meadow, River, Hidden, & Ridge Trails Loop, page 91, for details), is a half mile less than if you continue on the Ridge Trail to the Creamery Meadow Trail.

If you do continue on the Ridge Trail (6.3 miles, 730'), your route will follow a nearly level traverse until it descends south to the Creamery Meadow Trail junction. Turn right and hike the final mile to the parking lot.

CHAPTER ten

Pfeiffer Big Sur State Park

■ ■

At the name Big Sur, many picture a landscape of ancient redwoods along clear creeks that cascade down to the Pacific. Others immediately think of Pfeiffer Big Sur State Park, the region's most popular park, a top spot to camp, picnic, hike, and swim. Hikers come for redwood-lined gorges, oak woodlands, lush forests of sycamores, maples, alders and willows, open meadows blanketed in spring wildflowers, and a deep, narrow canyon along the Big Sur River that offers opportunities to swim and sunbathe. Although the park lies along Highway 1, it's more than a mile inland—a blessing for those hoping to escape the fog that blankets the coast most summer days.

Sweeping panoramas of jagged ridgetops slice the headwaters between the Carmel and Big Sur Rivers east of Manuel Peak.

Pfeiffer Big Sur State Park

This parcel belonged to John Pfeiffer, son of Michael and Barbara Pfeiffer, who in 1869 became the first European immigrants to permanently settle in the region. John's wife, Florence, launched the first resort in Big Sur after deciding to charge freeloading guests for room and board. The Big Sur Lodge stands on this site, while the couple's 1884 homestead cabin lies along the Oak Grove Trail. In 1930 a Los Angeles developer offered John Pfeiffer $210,000 for his 1200-acre property, with the intent to parcel it off as a subdivision. Fortunately, the offer was rejected, and in 1933 the State of California purchased 700 acres and named the new park in Pfeiffer's honor.

DIRECTIONS: The park is on the east side of Highway 1, 26 miles south of the Carmel Valley Road (County Road G16) junction in Carmel and 28 miles north of the Nacimiento-Fergusson Road junction near Kirk Creek Campground.

VISITOR CENTER: Big Sur Station: (831) 667-2315. The station is on Highway 1, a half mile south of the park entrance. Open daily 8 a.m.–6 p.m. Memorial Day through Labor Day, 8 a.m.–4:30 p.m. the rest of the year.

NEAREST CAMPGROUND: Pfeiffer Big Sur State Park (218 sites, $35/standard site, $45/river site; reservations recommended in summer and on holidays). For more information call Reserve America at (800) 444-7275 or visit ReserveAmerica.com.

INFORMATION: Open daily 9 a.m.–8 p.m. There's a $10/vehicle entrance fee. No dogs or bikes allowed on park trails. No overnight camping.

WEBSITE: parks.ca.gov

PHONE: (831) 667-2315

Trip 16

VALLEY VIEW TRAIL

LENGTH AND TYPE: 1.6-mile loop

RATING: Easy

TRAIL CONDITION: Well maintained, poison oak, good for kids

HIGHLIGHTS: Sweeping views of the Big Sur River gorge, Point Sur, and Andrew Molera State Park

TO REACH THE TRAILHEAD: Pass the park's entrance kiosk and turn left at the stop sign, following signs to Pfeiffer Falls. After 100 feet the road will fork. Veer right past Ewoldsen Memorial Nature Center to the parking lot at road's end. The Valley View Trail begins either 0.1 mile from the start of the Pfeiffer Falls Trail or from the base of the falls, 0.4 mile down the same trail.

TRIP SUMMARY: Beginning alongside Pfeiffer Redwood Creek, this semi-loop route meanders past some of the park's largest coast redwoods. Climbing above the canyon floor, the trail offers views down the Big Sur River gorge.

Trip Description

The Pfeiffer Falls Trail begins beneath old-growth redwoods alongside Pfeiffer Redwood Creek. The narrow, well-used path gently ascends the canyon, soon reaching the Valley View Trail junction (0.1 mile, 400'). From the junction, the Valley View Trail branches west, crosses a wooden footbridge, and ascends Pfeiffer Redwood Canyon.

Rising above the canyon floor, you'll pass beneath some of the park's grandest redwoods. Over thousands of years, creek sediments have formed the rich alluvial soils necessary to support these trees. Over the next 0.1 mile a trio of switchbacks leads out of the canyon. Farther from the creek, these drier slopes support an entirely different group of plants. Twisted live oaks, scraggly brush, and spring displays of deep purple wild iris blanket the hillside (0.2 mile, 570').

As the trail climbs to the ridge, you'll glimpse the **Big Sur River** gorge off to the west. Three more switchbacks lead to a trail junction—the route to the right leads 0.2 mile to **Pfeiffer Falls,** while the route left leads 0.3 mile to the **Valley View Vista** (0.5 mile, 630'). Veer left toward the vista, climbing to a ridge that offers oak-filtered views to the north, east, and west.

The **viewpoint** (0.8 mile, 700') rewards you with panoramic views of the **Santa Lucia Range** and down the Big Sur River gorge to the Pacific. **Point Sur** rises over the rolling hills of Andrew Molera State Park, 7 miles northwest. In the canyon and on the river flats, dark redwoods stand beside alders, sycamores, bigleaf maples, black cottonwoods, and willows, which boast vibrant greens in spring and deep hues of orange, red, and yellow in fall. Sprawling oaks dot hillsides and ridges of golden grass, while tanoaks, live oaks, madrones, and bays fill the cool, moist, north-facing slopes and ravines. Offering contrast on the hot, dry south-facing slopes are the velvety greens and browns of the chaparral, dominated by chamise, ceanothus, manzanita, and coffeeberry. Take in the view and return the way you came.

WORLD'S TALLEST TREE ■ ■ ■ ■ ■ ■ ■ ■ ■ ■ ■ ■ ■ ■ ■ ■ ■ ■

Exceeding 300 feet in height, coast redwoods (*Sequoia sempervirens*) are the world's tallest trees. Big Sur marks the species' southernmost range. These moisture-loving giants thrive in the region's narrow river gorges. Farther south, temperatures are too hot and precipitation too low to sustain them. The remaining trees represent a fraction of the original groves.

Coastal Indians were the first to make use of the trees, stripping the roots of their strong fibers for use as thread in basketry. In subsequent settler days the land was ill managed. Many old-growth groves were lost when the Ventana Power Company operated a sawmill here in the late 19th century. About the same time, John and Florence Pfeiffer opened Pfeiffer Ranch Resort. To supply guests with lodging and warmth, the Pfeiffers turned to the mill for their lumber needs. Decades later, when Highway 1 was being built, the mill supplied lumber for worker housing.

■ ■

Trip 17

PFEIFFER FALLS TRAIL

LENGTH AND TYPE: 1.4-mile round-trip

RATING: Easy

TRAIL CONDITION: Well maintained, good for kids

HIGHLIGHTS: Ancient redwoods flank this spectacular 60-foot waterfall.

TO REACH THE TRAILHEAD: Pass the park's entrance kiosk and turn left at the stop sign, following signs to Pfeiffer Falls. After 100 feet the road will fork. Veer right past Ewoldsen Memorial Nature Center to the parking lot at road's end.

TRIP SUMMARY: Unquestionably one of the most popular hikes in Big Sur, this short, easy 0.7-mile trail leads past ancient redwoods to the base of the 60-foot cascade. Expect crowds in summer, when the park campground often fills. The falls are most impressive during the winter wet season, when lush ferns, fungi, and mosses line the canyon.

Trip Description

Pfeiffer Falls Trail begins beside **Pfeiffer Redwood Creek,** shaded by the park's most magnificent redwoods. Once comprising some 2,000,000 acres of fogbound coast between Big Sur and southern Oregon, most of the old-growth redwood forests were heavily logged, and now only small stands of these ancient trees remain in an area of less than 300,000 acres. A 6-foot diameter cross-section of a 1000-year-old felled redwood rests beside the upper trailhead. Although enormous, it's an average size and age for this region. Throughout their range in central California, redwoods rarely exceed 1500 years old, 10 feet in diameter, or 250 feet in height. It's the celebrated redwoods in Northern California's Coast Ranges that commonly exceed 2000 years old, 15–20 feet in diameter, and 300 feet in height.

A gentle ascent up the narrow, well-used path beside **Pfeiffer Redwood Creek Canyon** leads to the **Valley View Trail junction** (0.1 mile, 400'), on your left. Both trails lead to the falls, but the Pfeiffer Falls Trail is less steep and a quarter mile shorter than the Valley View Trail. Pass this junction and you'll soon reach steps that ascend to the **Oak Grove Trail junction** (0.2 mile, 470'), which veers sharply south. Stay on course to reach the first of four scenic wooden footbridges that cross the creek.

A PFEIFFER ON EVERY HILL ■ ■ ■ ■ ■ ■ ■ ■ ■ ■ ■ ■ ■ ■ ■ ■

Still standing along the Oak Grove Trail, the Homestead Cabin was built in 1884 by homesteader John Pfeiffer. John was 7 years old when his family arrived in Big Sur in 1869, becoming the first European immigrants to settle here permanently. By the turn of the century, the Pfeiffers were operating a sawmill and boarding house on the property. In 1933, John and wife Florence Pfeiffer sold most of the surrounding land to the state, stipulating that it be preserved as a park. Florence and seven of her children are buried in a cemetery near the Homestead Cabin.

Pfeiffer Redwood Creek cascades 60 feet along its path toward the confluence of the Big Sur River farther downstream.

Soon after crossing the fourth footbridge, you'll reach the northern **Valley View Trail junction** (0.4 mile, 590'), which leads northwest across a fifth bridge. Once again, continue straight and follow the burbling creek through its narrow, steep-walled canyon. You'll ascend more than 40 steps to the base of the 60-foot falls, where visitors pause on a wooden platform to watch water plunging over the mossy granite cliff into the crystal clear pool below. Benches on the platform offer a great picnic spot, though you shouldn't expect solitude.

Trip 18

NATURE TRAIL

LENGTH AND TYPE: 0.6-mile out-and-back

RATING: Easy

TRAIL CONDITION: Well maintained, good for kids

HIGHLIGHTS: Stroll through oak woodlands and ancient redwood groves on this 30-minute self-guided nature tour.

TO REACH THE TRAILHEAD: From the park entrance, head to the stop sign, then continue straight past Big Sur Lodge. Immediately past the lodge, the road forks. Continue straight for 0.1 mile to the next fork, then veer left. Drive a quarter mile farther, bypassing the campfire center parking lot for the smaller lot beside a picnic area. The trailhead is opposite this lot.

TRIP SUMMARY: This self-guided, 30-minute stroll through oak woodlands and a magnificent redwood forest is the perfect way to experience the park's diverse plant life. Informative pamphlets at either end of the trail describe two of the five major resident plant communities. Your $0.25 donation supports the Big Sur Natural History Association.

Trip Description

You'll start on a level trail that meanders beneath sprawling **live oaks,** fragrant bay trees, and twisting sycamores, whose bark may remind you of a jigsaw puzzle. A dozen numbered posts correlate to brochure entries, helping you identify plants and animals common to these unique forest communities.

By the tenth post (0.2 mile, 300'), you'll have entered a **redwood grove,** marked by dramatic changes in vegetation. Little sunshine penetrates the dense redwood canopy, creating a dark, cool microclimate. These ancient giants lie at the southern limit of their range, in a much warmer, drier climate than that associated with Pacific Northwest redwood groves. Only along the small creeks and rivers that slice the Big Sur coast are they able to find adequate moisture to survive. The adverse conditions prevent these redwoods from obtaining the impressive size and lifespan of their northern counterparts. Nonetheless, redwoods have thrived along the **Big Sur River** for thousands of years, their broad shallow roots taking hold in rich deposits of alluvial soil along the riverbank.

The trail crosses the roadway just past the eleventh post (0.25 mile, 300') and leads to one of the park's largest trees, which towers nearly 300 feet. Most trees at the trail's end are 500–800 years old, hardly record-breaking for a species that can live more than 2000 years and exceed 300 feet in height. The trail emerges at the visitor lot beside park headquarters. Retrace your steps to the trailhead.

Trip 19

BUZZARDS ROOST TRAIL

LENGTH AND TYPE: 3.1-mile loop

RATING: Moderate

TRAIL CONDITION: Clear, poison oak

HIGHLIGHTS: Summit views overlook prominent ridgelines east to the Big Sur River gorge and west to Sycamore Canyon and the vast blue ocean.

TO REACH THE TRAILHEAD: From the park entrance, head to the stop sign, then continue straight past Big Sur Lodge. Immediately past the lodge, the road forks. Bear right on the two-lane bridge over the Big Sur River. The parking lot is on the left just past the bridge. The trail begins on the west bank beneath the bridge.

TRIP SUMMARY: This trail follows the south bank of the Big Sur beneath a canopy of redwoods and tanoaks before climbing Pfeiffer Ridge. Despite the promise of gorgeous over-looks of the Santa Lucia Range and Pacific, the trail is little used. You may find yourself alone at the top with large turkey vultures that roost in the redwoods below. In summer, fog envelops the coast, obscuring views. Fog is less likely in the spring and fall, while winter views between storms are often spectacular. Strong winds are always a factor atop the open ridge—bring a windbreaker or sweater year-round.

Trip Description

From the trailhead, the **Buzzards Roost Trail** crosses beneath the bridge to follow the banks of the **Big Sur River**. Autumn visits are highlighted by deep yellow and orange hues from the large sycamores, alders, bigleaf maples, and willows that flank the river. A short, gentle descent downstream brings you to a spur that leads straight 0.1 mile to a riverside group camp.

From this **spur junction** (0.2 mile, 310'), the main trail forks uphill toward **Pfeiffer Ridge**. A riparian woodland dominated by broadleaf deciduous trees quickly gives way to a dense, shady redwood-tanoak forest. The redwoods persist despite a drier environment than that found in their northern range. As a result, much of the expected dense understory of ferns and mosses is not present here.

At a sign marked BUZZARDS ROOST TRAIL (1.4 miles, 550'), the route forks to become a 1.7-mile loop. Bear right on the more direct, well-graded ascent to **Buzzards Ridge**. The shaded path passes beneath young redwoods and thin, dense stands of bay trees. Closer to the ridgeline, the redwoods are stunted, perhaps from nutrient-poor soil or lack of water. You'll encounter a dramatic vegetation shift atop the ridge (1.9 miles, 1000'), as you enter dry thickets of manzanita and chamise.

The path crosses the ridge to a narrow **spur junction** (2 miles, 1010'), which bears right and climbs 50 feet to the **summit,** topped by a large antenna. Turn your back to the obtrusive antenna for beautiful views down **Sycamore Canyon** to the Pacific. Gaze east to take in the steep narrow Big Sur River gorge and the **Manuel Peak Trail,** which switchbacks and ascends the gorge's sheer north walls.

Back on the main trail, you'll skirt the ridgeline south for 200 feet, then descend a few large steps to reenter dense stands of redwoods, bays, and tanoaks. The next 0.7 mile is a gradual descent with limited views across the river gorge. From the loop junction, retrace your steps 1.4 miles to the trailhead.

Atop Buzzard's Roost, keep an eye out for the 9-foot wingspan of the California condor.

Trip 20

MANUEL PEAK TRAIL

LENGTH AND TYPE: 10.8-mile out-and-back

RATING: Challenging

TRAIL CONDITION: Passable to difficult, poison oak

HIGHLIGHTS: Panoramic views from a secluded peak deep within the Big Sur watershed.

TO REACH THE TRAILHEAD: From the park entrance, head to the stop sign, then continue straight past Big Sur Lodge. Immediately past the lodge, the road forks. Bear left and drive 0.7 mile past the picnic areas. Bear left at the next fork and park across from the trailhead at the base of a closed road, labeled on the park map as the Gorge Trail.

TRIP SUMMARY: Offering an overview of the Ventana Wilderness, this steep trail averages an 11% grade, reaching 3379' in 5.4 miles at the peak's scenic viewpoint. You'll ascend past sun-scorched chaparral, cool redwood groves, and oak woodlands. From May through October, this is often a sunny, dry trek, so bring a wide-brimmed hat and plenty of extra water. Despite the hot climb, wear long pants for protection from ticks, brush, and poison oak. In summer, the coast is often fogbound, though views inland remain unobscured.

Trip Description

The trailhead for the **Gorge Trail, Manuel Peak Trail,** and south end of the **Oak Grove Trail** begins at the base of the closed paved road across from the parking lot. Climb the service road 0.1 mile till it curves north at a junction with a dirt road. The main road continues straight as the Gorge Trail. Turn left (west) on the dirt road past John Pfeiffer's **Homestead Cabin.** Follow the Oak Grove Trail 50 feet north of the cabin, where it narrows to a single lane and leads 0.4 mile farther to the Manuel Peak Trail junction.

The trail makes an initial switchback east to meet a **spur** (0.2 mile, 220') that leads down to one of the picnic area parking lots. Continue your moderate ascent beneath a dense canopy of gnarled live oaks, tanoaks, and bays. In summer this short stretch of shade provides welcome relief from the mostly exposed Manuel Peak Trail.

Past an enormous downed oak, you'll clamber up a minor ridge to a **fork** (0.6 mile, 560'). A sign warns that from here the Manuel Peak Trail is a strenuous climb that ascends nearly 3000 feet in 4 miles. While largely well graded to the summit, the last mile is overgrown and requires brushing past, at times, shoulder-high shrubs. In winter and spring keep watch for hitchhiking ticks.

Take the right fork upslope along the Manuel Peak Trail, which soon leaves the shade on a steady climb through fragrant coastal scrub past chamise, sage, poison oak, coyote brush, and toyon. You'll switchback five times and climb 400 feet before catching your first glimpse of the jagged Big Sur coast and glistening Pacific, spurring you to continue your ascent. Trail switchbacks stand out clearly against the south-facing slopes, while the narrow river gorge below drops precipitously, seemingly the result of landslides in places. The **Pine Ridge Trail** traces the cool, forested north-facing slopes across the gorge. In summer and early fall, fog envelops the valley, obscuring views.

After 2.5 miles the trail turns north and enters a canopy of live oaks, madrones, and stately redwoods. Traversing the redwood-lined gully, the route descends into a smaller but more significant **gully** (3.4 miles, 1720'), home to a small seasonal creek—though in dry months (April through October), this is little more than a muddy seep.

From this minor gully, you'll climb east and enter the **Ventana Wilderness**. After 0.3 mile (3.7 miles, 2200'), turn north for your first views toward the scraggly bald peaks of **Ventana Double Cone** (4853') and neighboring summits. The trail is not regularly maintained from here to the summit, though it's still easy to identify through the overgrown brush. You'll have to scramble across a few downed trees and dry washes.

Continue your ascent through dense, sometimes shoulder-high thickets of coastal chaparral (4 miles, 2200'). Dominating the trailside is wartleaf, which bears pungent sawtooth leaves. After 0.4 mile passage through this moderate overgrowth, the trail opens and climbs west across a north-facing ridge studded with oaks and madrones. You'll soon crest the ridge with views of the Pacific (or perhaps fogbanks in summer) to the west and the rugged **Santa Lucia Range** to the east.

MANUEL INNOCENTI ■

Manuel Peak is named for Manuel Innocenti, an Esselen Indian from Big Sur who was raised and educated at the Santa Barbara Mission in Southern California. In 1868 he returned to this area, purchasing land and a cabin near Manuel Peak for $50.

Tragically, though the land and the sea had provided Manuel's tribe with an abundance of all they needed to survive—deer, rabbits, fish, shellfish, wild flax, tule reeds, berries, acorns, bulbs, quail—his people had vanished. From 1770, when Father Junipero Serra and Captain Gaspar de Portola founded a mission and presidio at Monterey, the "pagan souls" of the coast had been brought into the mission system. Most either assimilated, succumbed to disease, or were killed in warfare.

Manuel became head vaquero at Juan B.R. Cooper's Rancho El Sur, at present-day Andrew Molera State Park. Manuel and wife Francisca had seven children, none of whom reached adulthood.

■ ■

The trail switchbacks up a steeper crest, then makes a short ascent on an easier grade to a spur for the **Manuel Peak viewpoint** (5.3 miles, 3379'), capped with white marble rubble and a small scraggly live oak. The open summit offers a nearly 360-degree view of the Ventana Wilderness and neighboring **Big Sur State Park**. For relief in the shade, retreat to a dense stand of Coulter pines past a conspicuous, yet camouflaged reflector a few paces north of the viewpoint. Once rested, head back down the trail.

For those headed to Bottchers Gap, 12.7 miles farther north, reverse the trail description in TRIP 42 Manuel Peak & Pfeiffer Big Sur State Park (page 169). Be forewarned: The trail from Manuel Peak to Launtz Creek Camp is heavily overgrown and not recommended.

Trip 21

GORGE TRAIL

LENGTH AND TYPE: 1-mile out-and-back

RATING: Easy to challenging

TRAIL CONDITION: Well maintained, poison oak

HIGHLIGHTS: This steep, narrow canyon features large granite boulders amid brisk, refreshing swimming holes.

TO REACH THE TRAILHEAD: From the park entrance, head to the stop sign, then continue straight past Big Sur Lodge. Immediately past the lodge, the road forks. Bear left and drive 0.7 mile past the picnic areas. Bear left at the next fork and park across from the trailhead at the base of a closed road.

TRIP SUMMARY: This short trail skirts the Big Sur River to some of the region's best swimming holes. The gorge is easy to traverse in summer, when campers and hikers descend en masse to lounge poolside and bask on sunny boulders. During heavy winter storms, however, the river can rise several feet in just a few hours, flooding the trail.

Trip Description

Head southeast up the paved fire road through the gate and gradually ascend to the **Homestead Cabin** (0.2 mile, 340'), built in 1884 by John Pfeiffer. Continue along the paved road and cross the large bridge over the **Big Sur River** into the northern section of the park campground (0.3 mile, 300').

Officially, the **Gorge Trail** ends here, though you have yet to enter the gorge. Starting beside the bridge, two trails lead upstream along either the east or west banks to the gorge. Passage is easiest in summer and fall, when water levels are low.

To avoid hiking through people's campsites, take the west bank, which leads upstream 0.1 mile to a refreshing pool, followed by a steep granite wall. On summer afternoons, the surrounding granite rocks make warm, smooth sunbathing platforms. Water temperatures on even the hottest summer day remain in the low to mid 60s Fahrenheit, while on warm fall and spring days, temps linger in the mid to high 50s. Despite the brisk water, dozens of swimmers frequent these pools in summer.

If you prefer more solitude, head farther upstream, though steeper walls allow only slivers of sunshine to reach the canyon floor. The park discourages climbing here due to loose rock and unstable soil. Clambering atop the slick granite boulders that line the canyon floor is equally dangerous. During winter storms, the river can swiftly rise several feet above its normal level. Be aware of the weather and never enter the gorge when storm clouds are approaching.

Trip 22

PFEIFFER BEACH

LENGTH AND TYPE: 1-mile out-and-back

RATING: Easy

TRAIL CONDITION: Well maintained, good for kids

HIGHLIGHTS: Stroll barefoot along one of Big Sur's finest windswept beaches to commune with the sea.

TO REACH THE TRAILHEAD: The road to Pfeiffer Beach lies at a saddle with two roads on the west side of Highway 1, a quarter mile south of Big Sur Station and 1.1 miles north of the Ventana Inn entrance. Turn west on Sycamore Canyon Road, a narrow, winding stretch that leads 2.2 miles to the beach parking loop. There's a $5 day-use fee. You'll find water and bathrooms at the trailhead.

TRIP SUMMARY: This hike leads to one of the region's most striking beaches. In spring the coastal bluffs boast a colorful tapestry of wildflowers, including California poppies, sticky monkeyflowers, yellow sand verbena, Indian paintbrush, and lupines. Foaming surf crashes through dramatic nearshore arches, highlighting the gorgeous sunsets.

Trip Description

From the west end of the parking lot, follow Sycamore Creek 0.1 mile down to the ocean. Redwoods, bays, and buckeyes line the stream, soon giving way to a wind-sculpted stand of Monterey cypress, whose roots anchor in the steep dunes.

At the creek mouth, the trail emerges on the wide beach. Leave your own footprints in the soft sand. Just offshore, waves crash against rugged rocky outcrops, some carved over time into natural arches. These dramatic formations offer a natural barrier from the crashing surf, sheltering shallow tide pools for waders of all ages. Water temps remain a nippy 50s Fahrenheit year-round.

Enjoy a barefoot beach stroll along Pfeiffer Beach, one of the most incredible wave-washed beaches of Big Sur.

PFEIFFER BEACH GEOLOGY ■ ■ ■ ■ ■ ■ ■ ■ ■ ■ ■ ■ ■ ■ ■ ■

Referred to as the Pfeiffer Beach Slab, these low bluffs and loosely consolidated cliffs expose the variegated hues of ancient deformed rocks. The predominant rock at Pfeiffer Beach is sandstone, ranging in color from tan or gold to gray. Carved with numerous arches, the nearshore rocks are remnants of massive sandstone blocks that continue to erode with each pounding wave.

While part of the Franciscan complex, they have been less heavily metamorphosed than similar formations farther north. Geologists believe these differences are due to the numerous northwest-trending faults associated with the San Andreas Fault, which rends the Big Sur region.

■ ■

Sea arches and sunsets are not to be missed along Pfeiffer Beach.

CHAPTER eleven

Julia Pfeiffer Burns State Park

Julia Pfeiffer Burns State Park epitomizes Big Sur's natural scenic grandeur. This exquisite 3.75-square-mile parcel preserves a dramatic convergence of coastal and mountain features. Rocky points rise thousands of feet above rich underwater canyons, streams flow down steep gorges shaded by ancient redwoods, and a ribbony waterfall plunges over a granite lip to the sand of a pristine cove.

Julia Pfeiffer Burns State Park

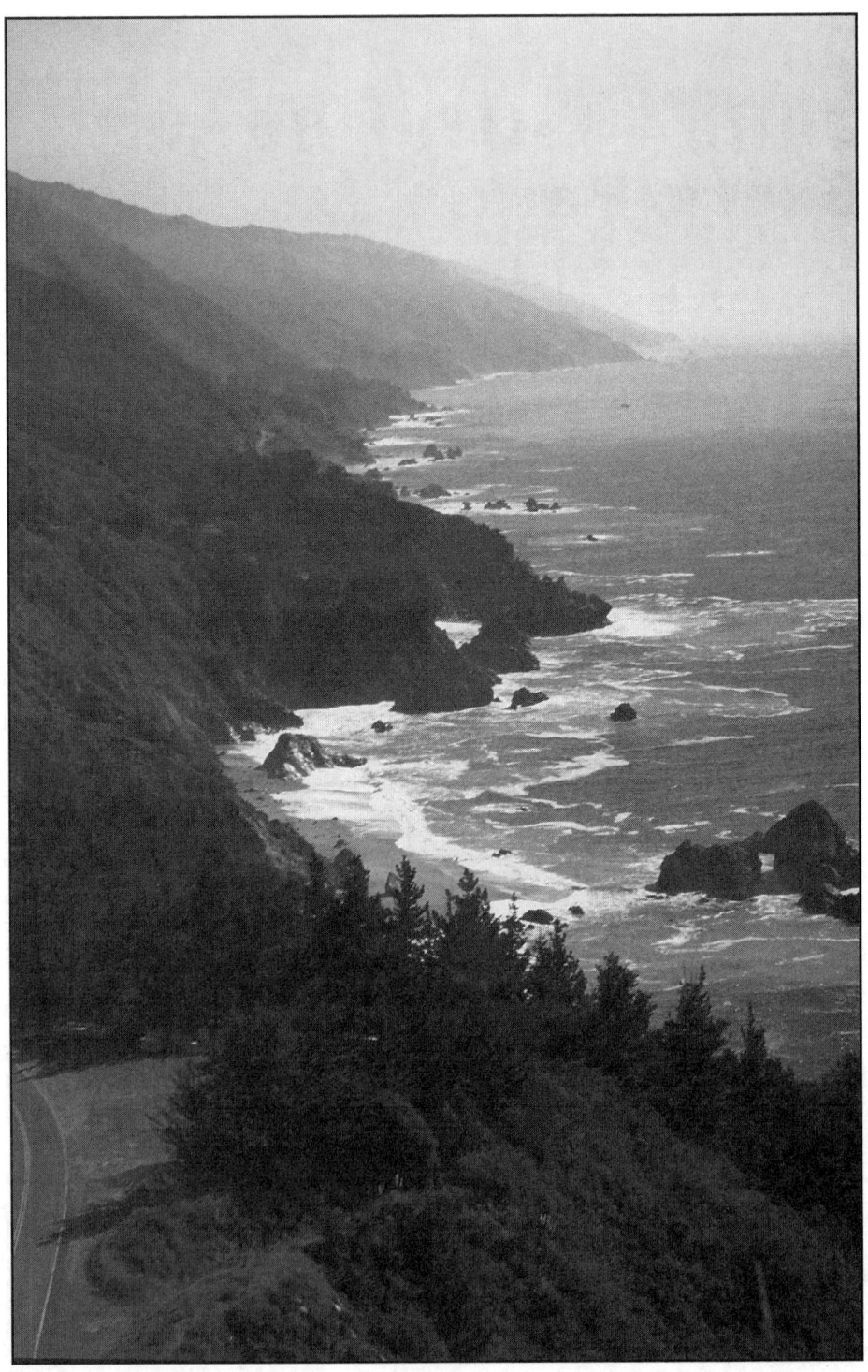

In addition to its 10 miles of coastline and 1860 acres of mountains, meadows, and valleys, the park also contains a 1680-acre underwater reserve that hosts diverse marine life. Scan the thick nearshore kelp beds to spot foraging seals, sea lions, and sea otters. You may also witness the annual winter migration of California gray whales, which journey south to breeding and calving grounds in Baja between November and January, then migrate north to Alaskan feeding grounds between February and April. In spring, females steer their calves close to shore for protection from predators. McWay Cove is an excellent vantage point.

The park is named for Julia Pfeiffer Burns, a respected Big Sur pioneer. She was less than a year old in 1869 when her parents, Michael and Barbara Pfeiffer, journeyed to this wild coast to become Big Sur's first permanent white settlers. The Pfeiffer family grew, prospered, and homesteaded so much of the surrounding land that it was often said, "There was a Pfeiffer on every hill."

In the late 1870s, Christopher McWay arrived to settle the adjacent canyon. Fifty years later, Lathrop Brown, a former New York congressman, and wife Helen Hooper Brown purchased McWay's Saddle Rock Ranch and built a home atop what today is the waterfall overlook. Helen Brown donated the ranch to the state of California in 1961, choosing to name the park in honor of Julia, the strong, self-sufficient pioneer.

DIRECTIONS: The park entrance is on the east side of Highway 1, 37 miles south of the Carmel Valley Road (County Road G16) junction in Carmel and 11 miles south of Big Sur State Park.

VISITOR CENTER: Big Sur Station: (831) 667-2315. The station is on Highway 1, 10 miles north of the park entrance. Open daily 8 a.m.–4:30 p.m. Memorial Day through Labor Day, 8 a.m.–6 p.m. the rest of the year.

NEAREST CAMPGROUND: The park's walk-in campground lies on the south side of the McWay Falls promontory, 0.3 mile from the parking lot. Two primitive sites ($30/night; reservations required) hold a maximum of eight people each. For more information call Reserve America at (800) 444-7275 or visit ReserveAmerica.com.

INFORMATION: Open 7 a.m.–10 p.m. There is a $10 day-use fee. Restrooms and water are available at the parking lot. No pets allowed except seeing-eye dogs.

WEBSITE: parks.ca.gov

PHONE: (831) 667-2315

Feel the raw elements of fog, wind, and sunshine along the jutting coastal cliffs within Julia Pfeiffer Burns State Park.

Trip 23

PARTINGTON COVE TRAIL

LENGTH AND TYPE: 0.6-mile out-and-back

RATING: Easy

TRAIL CONDITION: Well maintained, poison oak, good for kids

HIGHLIGHTS: Coastal access to a dramatic stretch of pounding surf, jagged granite rocks, and sheer cliffs

TO REACH THE TRAILHEAD: The trailhead is 2 miles north of the park entrance on Highway 1, at the west end of Partington Creek Bridge. There are small turnouts on either side of the bridge. A cattle gate on the ocean side of the road marks the trailhead. You won't find water or restrooms, save for two outhouses at Partington Cove.

TRIP SUMMARY: This short, steady descent traces Partington Creek's final yards to sea, emerging in a cove with stunning natural features and rich cultural history. In the 1870s the site served as a port from which tanoak bark was shipped to the tanning industry in San Francisco. Local legend has it the cove was also used as a booze smuggling port during Prohibition in the 1920s. Expect crowds in summer and on weekends.

Trip Description

From the cattle gate near the northwest end of **Partington Creek Bridge** (240'), you'll descend a steep grade 0.2 mile along a fire road to a small flat beside the creek. The trail narrows as you reach a **spur** (0.25 mile, 60') that leads upstream 100 feet toward an outhouse beside a dense stand of redwoods.

Continue downstream 100 feet to another **spur** (0.3 mile, 50'), which leads 200 feet to the narrow west cove at **Partington Point**. Taking this spur, you'll pass a cluster of grizzled redwoods that struggle against the salt spray and pounding surf.

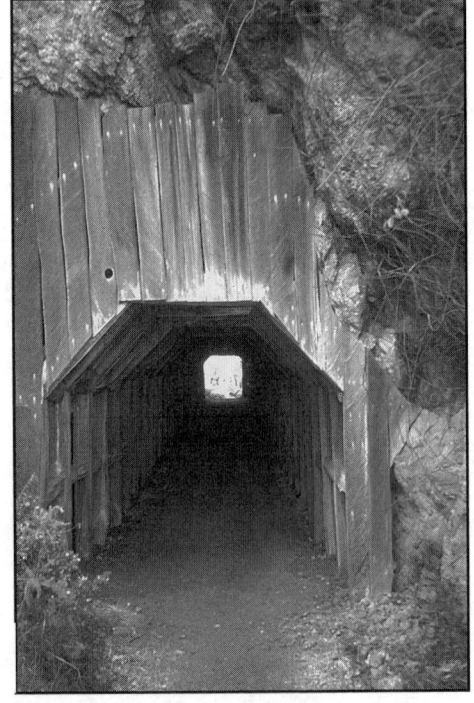

Local legend has it that the Partington Cove tunnel was used to smuggle booze during Prohibition.

The spur emerges on the beach, where you'll have to clamber over a few granite boulders onto coarse sand washed by exceptionally clear emerald water. Dominating the cove is Salinian block granite, formed 80 million years ago in Mexico and carried here along the San Andreas Fault. This granite is extremely erosion resistant, leaving the water largely free of sediments that cloud water elsewhere along the coast.

From the prior junction, the main trail bears left and threads through a 100-foot tunnel to the east cove. Built in the 1870s by John Partington, the hand-split redwood tunnel leads to **Partington Landing.** Here the canyon's redwoods and oaks were loaded onto waiting ships. Redwood was used to build homes, roofs, and fences in rapidly growing San Francisco, while tanoak bark was used to tan leather. Today, this is an ideal spot to have a picnic, watch for whales and sea otters, and soak up magnificent sunsets. Return the way you came.

Trip 24

TAN BARK TRAIL & FIRE ROAD LOOP

LENGTH AND TYPE: 6.6-mile out-and-back or 5.6-mile loop

RATING: Moderate to strenuous

TRAIL CONDITION: Clear, poison oak

HIGHLIGHTS: Old-growth redwoods and sweeping Pacific vistas.

TO REACH THE TRAILHEAD: The Tan Bark Trail starts at the east end of Partington Creek Bridge, 2 miles north of the park entrance on Highway 1. There are small turnouts on either side of the bridge. The Fire Road emerges near Vista Point at Mile 37 on Highway 1. The road lies 70 yards east of the parking area. Neither trailhead offers restrooms or water.

TRIP SUMMARY: Choose between a 6.6-mile out-and-back hike via the Tan Bark Trail or a 5.6-mile loop that traverses the Tan Bark Trail and Fire Road back to Highway 1. The 3.3-mile Tan Bark Trail is a longer, more scenic route to the Tin House and is better graded than the wide, steep Fire Road. That said, it starts lower and thus climbs more than 2000 feet versus the Fire Road's 1580-foot climb. The 2.2-mile Fire Road is a steep climb past sunny hilltops with coastal views. The following description starts on the Tan Bark Trail, ascends to the Tin House, then descends the Fire Road to Highway 1.

Trip Description

From the southeast end of **Partington Creek Bridge** (210'), the **Tan Bark Trail** follows **Partington Creek** as it tumbles over granite boulders beneath towering redwoods. In 0.1 mile a spur bears left across the creek on a **wooden bridge** (0.1 mile, 170'). This spur leads back downstream to the west end of the bridge. Continue straight along the south fork of Partington Creek, taking in the persistent cries of tiny brown winter wrens.

The trail follows the south bank in the cool shade of redwoods, tanoaks, and bays. After 0.3 mile the trail reaches another spur that darts upstream 100 feet to the creek. At this junction, the main trail turns east through the **Donald McLaughlin Memorial Grove** (0.3 mile, 350'). The trail then begins its major ascent, climbing a series of steep switchbacks past a minor gully that hosts a creek only during the wettest months. Glance across canyon at the sun-baked south-facing slopes, dotted with homes in the **Partington Ridge** subdivision.

The trail continues northeast, switching from redwoods amid lush sorrel and sword ferns to drier stands of oaks and bays. Sadly, most of these oaks are dead or dying from sudden oak death. The main trail is clearly marked and well trodden in contrast to the numerous spurs, remnants of trails once used to haul out batches of tanoak bark.

BIG SUR LUMBER ■

The redwoods along Partington Creek are among Big Sur's largest, survivors of a lumber industry that clear-cut whole stands along the Coast Ranges. Redwood is highly valued as a building material, but these gnarled old-growth trees were unsuitable for lumber and spared from the axe.

Tanoaks, however, were extensively harvested for the leather-tanning industry. The trees were clear-cut in this canyon, then shipped from Partington Cove to tanneries in Santa Cruz and San Francisco. The harvest was hard on the forest. Tanoaks didn't grow in pure stands, so loggers forged rough trails to reach the trees. Although tanoak wood is usable as a building material or firewood, loggers were only after the bark and left the trees to rot.

Yet today, extensive stands dominate Partington Canyon along the Tan Bark Trail. This recovery is due to tanoak's reproductive capacity to "stump sprout" from the roots of a felled tree. These sprouts grow at the same time, establishing multiple trunks from a common root system.

■ ■

Just past a minor confluence of the **south fork** (2 miles, 1550'), note the enormous old-growth redwoods, some nearly 10 feet in diameter. Continue your gentle ascent through the glade to a creek that flows in all but the driest months. Ignore the overgrown trail to the northeast and follow the main trail southeast to a bench beside the creek. Check the path for obvious stonework (2.3 miles, 1680'), remnants of **Swiss Camp,** built by settler Gunder Bergstrom in the 1920s. The most strenuous climbing is now behind you.

For the next 0.7 mile you'll climb a gentle grade, soon reaching a junction with a **spur** (3 miles, 2110') that climbs a prominent ridge on private property. Stay on the main trail and follow it downhill 200 yards till you merge with the wide Fire Road. From here you'll bear left and descend another 200 feet to the **Tin House** (3.3 miles, 1960'), perched on a ridge crest.

Built during World War II from tin scavenged from a defunct gas station, the Tin House is a peculiar structure with an obscure history. In wartime, tin was a tightly controlled material, so it's unusual to find so much tin in a house from that era. The previous landowner was Lathrop Brown, a politician who served in Congress and the Department of the Interior. Locals insist Brown built the house as a retreat for friend and college classmate Franklin D. Roosevelt. Others believe it served as the Browns' second home. Regardless, this is a beautiful spot for a picnic, atop a golden hilltop that offers sweeping views of the coast.

When rested, you can return the way you came or finish the loop via the **Fire Road,** a 2.2-mile descent to **Vista Point** on Highway 1, a mile north of Partington Creek Bridge. From the Tin House, head back uphill 0.2 mile to the Tan Bark Trail **junction** (3.5 miles, 1980'), then turn north to descend the canyon's east side. Over the next 0.6 mile the steep road switchbacks in the shade of tanoaks and redwoods. After 1.4 miles the road reaches a prominent **ridge** (4.7 miles, 1030'), with excellent views across steep, narrow **Partington Canyon.** Leaving the shade, the road emerges amid fragrant coastal scrub that flaunts colorful wildflowers in the spring, when abundant lupines, golden yarrow, and poppies paint the hillsides in yellow, purple, and orange hues.

The coastal views continue to impress as you descend the Fire Road, weaving past gullies to a minor spring flanked by redwoods and lush ferns. It's a 200-foot jaunt from here to the Fire Road gate and Highway 1.

If you parked at Vista Point, cross the highway and walk 200 feet north to the lot. If you parked at Partington Creek Bridge, continue walking a mile north on Highway 1. Use caution, especially when walking with children, as the shoulder narrows in places.

Trip 25

EWOLDSEN TRAIL

LENGTH AND TYPE: 5.7-mile loop

RATING: Moderate

TRAIL CONDITION: Restored in 2013 after the 2008 Basin Complex Fire, poison oak

HIGHLIGHTS: Wind past some of Big Sur's oldest, largest redwoods and admire coastal views from hillsides covered in wildflowers and oaks.

TO REACH THE TRAILHEAD: The trailhead is at the far end of the upper parking lot on the north side of McWay Creek. Restrooms and water are available at the trailhead.

TRIP SUMMARY: This hike is a semi-loop with gorgeous coastal views. You'll follow boulder-laden McWay Creek in the shade of redwoods before ascending a ridgetop more than 1600 feet above the sea. In winter and spring, gray whales skirt the shore on their migration route between Baja and Alaska. Watch for their blowholes and arching backs from the open bluffs.

Trip Description

The **Ewoldsen Trail** begins at the far end of the upper parking lot (260'), following **McWay Creek** through a lush canyon of redwoods to a creekside **picnic area** (0.1 mile, 280'). A few feet farther the trail skirts past a dilapidated barn and crosses the creek on a rustic wooden bridge, one of many along the creek.

You'll soon pass redwoods bearing fire scars at the base of their trunks. In 1985 the Rat Creek Fire raged through much of the canyon. Thanks to their thick, fire-resistant bark, these redwoods endured the heat and flames with only minor burns. This unique adaptation has enabled the trees to survive for thousands of years in fire-prone areas. Ecologists believe that prior to permanent European settlement, fires hit the Big Sur every 12–20 years, and as a result, the dominant vegetation evolved to adapt to fire.

CONDOR COMEBACK ■ ▓ ■ ▓ ■ ▓ ■ ▓ ■ ▓ ■ ▓ ■ ▓ ■ ▓ ■ ▓ ■ ▓

By the early 1900s, after decades of habitat loss, hunting, and poisoning, California condors were severely threatened. In 1987 researchers rounded up the last of the state's 27 remaining wild condors and laid the groundwork for a captive breeding and reintroduction effort. Under the auspices of the U.S. Fish & Wildlife Service, the California Condor Recovery Program is a multi-entity effort to recover the wild condor population. There are three release sites in California, including one in Big Sur, managed by the Ventana Wilderness Society, a nonprofit research, education, and restoration organization.

In 2012 the total California condor population reached 186 birds, 126 of those in the wild. Visitors and researchers regularly spot condors along the ridgeline atop the Ewoldsen Trail.

For more information about restoration efforts and how you can help, contact the Ventana Wilderness Society in Salinas: (831) 455-9514, info@ventanaws.org.

■ ■ ▓ ■ ▓ ■ ■ ▓ ■ ▓ ■ ▓ ■ ▓ ■ ▓ ■ ▓ ■ ▓ ■ ▓ ■ ▓ ■ ▓ ■ ▓ ■

A quarter mile up the trail, you'll reach the **Canyon Trail junction** (0.25 mile, 390'). This worthwhile spur leads 0.1 mile farther upstream along the south fork of McWay Creek. A few feet past a confluence with the main creek, you'll reach a bench that overlooks a waterfall.

From the Canyon Trail junction, the Ewoldsen Trail branches right and ascends the canyon. Switchbacks thread deep into the redwoods high above McWay Creek, often at eye level with the forest canopy. Watch for birds that rarely visit the canyon floor, such as the golden-crowned kinglet, which hovers to glean insects from the tips of branches. This tiny insectivore has a boldly striped face and bright yellow crown. Woodpeckers' raucous chatter permeates the silence, as they busily carve insects out of trees. Acorn woodpeckers store acorns in their bore holes, providing food for insects, which in turn provide the woodpecker a scrumptious meal of fattened grubs.

You'll exit the south fork canyon along four switchbacks, cross the creek on a stable bridge, and emerge from the shady groves amid dry, exposed chaparral. The vegetation switches back just as quickly once you hike 0.1 mile into the main fork watershed. As you approach the gurgling creek in the shade of redwoods, you'll reach the **loop junction** (1.5 miles, 800').

The loop is 2.1 miles. The left fork climbs a mile along an exposed trail to the viewpoint spur, while the right fork climbs 1.1 miles in the shade of oaks, bays, redwoods, and madrones to the same junction. Ascend the right fork along redwood-lined **McWay Canyon.** You'll soon turn west on a steep grade through dense oak woodland, then curl south to a minor ridge that offers stunning coastal views.

Continue across an oak-clad ridge to the spur in a shallow **saddle** (2.6 miles, 1700'). Follow the VIEWPOINT sign northwest up this 0.3-mile spur, which ends atop a marble-crested ridge with dramatic views north and south along the coast. Keep watch for red-tailed hawks, American kestrels, and, if luck is on your side, endangered California condors in search of tasty rotting flesh. When ready, head back to the spur junction.

The loop continues southwest on a gentle grade along a ridge crest of exposed marble, easily identified by its white to gray coloring and sugary texture. You'll soon emerge on bare golden hillsides that in spring display decadent carpets of wildflowers. The path plunges south and passes a huge, temporarily stabilized landslide scar above Highway 1. A mile farther you'll arrive at a bridge near the loop junction. From here retrace your steps to the trailhead.

Trip 26

MCWAY FALLS

LENGTH AND TYPE: 1-mile out-and-back

RATING: Easy

TRAIL CONDITION: Well maintained, poison oak, good for kids

HIGHLIGHTS: Unforgettable overlook of an 80-foot waterfall that drops from a granite precipice into a serene cove

TO REACH THE TRAILHEAD: The trailhead is on the east end of the main parking lot.

TRIP SUMMARY: This is one of Big Sur's shortest, most spectacular, and most popular trails. You'll follow McWay Creek a half mile to the viewpoint atop an open bluff for stunning views of the cove and open coastline. Summer crowds are elbow to elbow along this heavily used trail.

Trip Description

From the east end of the parking lot, the **Waterfall Overlook Trail** crosses a bridge over **McWay Creek** to a **spur junction** (0.1 mile, 250'). Turn left on this spur and walk 50 feet to see the Pelton Wheel, a vintage hydroelectric plant that once harnessed steep, low-volume McWay Creek to generate electricity. It supplied Saddle Rock Ranch (now part of the state park) with all of its power needs until 1952, when Pacific Gas & Electric brought in power.

McWay Falls plunges 80 feet over a granite precipice to pristine McWay Cove.

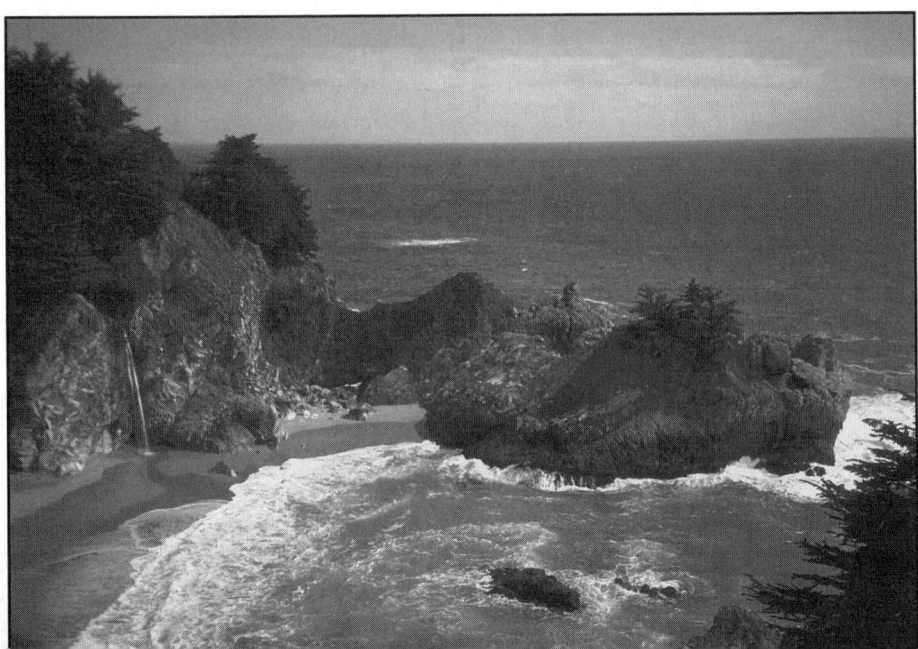

From the spur junction, the main trail heads southwest through a tunnel beneath Highway 1, emerging on the north end of **McWay Cove,** one of Julia Pfeiffer's favorite places to sit, wander, and explore. At one time, a trail descended to the cove, but access is no longer permitted down the rocky, unstable cliffs. Trespassing on the beach can also interrupt the feeding and breeding patterns of sea otters, peregrine falcons, and other protected species.

Bear right for the best vantage point of 80-foot **McWay Falls,** which plunges over a narrow notch in the granite cliff face to the wave-washed crescent of sand below. Fragrant coastal scrub flanks the trail, highlighted in spring by the orange and yellow blossoms of paintbrush, golden yarrow, and sticky monkeyflowers. Palms, bluegum eucalypti, and a number of other exotic species are remnants of a garden planted by the Browns, former owners of Saddle Rock Ranch.

In the 1920s, Lathrop and Helen Hooper Brown purchased the ranch from Christopher McWay, who had settled here in the late 1870s. The Browns built a simple redwood cabin on this overlook, replacing it in 1940 with a larger dwelling called the **Waterfall House.** Helen Brown donated the property for parkland in 1961, and the spectacular house was later demolished. The trail ends at the former homesite, a great spot to watch for the spouts of migrating gray whales.

WHALE-WATCHING

Don't miss some of the best opportunities for whale-watching along the Big Sur coast at the bend at the end of Overlook Trail. In December and January, the gray whales migrate southward to their breeding and calving grounds off the Baja California coast. Watch for their high, bushy, heart-shaped blow up to 15 feet and the occasional fluke lifted out of the water prior to a deep dive. These gray whales undertake one of the longest annual migrations of any mammal, traveling some 9,300–12,500 miles (15,000–20,000 km) round-trip. Many whales pass close to shore at this point, and occasionally one will come into the mouth of the cove. In March and April, they can be seen returning north to their summer feeding grounds in the North Pacific.

CHAPTER twelve

Limekiln State Park

■ ■   ■   ■   ■   ■   ■   ■   ■   ■   ■   ■   ■

CRUISING HIGHWAY 1, most visitors overlook Limekiln State Park. Yet the sheer, jagged cliffs that make coastal access so difficult along most of the Big Sur coast are not an issue at Limekiln, where you can step a few yards from a shady redwood canyon for a barefoot stroll on the beach.

Once exploited and then forgotten, the park boasts a rich history of homesteaders and entrepreneurs who tramped down the lonely, isolated coast in the late 1800s in search of opportunity. Today, hikers stroll in peaceful solitude amid forests that once supported timber harvesting and limestone extraction and a beach that once flanked a busy shipping port.

Added to the state park system in 1995, Limekiln comprises 716 acres and offers three short hiking trails that follow Limekiln Creek through redwood-lined canyons to a spectacular waterfall and historic limekilns that lend the park its name. The park is open for day use and overnight camping.

DIRECTIONS: The park entrance is on the east side of Highway 1, 56 miles south of Carmel, 2 miles south of Lucia, and 94 miles north of San Luis Obispo.

VISITOR CENTER: Big Sur Station: (831) 667-2315. The station is on Highway 1, 30 miles north of park entrance and just south of Pfeiffer Big Sur State Park. Open daily 8 a.m.–6 p.m. Memorial Day through Labor Day, 8 a.m.–4:30 p.m. the rest of the year.

NEAREST CAMPGROUND: The park campground (33 sites, $35/night; reservations recommended in summer and on holidays) offers developed sites with picnic tables and fire rings. Some sites accommodate RVs and trailers. There are showers, picnic areas, and flush toilets. For more information call Reserve America at (800) 444-7275 or visit ReserveAmerica.com.

INFORMATION: Open daily 9 a.m.–7 p.m. Memorial Day through Labor Day, 10 a.m.–5 p.m. the rest of the year. There is a $10 day-use fee. No dogs or bikes allowed on park trails.

WEBSITE: parks.ca.gov

PHONE: (831) 667-2403

Limekiln State Park

LIMEKILN TRAIL

LENGTH AND TYPE: 0.8-mile out-and-back

RATING: Easy

TRAIL CONDITION: Well maintained, good for kids

HIGHLIGHTS: Historic limekilns nestled in a peaceful redwood grove

TO REACH THE TRAILHEAD: Day-use parking is immediately past the kiosk, adjacent to the restrooms. Park your vehicle and stroll past the north end of the campground (sites 23–34), where all three of the park's trails begin.

TRIP SUMMARY: This hike meanders along Limekiln Creek's West Fork amid dense redwood groves, once home to a vigorous lumber and lime manufacturing industry. Early settlers used harvested trees to fuel kilns that purified, or "slaked," limestone extracted from rich deposits in the canyon. The lime was then loaded in barrels and hauled to Rockland Landing, near Limekiln Beach. Schooners transported the lime to Monterey and San Francisco, where it was used to make cement. Schooners also brought in heavy goods and supplies to sustain the growing population. Today, all that remains are four stone-and-steel furnaces from which the creek and park takes its name. The trail roughly follows an old wagon trail to the kilns.

FIFTY CENTS A DAY ■ ■ ■ ■ ■ ■ ■ ■ ■ ■ ■ ■ ■ ■ ■ ■ ■ ■ ■

Only the hardiest, most self-reliant settlers successfully homesteaded the seemingly impenetrable Santa Lucia Range. These early explorers, adventurers, and entrepreneurs forged a loose network of trails to cultivate flood-prone land and raise livestock, relying on one another for bartered goods and services. When there was a need for money, companies such as Rockland Lime & Lumber offered hard work. Whether they were harvesting redwoods to fuel the limekilns or building wagon trails along Limekiln Creek, men in 1920 made $.50 a day during a typical 10-hour workday.

■ ■

Trip Description

From the trailhead (70'), you'll cross a large wooden footbridge over **Hare Creek**. A few paces beyond the bridge, the trail passes a junction with the eastbound **Hare Creek Trail**. Bear left and climb above the confluence of Hare Creek and **Limekiln Creek,** which flow clear as glass past lush carpets of ferns and mosses. You'll soon pass the remains of an old-growth forest, logged to sustain the appetite of Rockland Lime & Lumber Company. Continue 150 feet past the confluence of the **West Fork** and Limekiln Creek to a junction with the **Limekiln Falls Trail** (0.25 mile, 110') on your right.

Skirting the west bank of the West Fork, the main trail continues straight, turns north, then crosses the creek on a **wooden bridge** (0.3 mile, 170'). A minute farther a split rail fence marks the site of the large stone-and-steel **kilns** (0.4 mile, 240'), built at the base of a natural limestone deposit. Take a moment to explore

A diverse array of fungi live within the damp, dark, dense redwood forests that shade Limekiln Creek.

the ruins before returning the way you came. Please don't hike off-trail, as canyon walls are steep, poison oak is abundant, and the kilns may be unstable.

Trip 28

LIMEKILN FALLS TRAIL

LENGTH AND TYPE: 1-mile out-and-back

RATING: Easy

TRAIL CONDITION: Well maintained, good for kids

HIGHLIGHTS: A 100-foot waterfall cascading down vertical limestone cliffs

TO REACH THE TRAILHEAD: Day-use parking is immediately past the kiosk, adjacent to the restrooms. Park your vehicle and stroll past the north end of the campground (sites 23–34),

where all three of the park's trails begin.

TRIP SUMMARY: This hike traverses the steepest coastal canyon in the Lower 48, where Limekiln Creek's headwaters pour down from Cone Peak, nearly a mile above sea level and just 3.2 miles from the Pacific. The short, easy trail leads to the base of the falls.

Trip Description

From the trailhead (70'), cross the large wooden footbridge over **Hare Creek**. Bear left past the **Hare Creek Trail junction** and climb past the remains of an old-growth forest. You'll soon reach the **Limekiln Falls Trail junction** (0.25 mile, 110'), 150 feet past the confluence of the **West Fork** and **Limekiln Creek**. Bear right and head northeast.

The trail descends a few steps, then crosses the creek on a narrow wooden

Limekiln Falls plunges 100 feet past limestone cliffs as it descends the steepest coastal canyon in the continental US.

footbridge. Follow the east bank, then turn northwest across another small **footbridge** (0.3 mile, 140'). The trail crosses the creek once more and climbs a small set of stairs past a wooden retaining **wall** (0.4 mile, 170'). Follow the sound of falling water 0.1 mile uphill to the base of these spectacular 100-foot falls. Visitors gaze in silence as water cascades down the moss- and fern-covered limestone cliffs. Rest and feel the mist on your face before heading back.

Trip 29

HARE CREEK TRAIL

LENGTH AND TYPE: 0.6-mile out-and-back

RATING: Easy

TRAIL CONDITION: Well maintained, poison oak, good for kids

HIGHLIGHTS: A fertile coastal river canyon lined with majestic old-growth redwoods

TO REACH THE TRAILHEAD: Day-use parking is immediately past the kiosk, adjacent to the restrooms. Park your vehicle and stroll past the north end of the campground (sites 23–34), where all three of the park's trails begin.

TRIP SUMMARY: This hike begins amid a narrow band of redwoods along Hare Creek. Though you'll find a few mature old-growth trees, most of the redwoods are relative toddlers. These stands are rebounding from heavy logging in the late 1800s, when Rockland Lime & Lumber harvested dozens of ancient trees to fuel nearby kilns used to purify commercial limestone. Today, the trail leads past quiet, undisturbed groves.

Trip Description

From the trailhead, you'll cross the large wooden footbridge over **Hare Creek**. Thirty feet beyond the bridge, the trail reaches the **Hare Creek Trail junction**. Turn right and head east along the north bank. The trail skirts the clear creek, sheltered by sheer canyon walls and a dense redwood canopy. Shrouded in darkness, your surroundings suggest a vast forest, but this narrow band of trees is restricted to the canyon floor.

The trail soon emerges on open slopes that support oaks, shrubs, and grasses, then ascends **rock steps** (0.2 mile, 160') past lush ferns, redwood sorrel, blackberries and thimbleberries. Steep cliff faces across the canyon are draped with a vibrant green tapestry of mosses and ferns. Head back when you reach the END OF TRAIL sign beside a large downed **redwood** (0.3 mile, 200'). Avoid hiking off-trail, as poison oak is abundant and the canyon walls are steep and unstable.

STEELHEAD MIGRATION ▦ ▦ ▦ ▦ ▦ ▦ ▦ ▦ ▦ ▦ ▦ ▦ ▦ ▦ ▦ ▦

Serving as a vital habitat for southern steelhead trout, the entire Limekiln and Hare watershed is free flowing (i.e., no dams). Slowly approach small trailside pools and you may spot an immature steelhead darting amid shadows along the creek bottom.

Part of the family *Salmonidae*, which includes all salmon and trout, steelhead are the anadromous form of rainbow trout, which means the fish are born in freshwater and migrate to the ocean as adults. They spend their first one to three years here before heading out to sea from Limekiln Beach. After one to four years in the Pacific, they return to their native creeks to spawn.

In California most steelhead spawn from December through April. Limekiln State Park supports a significant run of southern steelhead trout. Contact the California Department of Fish & Game for local fishing regulations: (831) 649-2870, dfg.ca.gov.

▦ ▦

Pacific Valley to San Simeon State Park

■　■　■　■　■　■　■　■　■　■　■　■　■　■

THIS CHAPTER DESCRIBES state and federal day-use lands from Pacific Valley south to Sand Dollar Beach, Jade Cove, Ragged Point, Piedras Blancas, Hearst Memorial State Beach, and San Simeon. This stretch of coast is a premier hiking destination. Trails meander through wind-sculpted pine forests, across slopes of fragrant coastal scrub and spring wildflowers, and down to driftwood-strewn beaches. You'll also find plenty of the trademark ocean views that draw people up and down Highway 1.

Pacific Valley to Jade Cove

Pacific Valley's rocky bluffs and rolling prairie overlook a prominent marine terrace punctuated by archways and pounding surf. Several intriguing trails cut through golden grasslands and dense coastal shrub to secluded coves and dramatic views. Farther south off Highway 1, Sand Dollar Beach and Jade Cove offer access to beachcombers, anglers, surfers, scuba divers, and rock hounds in search of the coveted green gemstone.

DIRECTIONS: This coastline is accessible via pullouts along Highway 1, some 60 miles south of Rio Road in Carmel and 30 miles north of Hearst San Simeon State Historical Monument (Hearst Castle).

VISITOR CENTER: Pacific Valley Station: (805) 927-4211. Open daily 8 a.m.– 5 p.m. The station is on the east side of Highway 1, 3 miles north of the Sand Dollar Beach Day-Use Area, 60 miles south of Carmel, and 30 miles north of Hearst Castle.

NEAREST CAMPGROUND: Plaskett Creek Campground (41 sites, $22/night; 3 group sites, $80/night; reservations recommended in summer and holidays) is on the east side of Highway 1, 0.1 mile south of the entrance to the Sand Dollar Beach Day-Use Area. There's a maximum of eight people per site. Each site includes a picnic

Pacific Valley Trail, Sand Dollar Beach and Jade Cove

table, fire ring, and pedestal grill. Drinking water is available. For more information call Reserve America at (800) 444-7275 or visit ReserveAmerica.com.

INFORMATION: Open 8 a.m.–sunset. There's a $10 parking fee at Sand Dollar Beach. If you're willing to hike 0.3 mile, you'll find free parking at turnouts on Highway 1 north and south of Sand Dollar Beach. Dogs must be leashed. No camping or fires permitted in Pacific Valley, Sand Dollar Beach, or Jade Cove.

WEBSITE: parksman.com

PHONE: USFS Pacific Valley Station: (805) 927-4211; USFS Monterey District Headquarters: (831) 385-5434

Trip 30

PACIFIC VALLEY TRAIL

LENGTH AND TYPE: 0.7-mile out-and-back

RATING: Easy

TRAIL CONDITION: Clear, poison oak

HIGHLIGHTS: Dramatic views of eroding coastal cliffs, jagged outcrops, and sculpted arches

TO REACH THE TRAILHEAD: The trail starts from a free turnout on the west side of Highway 1, directly across from the Pacific Valley Station (see Visitor Center, page 128).

TRIP SUMMARY: Despite its name, this is not a valley, but 3 miles of gently sloping marine terrace. The flat coastal expanse represents a dramatic change from the Big Sur's trademark steep topography and offers some of the easiest hiking and beach access in the area. Bluff trails lead to daunting cliffs and promontories with spectacular views of the boulder-strewn coastline. Keep watch for passing whales, as well as seals and otters amid the nearshore kelp forests.

Trip Description

From the Highway 1 turnout, you'll step up and over a cattle gate onto a broad flat terrace. The US Forest Service manages this land, which has been extensively grazed for decades. At any time, you may share the trail with roaming livestock.

The trail traverses the terrace past waste-high coyote brush amid an open meadow. In spring these grasslands are speckled with buttercups, lupines, and poppies that have survived the intense grazing pressure.

Continuing toward the ocean, the trail leads to another cattle gate up and over the fence. Beyond it, the vegetation shifts from open grasslands to native lupine, poison oak, sagebrush, coyote brush, and sticky monkeyflower, easily identified by its narrow leaves and bright orange flowers. You'll soon wander past small, wind-sculpted dunes stabilized by low-lying sand verbena, lupine, lizard tail, and more poison oak.

Past the dunes, the trail veers north and gently climbs the scalloped cliffs to a dramatic **rocky promontory** (0.5 mile, 40'). Behind you to the northeast, the rocky ridges above **Lime-kiln** and **Hare Creeks** climb toward **Cone Peak,** comprising the steepest coastal slope in the Lower 48. To the west, **Plaskett Rock** thrusts above the surf amid natural arches carved by the Pacific. Watch for sea otters, which float on their backs to crack open shellfish. Resting otters are often mistaken for floating logs, as they wrap themselves in kelp in order to hold position on the surface.

You'll eventually circle back to the main trail, recrossing the coastal bluffs toward the turnout.

Trip 31

SAND DOLLAR BEACH & JADE COVE

LENGTH AND TYPE: 1-mile out-and-back

RATING: Easy

TRAIL CONDITION: Clear, poison oak

HIGHLIGHTS: Rugged cliffs overlook wave-washed coves speckled with veins of jade

TO REACH THE TRAILHEAD: The Sand Dollar Beach Day-Use Area is on Highway 1, 32.5 miles south of Big Sur Station, 63 miles south of Carmel, 0.1 mile north of Plaskett Creek Campground, and 15.1 miles north of Ragged Point ($10 day-use fee). There are restrooms and water at the trailhead.

TRIP SUMMARY: This hike begins along open bluffs blanketed in fragrant coastal scrub and heads south to cliffs overlooking Jade Cove. A steep 100-foot spur descends to a beach brimming with jade that has been sculpted smooth by the pounding surf. The trail then doubles back north toward the horseshoe cove at Sand Dollar Beach.

Trip Description

From the west side of the parking lot (90'), clamber up and over a cattle gate in the fence, then head south beside the planted Monterey cypress trees that shade the lot. The trail soon

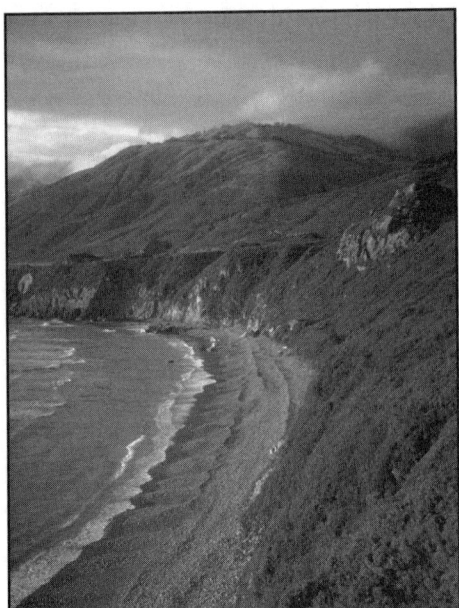

turns west toward the south end of **Sand Dollar Beach.** You'll stroll past open grasslands and low-lying coastal scrub to the dramatic cliffs above **Jade Cove** (0.2 mile, 60'). A short but steep and unstable spur leads down to the cove. Be aware of poison oak as you scurry down this spur.

Large green jade boulders and coarse gravel extend beyond the pounding surf into deep water. Just offshore is 100-foot **Cave Rock,** whose jade inner walls are continuously smoothed and polished by breaking waves.

A sweeping crescent of coarse white sand is home to one of Big Sur's most consistent surf breaks.

STONE OF HEAVEN ■ ■ ■ ■ ■ ■ ■ ■ ■ ■ ■ ■ ■ ■ ■ ■ ■ ■

Ranging in size from pebbles to large stones, jade lies scattered throughout Jade Cove, atop the sand, beneath overhangs, and just off the beach, accessible to both beach-combers and divers. The USFS prohibits jade collection above the mean high tide line.

Chinese consider jade the stone of heaven, and artisans have carved the gem into tools and art objects for thousands of years. The type of jade found here is the mineral nephrite. Pure nephrite is white, but impurities lend the local jade a range of brilliant shades, from light turquoise to deep emerald green. Jade is strong and durable, harder than some types of steel, and the most difficult gem to polish.

Jade Cove comprises a jumble of rocks known as the Franciscan complex, formed millions of years ago when a massive tectonic plate was driven beneath the continent. Colliding plates crushed the rocks, which were then sheared off by the massive Sur-Nacimiento Fault and squeezed upward to form the rocky cove. Covered by ocean sediments for millennia, jade formed as minerals in the sedimentary rock (probably sandstone). Buried deep in the earth, these minerals were exposed to high pressure at low temperatures, metamorphosing them into jade.

■ ■

Head back past the parking lot a few feet north to a trail **junction** (0.5 mile, 40') on the left that leads toward the beach. You'll soon reach a fork. The right branch leads to an overlook, an excellent spot to watch for migrating gray whales. In spring, mothers escort their calves close to shore for protection from such predators as great white sharks and orcas. This is also an excellent spot to bird-watch. Boasting black bodies and bright orange beaks, oystercatchers perch along the rocks, while plovers scurry through the surf, and pelicans skim nearshore waves.

The left branch leads down to Sand Dollar Beach, the longest contiguous stretch of sand along the Big Sur coast. At low tide, it's an ideal spot for a barefoot stroll, surf casting, or surfing. Winter surge strips sand from the beach and replaces it with small granite rubble.

Ragged Point

RAGGED POINT lies midway between LA and San Francisco, where the vast Pacific meets the towering Santa Lucia Range. Here, a private parcel welcomes tourists with a short, sheer trail that skirts Big Sur's tallest waterfall, plunging 300 feet to a black sand beach. Those willing to brave the trail are rewarded with exquisite views. In wet weather, the trail is often closed, while the owner may restrict access anytime.

DIRECTIONS: Ragged Point lies off the west side of Highway 1, 15 miles north of Hearst Castle and 44 miles south of Big Sur.

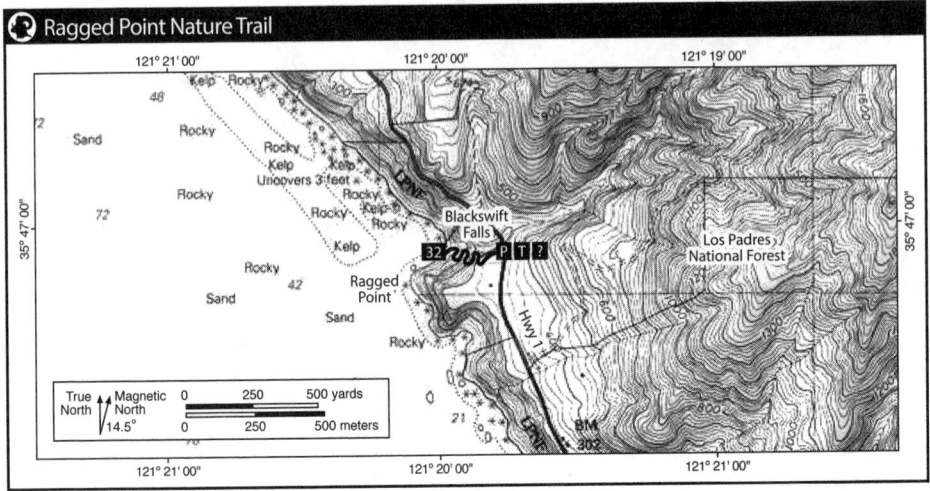

VISITOR CENTERS: Pacific Valley Station: (805) 927-4211. Open daily 8 a.m.–5 p.m. The station is on the east side of Highway 1, 16 miles north of Ragged Point. Hearst San Simeon State Historical Monument (Hearst Castle): (805) 927-2010. Open daily 8 a.m.–6 p.m. The visitor center is off Highway 1, 14 miles south of Ragged Point.

NEAREST CAMPGROUND: The nearest campground to the north is Plaskett Creek, while the nearest campgrounds to the south are in San Simeon State Park.

INFORMATION: This trail is on private land, and the owner may deny access at any time.

WEBSITE: raggedpointinn.com | **PHONE:** (805) 927-4502

Trip 32

RAGGED POINT NATURE TRAIL

LENGTH AND TYPE: 1-mile out-and-back

RATING: Moderate to strenuous

TRAIL CONDITION: Passable to difficult, poison oak

HIGHLIGHTS: In winter this tallest tiered waterfall in Big Sur cascades 300 feet into the surf off Ragged Point.

TO REACH THE TRAILHEAD: Ragged Point is off Highway 1, 23 miles north of Cambria and 44 miles south of Big Sur. Turn west into the Ragged Point Inn & Restaurant parking lot. The trail begins at the gazebo, just past the coffee shop and gift shop.

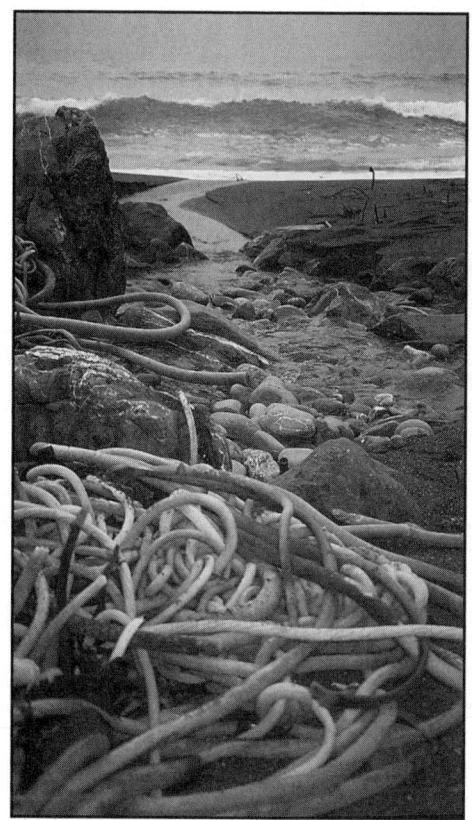

Blackswift Creek plunges 300 feet before disappearing into the surging tide.

TRIP SUMMARY: This hike descends the steep canyon beside Blackswift Falls, which plunges hundreds of feet onto the soft black sand of a secluded cove at the edge of the Pacific. This short, steep hike is subject to washouts each winter and is moderately overgrown with coastal brush in the spring. Watch for poison oak and ticks, which cling to trailside plants.

Trip Description

From the trailhead (380'), you'll switchback along the steep, eroding canyon walls beside **Blackswift Creek**. Views from the top bear witness to a dramatic topographical change, from gentle slopes and broad marine terraces south of the point to Big Sur's trademark rocky bluffs north of the point.

The trail drops 0.2 mile to a small wooden bridge at the base of **Blackswift Falls**. Stop on the bridge to admire the 300-foot tiered waterfall as it tumbles to the beach and mingles with the churning surf. Wander amid the granite boulders atop black sand before returning up the trail.

Piedras Blancas

TRUE TO ITS NAME, *Piedras Blancas* (Spanish for white stones) is named for a trio of treacherous white rocks just off the point. In 1875, a lighthouse was built to guide mariners along this lonely, fogbound coast. Today, the lighthouse is automated, and the only residents are thousands of noisy, boisterous seals, including massive elephant seals, which beach just south of the light.

The Bureau of Land Management (BLM) manages Piedras Blancas and is restoring the site. Guided tours offer insight into a bygone era of maritime travel. For tour information, see page 138.

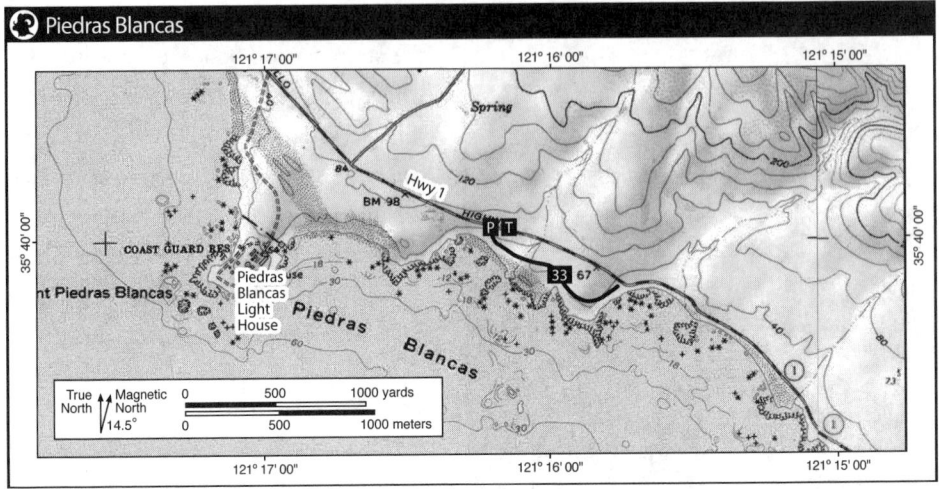

DIRECTIONS: Piedras Blancas is off Highway 1, 7.7 miles north of San Simeon.

VISITOR CENTER: Hearst San Simeon State Historical Monument (Hearst Castle): (805) 927-2010. The visitor center is a mile west of Highway 1, 5 miles north of San Simeon State Park, directly across the street from W.R. Hearst Memorial State Beach. Open daily 8 a.m.–sunset.

NEAREST CAMPGROUND: See San Simeon State Park (page 142).

INFORMATION: The BLM prohibits entry to the access roads, grounds, or lighthouse outside of designated times unless you're part of a scheduled tour. For information about docent-led guided tours visit piedrasblancas.org or call (805) 927-7361.

WEBSITE: blm.gov, piedrasblancas.org, or hearstcastle.org

PHONE: BLM, Piedras Blancas Light Station: (805) 927-7361.

Trip 33

PIEDRAS BLANCAS

LENGTH AND TYPE: 0.8-mile out-and-back

RATING: Easy

TRAIL CONDITION: Well maintained, good for kids

HIGHLIGHTS: Thousands of elephant seals spar for dominance, mate and give birth, or merely bask in the sun, flip sand on their backs, and snort at gaping tourists.

TO REACH THE TRAILHEAD: The Piedras Blancas elephant seal rookery is on the west side of Highway 1, 7.7 miles north of San Simeon. The parking lot is at Vista Point. There are no facilities or water at the trailhead.

TRIP SUMMARY: This short, easy trail skirts a broad marine terrace to a small sandy cove inhabited by thousands of noisy northern elephant seals.

BASKING & BARKING & BELCHING, OH MY!

The best time to view Piedras Blancas's elephant seals is December through March. Arriving in early December, enormous bulls wage violent, often-bloody battles to establish dominance. The successful bull becomes the alpha male and has the best chance of mating. When females arrive in late December, this bull establishes and guards his harem.

Days after the females arrive, they give birth and produce thick, rich milk that is 55% fat. Newborn pups suckle for a month, growing from about 70 pounds at birth up to 300 pounds. Weaned pups are lovingly nicknamed "weaners." By late March most of the adult females have mated with either the alpha male or competing beta bulls.

Females soon return to the ocean alone, leaving weaners to fend for themselves and learn how to swim and feed. They remain on the beach until the end of April, wading in tide pools, snorting at tourists, molting their black baby fur, and growing shiny new silver coats.

All elephant seals return to shore to molt in spring and summer. Females and juveniles land in April and May, subadult males in May and June, and enormous males in July and August. You'll recognize adult males by their enormous size (more than twice the weight of adult females) and large proboscis (reminiscent of an elephant's trunk).

These weaned elephant seals will snort at tourists, molt their black fur, and wade in the tidepools before venturing for months alone in the open ocean.

Trip Description

From the parking lot, follow the raucous barking sounds south. You'll skirt the open bluffs 0.1 mile, enjoying sweeping views of the sea and rocky shore. The trail quickly reaches a small cove packed flipper to flipper with elephant seals.

Turn your attention from the rookery to the **Piedras Blancas lighthouse**, built in 1875 to guide ships between the lights at Point Conception to the south and Point Piños to the north. The original tower was 115 feet tall and housed a first-order Fresnel lens. Today, technology has eased navigation and the light is now automated. The original Fresnel lens is on display at the Veterans Building on Main Street in Cambria, 13 miles south.

Guided tours of the lighthouse are offered Tuesday, Thursday, and Saturday September 1–June 14 and Monday–Saturday June 15–August 31 ($10/adults, $5 children ages 6–17, free/children age 5 and under). Contact the Piedras Blancas Light Station for further information: (805) 927-7361, piedrasblancas.org.

Hearst Memorial State Beach

THIS SANDY COVE was once part of the 24,000-acre Hearst property at San Simeon, a playground for the family, friends, and guests of media tycoon William Randolph Hearst. In 1953 the Hearst Corporation, which owns Hearst Castle and the surrounding acreage, donated the park grounds in memory of its founder.

San Simeon remains a popular year-round destination for visitors interested in hiking, swimming, fishing, kayaking, picnicking, and whale- and bird-watching. In May the park hosts "A Day in Old San Simeon," a celebration of the area's 19th-century heyday.

The Neptune Pool at Hearst Castle is 104 feet by 58 feet and holds 345,000 gallons of water.

ONE MAN'S CASTLE ■ ■ ■ ■ ■ ■ ■ ■ ■ ■ ■ ■ ■ ■ ■ ■ ■ ■

Perched high atop the San Simeon hills, Hearst Castle was the collaborative vision of eccentric news baron William Randolph Hearst and architect Julia Morgan. Transformation of the ranch and campsite into the lavish 165-room castle began in 1919 and dragged on nearly 30 years. It remains unfinished. A showcase for Hearst's international collection of antiques and art pieces, the 250,000-acre estate also included guesthouses, elaborate gardens and pools, tennis courts, and a zoo. Famous guests through the years included President Calvin Coolidge, Winston Churchill, Charlie Chaplin, and myriad other bigwigs and Hollywood celebs.

On most Friday and Saturday evenings from September through December, Hearst Castle offers two-hour living history tours ($30/adults, $15/children ages 6–17) that capture the bygone lifestyle of this great estate. Docents dress in elegant vintage clothing, discuss the social life of Hearst's guests, and lead visitors on enchanting strolls around La Cuesta Encantanda (The Enchanted Hill). For more information, visit hearstcastle.org.

■ ■

DIRECTIONS: Hearst Memorial State Beach is directly across Highway 1 from the Hearst Castle entrance, 8 miles north of Cambria and 60 miles south of Big Sur. Turn west on San Simeon Road and continue 0.2 mile to the large parking area.

VISITOR CENTER: Hearst San Simeon State Historical Monument (Hearst Castle): (805) 927-2010. The visitor center is a mile west of Highway 1, 5 miles north of San Simeon State Park, directly across the street from W.R. Hearst Memorial State Beach. Open daily 8 a.m.–sunset.

NEAREST CAMPGROUND: San Simeon Creek Campground, within San Simeon State Park, is 5 miles south of San Simeon (134 sites, $35/night; reservations recommended in summer and first come, first served October 1–March 14). On a plateau overlooking the Pacific, this campground includes showers and RV sites (no hookups). For more information call (800) 444-7275 or visit parks.ca.gov. Washburn Campground, within San Simeon State Park, 5 miles south of San Simeon (68 sites, $22/night; reservations recommended in summer; no showers), is a mile inland on a plateau overlooking the Santa Lucia Range. For more information call (800) 444-7275 or visit parks.ca.gov.

INFORMATION: The beach is open until sunset. There is no entrance fee. The day-use area offers 150 parking spaces, restrooms, water faucets, 24 picnic tables, barbecue grill stands, and a concession stand. Dogs must be on a leash. No overnight camping. Easy beach access makes this a great spot for fishing, beachcombing, swimming, and boat launching. In summer the concession stand sells bait and rents fishing poles, kayaks, and boogie boards. Licenses are not required when fishing from the pier, but limits are enforced.

WEBSITE: parks.ca.gov | **PHONE:** (805) 927-2020

Trip 34

HEARST MEMORIAL STATE BEACH

LENGTH AND TYPE: 2.5-mile out-and-back

RATING: Easy

TRAIL CONDITION: Clear, poison oak

HIGHLIGHTS: Soothing views of the Pacific from atop open bluffs

TO REACH THE TRAILHEAD: The trail begins from the north side of the main parking lot.

TRIP SUMMARY: This hike explores the half-mile coastal crescent that curls toward San Simeon Point. You'll stroll the soft white sand above open bluffs of coastal scrub, through forests of eucalyptus, pine, and cypress to tide pools teeming with life. Foxes, coyotes, and bobcats slink along the bluffs, while red- and white-tailed hawks and northern harriers scour the brush for the rabbits, mice, and voles. Watch nearshore kelp beds to spot sea otters, harbor seals, and sea lions as they frolic, feed, or happily float by.

Trip Description

From the parking lot, walk toward the beach through a stately eucalyptus grove to a small picnic area. Heading west, the route crosses **Arroyo del Puerto Creek** (0.1 mile, 10'), an ankle-deep wade in all but the wettest months.

CONTENDER FROM DOWN UNDER ■ ■ ■ ■ ■ ■ ■ ■ ■ ■ ■ ■ ■

> Early California settlers planted introduced Australian bluegum eucalyptus trees as windbreaks, ornamentals, and for firewood. The species adapted so well to wood-land areas along the central coast, that it quickly outcompeted native plants. Turns out, the trees secrete certain pathogens that inhibit the growth of native plants and discourage wildlife. As a result, the eucalyptus stands have little to no understory and are considered extremely invasive.

The path curves south to a **junction** (0.5 mile, 20'), where you'll bear right on a distinct trail toward the eroding bluffs. Atop the bluffs, you'll stroll past eucalypti and brief glimpses of glistening **San Simeon Bay**. The trail soon merges with a dirt road to **San Simeon Point** that passes numerous coastal overlooks. Pause at the point (1.2 miles, 20') to appreciate this pristine coastline before returning the way you came.

If you wish to hike farther, the trail leads west through a dense cypress forest to emerge on windswept dunes west of the point.

William Randolph Hearst bought out his coast-side neighbors to secure his private beach to host family, friends, and guests.

San Simeon State Park

OFFERING EXCEPTIONAL BEAUTY and respite from the everyday bustle, San Simeon was the perfect location for William Randolph Hearst to build his 165-room castle. It began as a rancheria during the mission era, serving as a coastal access point for supplies shipped to and from Monterey's Mission San Antonio. The park's Washburn Day-Use Area served as a gravel quarry through the late 1920s.

Set aside in 1932, San Simeon State Park is one of California's oldest reserves. Its 541 acres comprise miles of sandy beaches and rocky shorelines, as well as Monterey pine forests, rolling grasslands, and seasonal wetlands, creeks, and bogs.

DIRECTIONS: The park is off Highway 1, 35 miles north of San Luis Obispo and 65 miles south of Big Sur. Turn east on San Simeon Creek Road, drive a quarter mile, then turn right at the park entrance.

VISITOR CENTER: Hearst San Simeon State Historical Monument (Hearst Castle): (805) 927-2010. The visitor center is a mile west of Highway 1, 5 miles north of San Simeon State Park, directly across the street from W.R. Hearst Memorial State Beach. Open daily 8 a.m.–sunset.

NEAREST CAMPGROUNDS: Both the Washburn and San Simeon Creek Campgrounds lie within the park. San Simeon Creek Campground (134 sites, $35/night) provides a picnic table and fire ring at each site, restrooms with flush toilets and showers, pay phones, and a dump station and water fill-up for RVs. The adjoining Washburn Campground (68 sites, $22/night) provides a picnic table and fire ring at each site and vault toilets. Reservations are required between March 14 and September 30. For more

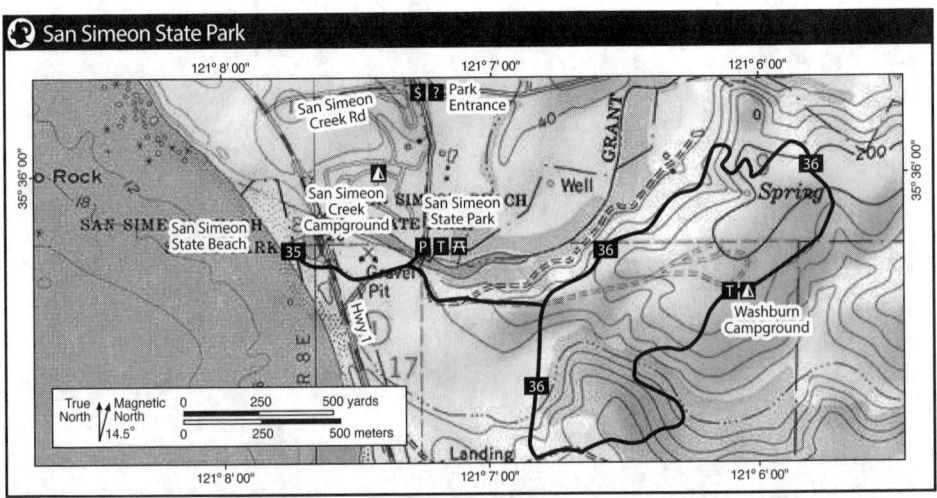

information call Reserve America at (800) 444-7275 or visit ReserveAmerica.com. The rest of the year, sites are available on a first-come, first-serve basis.

INFORMATION: San Simeon State Beach is open from sunrise to sunset. No dogs or bikes allowed on park trails. The San Simeon Nature Trail is wheelchair-accessible from the footbridge crossing San Simeon Creek to the beach and along the seasonal wetlands.

WEBSITE: parks.ca.gov | **PHONE:** (805) 927-2020

Trip 35

SAN SIMEON STATE BEACH

LENGTH AND TYPE: 1-mile out-and-back

RATING: Easy

TRAIL CONDITION: Well maintained, poison oak, good for kids

HIGHLIGHTS: Follow San Simeon Creek through seasonal wetlands to the beach and watch for elephant seals, sea otters, and gray whales.

TO REACH THE TRAILHEAD: The trailhead is adjacent to the Washburn Day-Use Area off Highway 1, immediately past the small bridge over San Simeon Creek. Head east on San Simeon Creek Road, drive a quarter mile, then turn right into the park. Water and restrooms are available.

Follow San Simeon Creek through seasonal wetlands as it deposits fine sand and gnarled driftwood along San Simeon State Beach.

TRIP SUMMARY: This easy hike begins on an elevated boardwalk through San Simeon Creek's unique seasonal wetland and riparian habitat. From the end of the boardwalk, stroll the beach barefoot in either direction. Bring binoculars for a chance at spotting migrating gray whales.

Trip Description

From the parking area, head north along the raised wooden boardwalk toward the mouth of **San Simeon Creek** (20'), which shelters a healthy population of turtles, frogs, snakes, and fish. This boardwalk shields the surrounding seasonal wetlands, which offer habitat to several endangered species. Winter rains fill the wetlands with 1 to 2 feet of nutrient-rich water, nourishing a multitude of small organisms waiting in the mud. As you stroll, listen to the chorus of chirping frogs and watch ducks, egrets, and herons descend on the marsh to feed.

Wheelchair access ends where the boardwalk stops, while the trail continues west under Highway 1 (0.1 mile, 10') to **San Simeon Beach**. Endangered snowy plovers nest along the south end of the beach directly west of the bridge, leading to seasonal closures between February and September. If the beach is closed, head north toward the creek to watch the tides roll in and out. Return the way you came.

POND TURTLE PRIMER ■ ■ ■ ■ ■ ■ ■ ■ ■ ■ ■ ■ ■ ■ ■ ■

By late spring, female Southwestern pond turtles leave San Simeon Creek in search of nesting sites on nearby hills. After digging a hole, they deposit several eggs and return to the creek. When the rainy season arrives, turtle hatchlings instinctively make their way to the creek, where they feed, grow, and spawn, renewing the life cycle. The creek is home to some 50 Southwestern pond turtles. Try to spot them basking on logs or swimming and diving in the shallows.

■ ■

Trip 36

SAN SIMEON NATURE TRAIL

LENGTH AND TYPE: 3.2-mile loop

RATING: Easy

TRAIL CONDITION: Well maintained, poison oak, good for kids

HIGHLIGHTS: A rural landscape wedged between the sheer Santa Lucia Range and the mighty Pacific

TO REACH THE TRAILHEAD: Choose between two trailheads. The northern trailhead is in Washburn Campground, across from Site 213 at the end of Washburn Campground Road. The southern trailhead is 0.1 mile east of the Washburn Day-Use Area, beside a footbridge over San Simeon Creek. Water and restrooms are available at both trailheads.

TRIP SUMMARY: San Simeon Creek ripples through a rolling landscape that's lush green after winter rains, blanketed with wildflowers in spring, and studded with gnarled coast live oaks and wind-sculpted Monterey pines year-round. Diverse habitats shelter a range of wildlife, including woodpeckers, elusive bobcats, coyotes, wintering golden eagles, and wild turkeys. Interpretive signs describe the seasonal wetlands, vernal pools, an 1800s ranch site, and prehistoric cultural sites of the Chumash and Salinian peoples.

Trip Description

From the southern trailhead at the **Washburn Day-Use Area** (30'), a raised wooden boardwalk leads east amid seasonal wetlands, home to endangered Southwestern pond turtles and red-legged frogs. You'll soon cross **Washburn Campground Road** (0.1 mile, 40') and skirt the road for 0.4 mile before reaching an unmarked junction (0.5 mile, 80'). Turn left and hike past eucalyptus trees to the **Whitaker Homesite** (0.8 mile, 40'), an 1800s ranch. A spur to your right leads 0.2 mile to **Washburn Campground**.

Instead, bear left along the trail, which gradually descends to **Whitaker Flats** through introduced Australian bluegum eucalypti amid a thick understory of German ivy from South Africa. These exotic plants invade woodlands throughout California and choke out native plants, threatening the natural ecosystem.

A mature forest of gnarled live oaks and wind-sculpted Monterey pines shades the trail along San Simeon Creek.

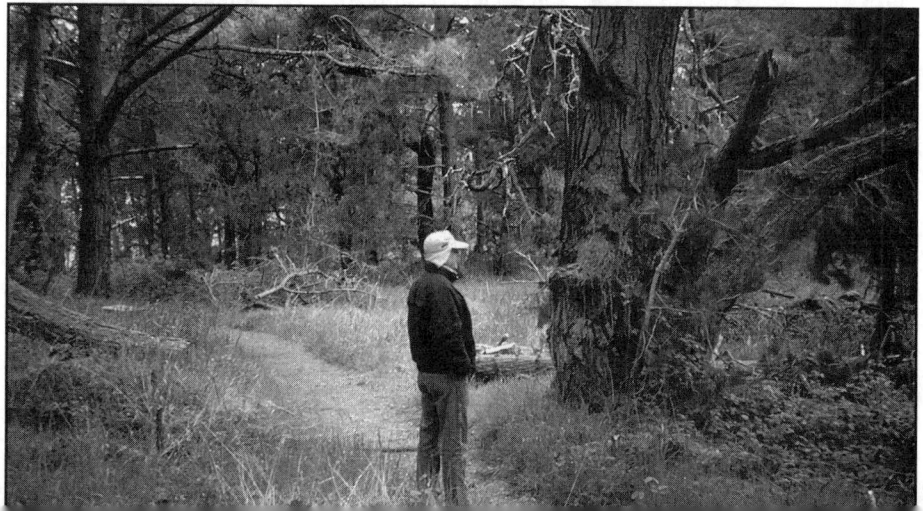

Your only major climb begins and ends in 0.2 mile at the next unmarked junction (1 mile, 180'). The right branch leads 0.3 mile to an open grassy knoll that offers views of the shore inland to the **Santa Lucia Range**. Your route continues along the left branch, descending 100 feet and then climbing 120 feet to a bench and overlook adjacent to the **vernal pools** and **mima mounds**.

VERNAL POOLS & MIMA MOUNDS ■ ■ ■ ■ ■ ■ ■ ■ ■ ■ ■ ■ ■

The uplands of San Simeon State Park contain small puddles called vernal pools amid scattered humps of soil called mima mounds—one of few places they occur together. At first glance, these pools and mounds may look like little more than stagnant water in a muddy field. But this landscape teems with life in winter and supports rings of brilliant wildflowers in spring.

When rain falls, the ground absorbs some water, while the rest flows overland as runoff. In a vernal pool grassland, this runoff accumulates in shallow depressions atop the hardpan, a layer of impermeable clay or minerals. The hardpan contains the water like a bathtub. The only way for vernal pools to empty is by evaporation, a process that can take days, weeks, or months, depending on rainfall, temperature, and the size of the pool.

Exactly how mima mounds form is a subject of debate. One of the more interesting theories is that the mounds are a byproduct of generations of industrious pocket gophers. Gophers prefer to build nests in deep soil. If the soil is shallow, gophers will carry in dirt from surrounding slopes, thereby creating mounds.

■ ■

From the pools and mounds, descend toward **Fern Gully**. Just past a wire fence, you'll reach a junction with the westbound and southbound **Nature Trail** (1.5 miles, 180'). Turn left on the southbound route past **Huff & Puff Hill** and cross Fern Gully on slotted wooden **Willow Bridge** (2.2 miles, 40'). Pause here to listen to warblers, thrushes, winter wrens, and dozens of other songbirds in the surrounding riparian woodland.

Leaving the bridge, you'll climb **Pine Ridge,** where wildlife includes bobcats, coyotes, deer, skunks, and foxes, as evidenced by plentiful scat. Though wind hushes through the open pines, calling to mind the Sierra Nevada, the glistening Pacific is in sight less than a mile west.

Continue through the pine and oak woodland and descend to a long **wooden bridge** (2.9 miles, 40') amid the wetlands. From this bridge, wheelchair-accessible platforms return 0.3 mile to the trailhead beside the footbridge, 0.1 mile east of the Washburn Day-Use Area.

PART TWO

■　　■　　■　　■　　■　　■　　■　　■　　■　　■　　■　　■

Ventana & Silver Peak Wildernesses

E NCOMPASSING MORE THAN 200,000 acres, the Ventana and Silver Peak Wildernesses lie within Los Padres National Forest, a place of exquisite beauty and profound isolation. Here rugged coastal ranges offer hikers unparalleled opportunities to explore more than 300 miles of trails and closed roads. Here, just a few miles from the vast Pacific, you'll find fog-shrouded redwoods, oak-studded grasslands, jagged marble peaks, waterfalls, thermal pools, and brisk swimming holes—a rejuvenating escape from the confinements of city life.

CHAPTER fourteen

Bottchers Gap

■ ■ ■ ■ ■ ■ ■ ■ ■ ■ ■ ■ ■

P ERCHED AMID THE HIGHEST PEAKS of the northern Ventana Wilderness, Bottchers Gap is a 2050-foot ridge saddle created by the Palo Colorado Fault. Following the uplift of the Santa Lucia Range, this northwest-trending fault carved the bed of the Little Sur River. The main fork of the Little Sur flows west for most of its course, until it meets the fault, which forces it into a sharp northwest turn to join the South Fork Little Sur River.

The gap welcomes almost year-round hiking and camping, except during severe winter storms and prolonged summer droughts. It features two trails that lead through dramatically different environments. The eastern Skinner Ridge Trail climbs one of the region's highest viewpoints, while the Little Sur Trail descends deep into the riparian forests and mystical redwoods along the Little Sur River.

> **DIRECTIONS:** To reach Bottchers Gap from Highway 1, turn east on narrow, paved Palo Colorado Road. The junction lies 2 miles north of Bixby Creek Bridge and 11.4 miles south of the Carmel Valley Road (County Road G16) junction in Carmel. *Palo Colorado* (Spanish for red wood) winds through a redwood-lined canyon, climbs through oak woodlands and chaparral, and ends at Bottchers Gap, 7.7 miles inland.
>
> **VISITOR CENTER:** Big Sur Station: (831) 667-2315. The station is on Highway 1, a half mile south of Pfeiffer Big Sur State Park. Open daily 8 a.m.–6 p.m. Memorial Day through Labor Day, 8 a.m.–4:30 p.m. the rest of the year.
>
> **NEAREST CAMPGROUND:** Bottchers Gap Campground (12 sites, $12/night) provides a picnic table, fire ring, and pedestal grill at each site. There's a maximum of eight people per site, and sites are granted on a first-come, first-serve basis. No water is available. For more information call Parks Management Co. at (805) 434-1996 or (805) 434-9199, or visit campone.com.
>
> **INFORMATION:** Fire permits (available from the campground host) are required for all stoves. Dogs are permitted and allowed off leash, except in designated campgrounds, where a 6-foot or shorter leash is required. There's a $5 day-use fee to park your car at the trailhead.
>
> **WEBSITE:** www.fs.usda.gov/lpnf | **PHONE:** Los Padres National Forest Headquarters: (805) 968-6640; Parks Management Company: (805) 995-1976

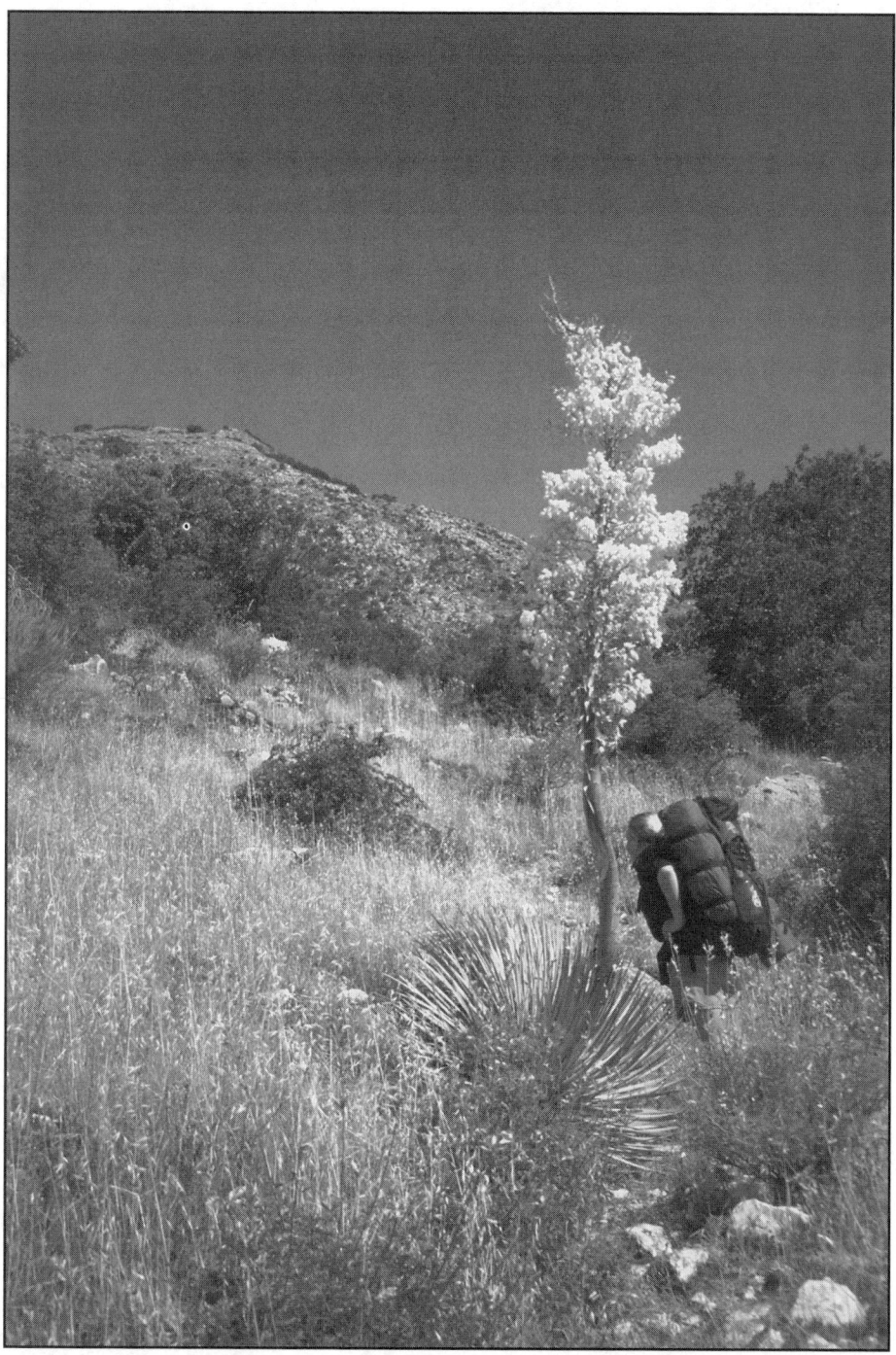

On Pico Blanco, lush redwood canyons are adjacent to desert-like settings with succulents such as Our Lord's candle.

Trip 37

DEVILS PEAK & MT. CARMEL

LENGTH AND TYPE: 9.4-mile out-and-back

RATING: Strenuous

TRAIL CONDITION: Passable, poison oak

HIGHLIGHTS: Spectacular vistas atop Devils Peak and Mt. Carmel stretch from Monterey Bay to Big Sur.

TO REACH THE TRAILHEAD: The Skinner Ridge Trail begins at the trailhead sign on the northeast corner of the parking lot.

TRIP SUMMARY: You can approach this as either moderate to strenuous day hikes or an overnight trip to Apple Tree or Turner Creek Camps.

Day hikes to Devils Peak and Mt. Carmel are rewarding ascents that overlook the entire rim of the Little Sur watershed. To the north, peaks of the Santa Lucia Range fold in on themselves as they meet the Carmel and Salinas Valleys. Clear days promise views of Monterey Bay and the Santa Cruz Mountains, more than 40 miles away. The best times to

Challenging ascents lead to spectacular vistas atop Skinner Ridge.

hike are clear days in spring, fall, or between winter storms. Fog often shrouds the coast in summer, obscuring most views.

If you're willing to haul gear, you'll find two camps just off Skinner Ridge Trail. The closest is Apple Tree Camp (3.2 miles from Bottchers Gap), a pleasant spot in all but the driest months (July–October) and perfect for novice backpackers seeking solitude but not a strenuous hike. Just 1.5 miles farther, Turner Creek Camp lies alongside the wildflower-strewn banks of Turner Creek, a gorgeous spot in spring.

Trip Description

The **Skinner Ridge Trail** begins along a singletrack path (2080') and quickly climbs north above **Bottchers Gap**'s oaks, madrones, and bays to a mosaic of chaparral. As you climb, look north to pick out the **Palo Colorado Fault,** which forms the **Little Sur River** drainage to the north and the **Mill Creek** drainage to the south. The gap is a saddle where the fault crosses a ridge separating the two drainages. West of the fault lie metamorphic rocks such as schist, marble, and gneiss, while quartz diorite lies to the east.

There's no mistaking **Pico Blanco** to the south, an enormous marble outcrop that towers over the Little Sur like a great pyramid, separating the north and south forks. *Pico Blanco* (Spanish for white peak) holds one of the West Coast's largest remaining deposits of pure limestone and marble. Some 525 feet thick and 2.5 miles long and containing an estimated 640 million tons of limestone, the deposit is privately owned. Fortunately, there's strong opposition to any attempts to quarry here, due to the adverse environmental impact it would have on adjacent national forest and state park lands.

As the trail climbs toward **Skinner Ridge,** it roller coasters through minor gullies, crossing three small seasonal springs in the Mill Creek drainage. The first is the largest, and if you're not bound for **Apple Tree** or **Turner Creek Camps,** this is the last water you'll see for at least 5 miles in summer and fall. The route from here is shady and viewless due to dense, 10- to 15-foot-high thickets of brush, dominated by different species of ceanothus.

After 2 miles of steep ascents and descents, the dense growth abruptly gives way to an open grassy knoll atop Skinner Ridge, highlighted by bracken ferns and seasonal wildflowers. The **Skinner Ridge viewpoint** (2.1 miles, 3370') lies just off the trail to the left. Vibrant wildflowers and green budding plants explode from the hillsides following winter rains. In summer, sprawling oaks and madrones offer a shady spot to rest. Some of the largest madrones in Big Sur grow along this ridge.

All too soon you must leave the ridge and begin a steep, 280-foot drop in less than a quarter mile to a saddle and the **Turner Creek Trail junction** (2.8 miles, 3180').

SIDE TRIP ■

Turner Creek Trail descends into a broad gully that closely follows the **Church Creek Fault**. A dense canopy of madrones shelters a sparse understory, except for the poison oak that grows aggressively alongside and sometimes on the trail. A quarter mile farther you'll arrive at **Apple Tree Camp** (3.1 miles, 2920'), which offers two small sites. To the right, the first site lies amid the shade of bays and white alders a few yards from **Turner Creek**'s seasonal headwater stream. The second site is nestled alongside the stream, and in wet season, the water gurgles along small mossy pools. Out of season, this creek may run dry, and to find water, you must continue down to **Turner Creek Camp** (4.8 miles, 2790').

Unfortunately, the trail from Apple Tree to Turner Creek is heavily overgrown. Just past Apple Tree's second campsite, you'll cross the creek and battle through a dense understory of blackberries, cow parsnip, thimbleberries, and tangles of poison oak. The gradual 1.5-mile descent crosses the creek three more times, then follows the north bank to the camp. The first site lies in the shade of white alders and an atypical walnut tree. The lush understory boasts spectacular spring wildflowers and bountiful berries by late summer. Also beware the mosquitoes and flies that flourish this time of year.

■ ■

From the Turner Creek Trail junction, the main route heads northeast along the **Big Pines Trail**. This trail is well cleared of brush, though that could change in the future. The route skirts the ridgetop, crossing a firebreak that was bulldozed during fires in the late 1990s. The subsequent passage of many hikers has created a clear trail that climbs **Devils Peak** through open oak woodlands. Live and black oaks offer well-deserved shade to hikers on this sunny stretch through chamise and manzanita.

Continue uphill to a switchback labeled simply TRAIL, pointing north toward the summit. An unofficial campsite lies a few yards past this sign, atop an exposed ridge with expansive views of rolling grasslands, forested canyons, ravines, and beaches that are typically shrouded in fog in summer. Devils Peak viewpoint is only a few hundred feet past this switchback.

To reach the summit, veer left at the unmarked **Mt. Carmel–Devils Peak Trail junction** (3.8 miles, 4130') that branches north off the Big Pines Trail. Along this trail, another unmarked trail veers left to the summit of **Mt. Carmel**, just past a notable sprawling black oak. If you miss this junction, you'll continue southeast to an unofficial **campsite** (3.9 miles, 4154'). Although void of water, this site boasts magnificent views of the Little Sur watershed.

If you're headed to Mt. Carmel, veer left on the aforementioned unmarked trail less than 100 feet past the Big Pines Trail–Devils Peak junction. You'll clearly see Mt. Carmel just to the north, well worth the 20- to 30-minute uphill hike. The trail descends to a minor saddle topped by a few large fallen black oaks before climbing toward the summit. Consider wearing a long shirt and pants, as the narrow trail scrapes past encroaching manzanita, scrub oak, and coyote brush. Fortunately, the trail is virtually devoid of poison oak.

At the **summit** (4.7 miles, 4417'), a telephone pole that was lugged in and erected for enhanced views is now split in two and leaning precariously. Were it not for the existence of a large granite outcrop, you might never see above the chaparral. Once you climb these boulders, the panorama comes into view.

About 20 miles southeast of Carmel, this is one of the northernmost summits in the Ventana Wilderness. On a clear day, you can see the sparkling blue **Pacific** and all of **Monterey Bay**. Moss Landing lies due north, just above the tip of the Monterey Peninsula, 19 miles away. Flat-topped **Palo Escrito Peak** (4465') lies some 16.5 miles to the east, rising amid the **Sierra de Salinas** (Salt Marsh Mountains), an eastern component of the Santa Lucia Range that flanks the west side of Salinas Valley. Just east of Palo Escrito is the city of Salinas itself, about 21 miles away, named for salt marshes at the mouth of the Salinas River, from which the Spanish commercially extracted salt. On a day with excellent visibility, you may be able to spot Santa Cruz, some 43 miles away on the north shore of Monterey Bay.

As at most peaks along this dramatic coast, the best times to hike are between mid-November and April, taking advantage of cooler temperatures, fogless days, and fewer pesky mosquitoes and flies. Be prepared for rain and snow if you hike in winter, when snow levels can drop to 2000 feet. Take in the view and return the way you came. If you're hiking farther, skip to the following trip.

Trip 38

VENTANA DOUBLE CONE VIA VENTANA TRAIL

LENGTH AND TYPE: 29.8-mile out-and-back

RATING: Challenging

TRAIL CONDITION: Passable (with brush, poison oak, and deadfalls), tread evident

HIGHLIGHTS: Unobstructed views from wildflower-strewn oak woodlands, golden grassland ridges, and atop nearly mile-high Ventana Double Cone

TO REACH THE TRAILHEAD: See TRIP 37 Devils Peak & Mt. Carmel (page 152) for the first 3.8 miles of this route to the unmarked Mt. Carmel–Devils Peak trail junction.

TRIP SUMMARY: This book describes several routes to the remote 4853-foot summit of Ventana Double Cone, in the heart of Ventana Wilderness. The most popular options

Views west toward Pico Blanco at the summit of Ventana Double Cone

include this route from Bottchers Gap, as well as routes from Los Padres Dam along the Carmel River Trail (page 185) and the Big Pines Trail (page 187), and from China Camp via Pine Valley (page 205). Each route has its advantages and disadvantages. Read on for general details, but see each trip description for specifics.

No matter which way you approach Ventana Double Cone, expect a long hike with ample opportunities to commune peacefully with nature—that is, if the flies, ticks, encroaching brush, and poison oak don't wear you down! Rising nearly a mile above the Pacific some 6 miles distant, the summit offers unobstructed 360-degree views of deep gorges, diverse ecosystems, and isolated peaks along the northern Santa Lucia Range.

This route promises incredible ridgetop views (particularly in winter and spring) and the shortest hike, but it also involves the greatest elevation gain. Although the Ventana Trail junction is just 6.3 miles from Bottchers Gap (versus 9.1 miles from Los Padres Dam), this route requires an additional 1000 feet of climbing as it roller coasters along Skinner Ridge and Devils Peak.

If you can arrange a shuttle vehicle, consider combining trips for an excellent point-to-point backcountry excursion. Begin from Bottchers Gap and tackle the 14.9 miles to Ventana Double Cone, then hike out 15.5 miles to Los Padres Dam via the Puerto Suelo and Carmel River Trails (see TRIP 46 Ventana Double Cone via Carmel River Trail, page 185).

As at most peaks along this dramatic coast, the best times to hike are between mid-November and April, taking advantage of cooler temperatures, fogless days, and fewer pesky mosquitoes and flies. Be prepared for rain and snow if you hike in winter, when snow levels can drop to 2000 feet. During the driest months (August through November), you may not find water until Big Pines Camp (upper Danish Creek) or Pat Spring. In drought years there's even a chance these two water sources could run dry. In such conditions, consider one of the alternative routes.

Trip Description

From the unmarked **Mt. Carmel–Devils Peak Trail junction** (3.8 miles, 4130'), you'll continue southeast along the **Big Pines Trail** on a gentle descent across meadows dotted with sprawling oaks and madrones. This stretch promises fantastic views of the **Little Sur River** drainage, including its headwaters below **Ventana Double Cone** (4853'). Notice the different colors and textures that distinguish each ecological community. Velvety light and dark green chaparral line the dry south-facing slopes, golden grasslands dotted with oaks and pines cap the knolls and ridges, dark green hardwood forests flourish on cool north-facing slopes, and emerald redwood canopies shelter the deepest valleys and narrow stream courses.

The trail descends a yucca-flecked slope, followed by a 500-foot drop to a clearing atop a minor saddle. Pause here to picnic beneath impressive black oaks and madrones, the latter identified by peeling paper-thin bark. The trail rises to round a small summit (3682'), then descends to two smaller saddles. At the second saddle, you'll reach the **Big Pines Trail junction** (5.1 miles, 3500'), which connects the southbound **Comings Camp Trail** and northbound **San Clemente Trail** and leads to the eastbound **Ventana Trail**.

SIDE TRIP ■

From the Big Pines Trail junction, the **Comings Camp Trail** descends southeast for half a mile into a mature forest dominated by oaks, madrones, and the occasional massive ponderosa pine. This shady, viewless trail reaches a minor gully before the final descent to **Comings Camp** (5.6 miles, 3200'). Nestled beneath several enormous trees, the first campsite is big enough to accommodate a large group, perhaps as many as 10 tents. A smaller second site lies about 100 yards down the trail alongside willows and a large black oak. The camp offers little other than stone fire rings. Water is not provided, though in wet months, a small creeklet may trickle past the willows at the second site.

For a second side trip: From the Big Pines Trail junction, the faint **San Clemente Trail** branches left and descends 1.5 miles northwest to **Pine Creek Camp**. This trail is so overgrown with poison oak and brush, you'd be better off skipping it altogether.

■ ■

From this four-way junction with the San Clemente and Comings Camp Trails, the Big Pines Trail continues straight, climbing east to a minor ridge, then descending to a saddle with impressive views north across the **Carmel** and **Salinas Valleys.** Passing live oaks and a few massive black oaks, the trail emerges amid ponderosa pines and an open grassy knoll atop a 4052-foot ridge. From here steep switchbacks drop to a major saddle and the **Ventana Trail junction** (6.3 miles, 3620').

You'll veer right onto the Ventana Trail along a well-graded slope past tanoaks, madrones, and lone ponderosa pines to the headwaters of the south fork of **Danish Creek** (7 miles, 3560'). From here a spur darts left across the creek and returns downstream a half mile to the Big Pines Trail. Pass the spur and continue upstream 0.1 mile to a spacious, **unnamed camp** that many mistake for Pat Spring Camp. The first campsite lies beneath an impressive madrone amid scattered ponderosa pines and oaks. Another site sits across Danish Creek atop a flat saddle 50 yards northeast of the first site. In summer and fall the creek may run dry. To find water, head downstream a half mile toward **Big Pines Camp** or upstream toward **Pat Spring,** 0.3 mile past the divide.

Past the camp, the route rises 0.2 mile southeast to a prominent saddle and a four-way junction with the **Pat Spring Camp Trail** and **Pat Spring Trail** (7.3 miles, 3740'). Pay attention at this potentially confusing junction. The trail straight ahead leads 100 yards downslope to **Pat Spring**—but this is *not* the Ventana Trail. Many hikers mistakenly think Pat Spring is along the Ventana Trail, which is how it appears on US Forest Service maps. To continue on the Ventana Trail, you'll turn left past the junction and climb northeast toward a minor ridge. The trail to **Pat Spring Camp** branches right.

SIDE TRIP ■

Pat Spring Camp is among the most scenic in the Ventana Wilderness. From the Ventana Trail junction, turn right on the **Pat Spring Camp Trail** and climb west along a minor ridge. Within 50 feet you'll reach the first campsite on your left, while the second site (9.8 miles, 3880') lies atop a minor summit with views of marble-capped **Pico Blanco** and the Pacific. Past the second site, a narrow trail leads 0.1 mile farther to a dramatic outcrop overlooking the Little Sur watershed.

To obtain water, return to the Ventana Trail junction, turn right on the eastbound **Pat Spring Trail,** and continue downhill 100 yards to the spring—a reliable water source in all but the driest years.

■ ■

Fifteen feet past the four-way junction, the Ventana Trail veers left on a moderate climb to a **ridge** (7.6 miles, 4180') topped with ponderosa pines, madrones, and live oaks, where you'll catch glimpses north across Carmel Valley to the **Sierra de Salinas.** A gradual climb leads southeast to a **saddle** (8.4 miles, 3940') that offers views southwest across the Little Sur drainage to Pico Blanco, which splits the river's south and main forks. Beyond lies the broad Pacific.

It's a moderate climb from the saddle to **Little Pines** summit (9.1 miles, 4189'), beyond which lies the **Little Pines Camp Trail junction** (9.4 miles, 3970'). This easily missed unmarked spur branches left 100 feet to the camp, a dry, undesirable spot that's littered with multiple fallen snags.

Past this spur, you'll cross open pine, oak, and madrone woodland, then descend grassy slopes along the western flank of **Uncle Sam Mountain,** which boasts stunning views south toward Ventana Double Cone and its unnamed 4653-foot neighbor. Onward 0.3 mile, the trail crosses the first of four ephemeral creeklets (9.7 miles, 3720'), which typically only flow in wet season.

Past the fourth creeklet (10.3 miles, 3620'), the trail descends to the signed **Puerto Suelo Trail junction** (11.2 miles, 3520'). The only major saddle along this ridge, Puerto Suelo lies along the fractured path of **Church Creek Fault,** which runs northwest out to sea. The Puerto Suelo Trail descends southeast 2.6 miles to **Hiding Canyon Camp,** along the **Carmel River Trail.**

Continue along the Ventana Trail, which climbs 0.2 mile to a westbound switchback on your right. (If you miss the switchback, you'll wind up descending a granite-lined gully on a rapidly diminishing deer trail.) Beyond the switchback, the well-graded trail climbs a 4366-foot ridge, crosses a southeast ridge, and gradually descends to a saddle and the **Lone Pine Camp Trail junction** (12.6 miles, 4300'). A sign marked WATER points southeast along a spur on your left.

The spur descends a few feet past the remains of **Lone Pine Camp,** since reclaimed by overgrowth and large fallen snags. In winter you'll find water less than 0.1 mile down a shallow gully from the junction, while in summer you may have to descend cross-country several hundred feet to find the merest trickle. Don't expect to find water from late summer till the first winter rains.

Beyond the saddle, the Ventana Trail climbs a series of moderate switchbacks along exposed slopes blanketed in fragrant shoulder-high chaparral. Take in outstanding views south toward Ventana Double Cone, which separates the Carmel, Big Sur, and Little Sur River watersheds. Near the summit, vegetation switches to mature stands of live oaks, madrones, and lone Coulter pines, distinguished from ponderosas by their foot-long cones with hook-like scales.

Less than a mile from the peak, the narrow trail follows a granite ridge to a minor saddle, then bypasses the north summit. Here you'll find the rare Santa Lucia fir, endemic to the northern Santa Lucia Range.

SANTA LUCIA FIR ■ ■ ■ ■ ■ ■ ■ ■ ■ ■ ■ ■ ■ ■ ■ ■ ■ ■ ■

Found both in deep canyons and perched high atop the Santa Lucia Range lives the rarest and most narrowly distributed of all fir species, the endemic Santa Lucia fir. The species' seemingly disparate habitats share one attribute: Each is relatively fire resistant. For although the range is subject to periodic blazes, this fir has not developed resistance to fire.

Fossil evidence suggests that Santa Lucia firs were once widely distributed throughout western North America. The tree thrived during the Miocene epoch (24 million to 5 million years ago), as the climate was much warmer and wetter than today, including regular summer rainfall. But during the Pliocene epoch (5 million to 1.6 million years ago), the climate began to cool, ushering in the ice ages of the Pleistocene (1.6 million to 11,000 years ago). The fir could not withstand the colder, drier conditions and thus retreated to milder climates amid the coastal mountains.

Ventana Double Cone supports a small, isolated grove of Santa Lucia firs, easily identified by droopy, densely foliated crowns that extend from the base of the tree with lower branches that nearly touch the ground.

■ ■

From a saddle (14.8 miles, 4640') between the two summits, hike the remaining 0.1 mile to the main **summit** (14.9 miles, 4853'), capped by the foundation of a fire lookout station and a logbook filled with the musings of fellow hikers.

On clear, fogless days, the views encompass all major peaks and watersheds along the northern Santa Lucia Range. To the northwest, the Little Sur River drainage crouches beneath the sheer marble cliffs of Pico Blanco. The Carmel River drainage lies northeast, its headwaters due east. Off to the south, the Big Sur River drainage leads west to Highway 1, joined by small tributaries all along the way.

Notice how Ventana Double Cone is connected to its sister peaks by steep, narrow ridgelines. One conspicuous ridge extends 2 miles southeast from this summit to 4727-foot **Ventana Cone,** while to the left and just above Ventana Cone, another ridge continues 2.5 miles east-southeast to 4965-foot **South Ventana Cone.**

Scratching the horizon to the right of Ventana Cone is 5862-foot **Junipero Serra Peak,** the highest mountain in central California's Coast Ranges. Though nearly 20 miles distant, it towers higher than any neighboring summit or cone. To its right rises 5155-foot **Cone Peak,** 21 miles away and only 3.2 miles from the Pacific. Its rise from shore represents the steepest gradient in the continental United States.

Celebrate your accomplishment before heading back down the trail.

Trip 39

LITTLE SUR & JACKSON CAMPS

LENGTH AND TYPE: 10.2-mile out-and-back

RATING: Moderate

TRAIL CONDITION: Passable (with brush, poison oak, and deadfalls), tread evident

HIGHLIGHTS: Enjoy mountain views en route to camps nestled amid redwoods beside the Little Sur River.

TO REACH THE TRAILHEAD: At Bottchers Gap, the trail begins 30 feet west of the parking lot at the gated dirt Pico Blanco Road.

SACRED MOUNTAIN ■ ■ ■ ■ ■ ■ ■ ■ ■ ■ ■ ■ ■ ■ ■ ■ ■

The region's native Esselen people revered Pico Blanco as a sacred mountain from which all life originated. According to Esselen legend, three creatures—eagle, coyote, and hummingbird—rode out the great flood atop this mountain and went on to recreate the world.

The present owners value the peak in a less sacred light. The Granite Rock Company of Watsonville bought Pico Blanco in the late 1960s, intending to mine the peak for limestone, an essential ingredient in concrete. Fortunately, their plans to lop off the top several hundred feet of the mountain were met with a groundswell of opposition. The resulting environmental lawsuits went all the way to the U.S. Supreme Court and put an end to mining plans on Pico Blanco.

■ ■

TRIP SUMMARY: You can approach this as either a moderate day hike or an overnight backpacking trip. Little Sur Camp lies 2.6 miles from Bottchers Gap, while Jackson Camp is 5.1 miles from the trailhead. The hike takes you from redwood-lined gullies along Pico Blanco Road into dry mountainous terrain that overlooks marble-capped Pico Blanco. The road winds along the Little Sur River through Pico Blanco Boy Scout Camp, on land donated to the scouts in 1948 by William Randolph Hearst. Hearst first purchased the land in 1921 in order to preserve the redwoods from intense logging pressure. Scouts descend on the camp between mid-June and mid-August, thwarting any plans for a wilderness escape. Crossing the river, the Little Sur Trail heads east toward Jackson Camp, home to two riverside sites.

Trip Description

From the west side of the parking lot at **Bottchers Gap** (2080'), head south along the gated dirt road toward **Pico Blanco Boy Scout Camp.** After a gradual quarter-mile descent, you'll reach the first switchback and views of **Pico Blanco, Marble Peak,** and **Ventana Double Cone.** You'll also see evidence of the 1977 Marble–Cone Fire, which consumed thousands of acres. Covered in chaparral, the dry south-facing slopes burned more completely than the damp, tree-lined north-facing slopes.

Past the first switchback, the trail leads north into a stand of redwoods, hairpins south, then reaches another switchback and the **Little Sur Camp Trail junction** (1.8 miles, 1230'), on the east side of the road. Pause for views of the **Little Sur River** drainage and 3709-foot **Pico Blanco,** the largest single mass of limestone west of the Rocky Mountains.

SIDE TRIP ■

To reach **Little Sur Camp,** take the 0.8-mile spur on your right, which leads south along a shady ridge, plunging nearly 600 feet to the banks of the Little Sur. As you meander past live oaks and Douglas firs, keep an eye on the trail for encroaching poison oak. A series of moderate to steep switchbacks drop east into a dense forest of bays, oaks, and madrones. Consider bringing protective head netting once temperatures rise above 70°F, as flies make their presence known. After descending west on an easier grade, you'll arrive in camp (2.6 miles, 670'), which provides two small riverside sites.

Use caution when scrambling over a couple of large fallen trees across the trail. Due to the camp's proximity to both Bottchers Gap and Pico Blanco Boy Scout Camp, these sites fill up quickly during spring vacation and between mid-June and mid-August when the scouts arrive.

■ ■

Past the Little Sur Camp Trail junction, the main route descends north 0.3 mile, returning to the welcome shade of a redwood forest. The next switchback crosses a fault-line creek beside a small waterfall and weaves through several gullies past welcoming signs for the Pico Blanco Boy Scout Camp. The camp's **ranger station** is on the west side of the trail, 100 yards past the first sign. Follow signs toward the main camp, as spur roads and trails only lead to camp structures and sites. The road gently roller coasters down to the Little Sur, then crosses it on a wooden footbridge into Pico Blanco Boy Scout Camp proper (3.6 miles, 820').

Just past the bridge and quartermaster's store, the road forks into three branches. The left branch leads to **Camp Geronimo,** where it parallels the river upstream to a crossing. The right branch leads through camp to a gravel beach with a refreshing waist- to chest-high wading pool. Instead, follow the middle branch, which soon passes the central kitchen and quickly climbs, passing a small sign for the start of the **Los Padres National Forest Trails** and a spur on the right marked simply TRAIL (3.7 miles, 950').

You may either follow this spur or continue on the road—both climb roughly 250 feet in 0.3 mile. The road makes a hairpin turn right and then snakes steeply westward, passing a ruin marked by a lonely chimney. The spur climbs more gradually, veering west and then looping around to join the road. From that point, you'll ascend 25 yards farther to the **Little Sur Trail junction** (4 miles, 1080').

The eastbound **Little Sur Trail** to **Jackson Camp** is essentially a viewless trail that leads south-southeast 200 feet above the Little Sur River in the shade of tanoaks and redwoods. Half a mile from the junction, you'll reach a seasonal spring that's little more than a mud puddle in summer. A few hundred yards farther the trail narrows at a small washout. Be especially careful if you're lugging heavy gear, as this section could erode further over time.

Past the washout, the trail makes a hairpin turn east across a creeklet in a redwood-lined gully blanketed in sword ferns, redwood sorrel, and trillium (4.6 miles, 1120'). Here the trail leaves Boy Scout territory and enters the Ventana Wilderness. You'll climb another 100 yards, then make the final half-mile descent into **Jackson Camp** (5.1 miles, 930'), whose two sites lie along the south bank of the Little Sur.

You'll literally emerge at the first site, while the second site lies just 20 yards downstream. Enjoy the serene backcountry and return when you're rested. A trail from the Boy Scout camp climbs the river to Jackson Camp, so expect badge-carrying visitors in July and August.

Trip 40

COAST ROAD TO PICO BLANCO CAMP

LENGTH AND TYPE: 12-mile out-and-back or 12.4-mile point-to-point

RATING: Strenuous

TRAIL CONDITION: Passable (some brush and/or deadfalls), tread evident to faint along the private property boundary

HIGHLIGHTS: Stroll along the redwood-flanked Little Sur River to a crystal clear swimming hole near Pico Blanco Camp.

TO REACH THE TRAILHEAD: The south end of Coast Road emerges on Highway 1 opposite the entrance to Andrew Molera State Park, 4.5 miles north of Pfeiffer Big Sur State Park and 22 miles south of Carmel. The north end of Coast Road emerges on Highway 1 at the north end of the Bixby Creek Bridge, 2 miles south of the Palo Colorado Road junction, and 13.4 miles south of the Carmel Valley Road (County Road G16) junction. In wet months the 10.3-mile road may be impassable for two-wheel-drive vehicles.

The best route to the trailhead is via the south end of Coast Road, as this stretch is shorter than the north end (3.8 miles versus 6.5 miles), usually in better condition, and the grade is more consistent. You'll find mileage markers at half-mile intervals along Coast Road. The trail begins at a gate on the east side of the road, 100 feet north of Mile 6.5. Watch for the fire warning sign. Unlatch and close the gate behind you to begin the descent to the Little Sur's South Fork.

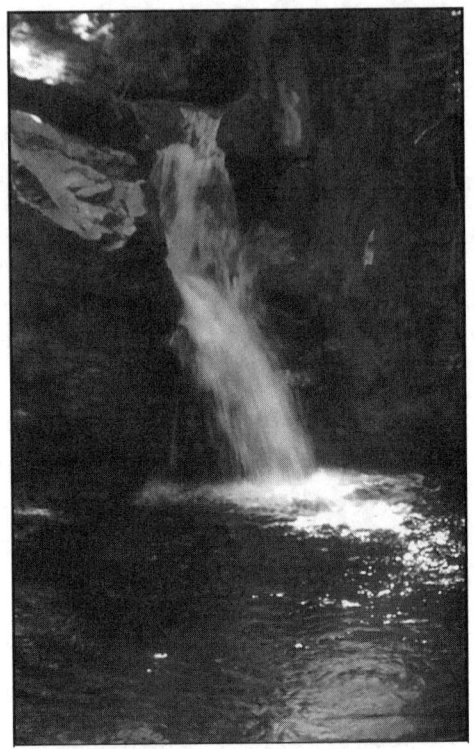

TRIP SUMMARY: You can approach this as either a strenuous day hike or an overnight trip. The camp is also accessible from Bottchers Gap via the Little Sur Trail (see TRIP 41 Pico Blanco, page 167). Although this trail is the shorter route (6 miles versus 7.4 miles), tangled overgrowth, persistent poison oak, and dangerous washouts make it tough going. If you have time, choose

After a strenuous hike, the respite of the refreshing emerald swimming pool at the end of Pico Blanco Camp is not to be missed.

the overnight option, as you'll want time to enjoy the swimming hole at trail's end.

The camp lies amid redwood groves and open oak woodlands along the sun-drenched south-facing canyon walls of the Little Sur. Just upstream, the South Fork has carved into Pico Blanco's marble flanks, creating a redwood-shaded grotto highlighted by a waterfall and swimming hole.

The 12.4-mile point-to-point trip from Bottchers Gap to Coast Road is an ideal weekend trip (see TRIP 41 Pico Blanco, page 167). Watch for ticks in spring, when brush encroaches on the trail, particularly beneath Pico Blanco on the last 3 miles of the route.

Trip Description

From the trailhead gate (290'), descend the lightly used **Little Sur Trail** through redwood groves to the **South Fork** of the **Little Sur River.** You'll follow its banks upstream 1.5 miles past small unofficial campsites nestled beneath the lush riparian and redwood forest. During the wet season (November through April), fragile wildflower blooms paint the trail. Redwood sorrel, western starflower, Douglas' iris, and Solomon's seal thrive in the cool, damp understory and continue to bloom through June. A vigorous secondary forest rises above the stumps of redwoods that inhabited these banks for thousands of years.

You may also notice several downed and dying tanbark oaks, victims of sudden oak death. Hikers toting heavy packs will find these fallen oaks a particular nuisance, as they must clamber over or crouch to get through the tangle.

TREE KILLER

Responsible for killing California oaks in epidemic proportions, sudden oak death is caused by the fungus-like pathogen *Phytophthora ramorum*. Since it first appeared in 1995, the disease has killed hundreds of thousands of tanoaks, coast live, black, and Shreve oaks in Northern California. Though left unharmed, neighboring species such as Douglas fir, rhododendron, buckeye, madrone, manzanita, bigleaf maple, bay laurel, and evergreen huckleberry may serve as "carriers" of the pathogen, which may then spread aerially via windblown rain. Mortality is most common where oaks and these carriers grow side by side.

Until the disease is better understood, researchers ask hikers to help prevent the spread of *P. ramorum.* Before leaving the area, thoroughly clean your tires, shoes, and your pets' feet.

You'll soon leave **Los Padres National Forest** and cross private property, skirting the river 0.3 mile farther upstream to a **campsite** for one to two tents (1.8 miles, 425'). From

Nestled along the edge of a redwood-forested gorge, Pico Blanco Camp is just a short walk upstream from one of Big Sur's most magnificent swimming pools.

here the Little Sur Trail fords the South Fork and crosses a creek. This is usually an easy boulder-to-boulder hop, except during winter storms, when a knee- to waist-high wade is inevitable. During intense rainfall, the river may be too swift and deep to cross.

Onward, the route begins its first major ascent, climbing from the cool redwood canopy into fragrant coastal scrub. Trail conditions deteriorate from this point, largely due to aggressive brush. A crew from the Ventana Wilderness Alliance restored some of the trail but reported many sections still in need of work.

You'll continue climbing east amid dense northern and southern coastal scrub and chaparral species. South-facing slopes allow the southern species to tolerate hot, dry summers, while ocean fog creeps up the canyon, providing moisture to the northern scrub. The trail leads through a fragrant tapestry of black sage, bush lupine, coyote brush, sagebrush, and poison oak to a seeping spring that supports a small grove of redwoods. From here the trail meanders 150 feet to a switchback across the private dirt **Granite Rock Road** (2.2 miles, 760').

Continue east, ducking through two minor gullies that host seasonal creeks. Though passable, the trail is narrow and slippery with several brush-covered washouts. Past the second gully, the trail parallels Granite Rock Road for 0.6 mile to another **switchback** (2.8 miles, 840'). This marks the start of a steep climb of more than 1000 feet in 2 miles.

The trail first climbs north, then switchbacks, reentering the US Forest Service land along the south flanks of **Pico Blanco**. Hardwoods and redwoods are limited to the ravines, while the scrub-clad slopes and grassy ridgelines are studded with such drought-tolerant species as Our Lord's candle, a yucca that shoots forth a large stalk of cream-colored blossoms.

Among the oldest known rocks along the Coast Ranges, Pico Blanco's limestone and marble outcrops create dramatic vegetation zones. Though the area often receives more than 60 inches of rainfall per year, the runoff drains into the marble and limestone rather than remaining in the overlying soil. Thus the slopes are dominated by drought-tolerant species.

Past these blinding outcrops, the trail meanders through hardwood-lined ravines, crosses a broad meadow, and climbs to an oak-clad **ridge** (4.8 miles, 1840') with views up and down the South Fork drainage. Beyond the ridge, you'll begin the descent into camp.

The trail crosses open slopes and a series of shallow gullies. Past the third gully, home to a small seasonal tributary, you'll reach the **Pico Blanco Camp Trail junction** (5.9 miles, 1385'). Descend this 0.1-mile trail past sprawling oaks and a grassy slope into **Pico Blanco Camp** (6 miles, 1300'). The camp offers four sites with fire rings. Three lie on the perimeter of a sundrenched grassy slope, while the fourth lies 20 yards south of the first site you reach along the trail. Be on your guard for poison oak.

A quick 100-foot stroll upstream from camp lies a **waterfall oasis**, widely considered one of the most beautiful spots in the Ventana Wilderness. You'll arrive at a deeply eroded marble gorge that enfolds a deep emerald swimming hole. At best, the water reaches the mid-50s Fahrenheit, making your swim brisk, refreshing, and likely brief. The midday to early afternoon sun warms the pool and adjacent boulders, though this may not be sufficient heat following your chilly swim. Return to camp to warm up.

If you're venturing farther along the Little Sur Trail to **Bottchers Gap** or the **Manuel Peak Trail,** refer to the following trip description. To reach the **Manuel Peak Trail junction,** continue 1.2 miles past the camp along the Little Sur Trail (see TRIP 42 Manuel Peak & Pfeiffer Big Sur State Park, page 169).

Trip 41

PICO BLANCO

LENGTH AND TYPE: 14.8-mile out-and-back or 12.4-mile point-to-point

RATING: Strenuous

TRAIL CONDITION: Passable (with brush and poison oak encroachment and deadfalls), tread evident

HIGHLIGHTS: Follow a magnificent, steep-sided canyon through redwood groves to a perfect swimming hole at Pico Blanco Camp.

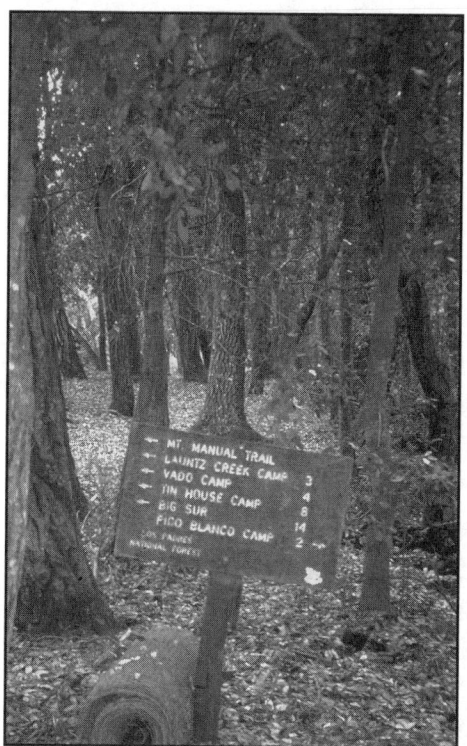

The Manuel Peak Trail junction leads to remote and isolated areas of Ventana Wilderness.

TO REACH THE TRAILHEAD: At Bottchers Gap the trail begins 30 feet west of the parking lot at the gated dirt Pico Blanco Road.

TRIP SUMMARY: This route leads 7.4 miles to Pico Blanco Camp. You can approach it as a strenuous day hike, a one- to three-night out-and-back, or a point-to-point trip. On a two- to three-night trip, consider staying at Little Sur Camp (2.6 miles from Bottchers Gap) or Jackson Camp (5.2 miles from Bottchers Gap), then hiking on to Pico Blanco Camp (see TRIP 39 Little Sur & Jackson Camps, page 161). For a rewarding 12.4-mile point-to-point passage, leave a shuttle vehicle at the trailhead along Coast Road (see TRIP 40 Coast Road to Pico Blanco Camp, page 163).

The hike descends into the Little Sur drainage via Pico Blanco Road, promising panoramic views of Pico Blanco, the largest marble and limestone deposit in the Lower 48. The road follows the banks of the Little Sur into Pico Blanco Boy Scout Camp. Scouts descend en masse between mid-June and mid-August, thwarting any plans for a wilderness escape. Past the camp, you'll join the Little Sur Trail, which leads east 1.2 miles to Jackson Camp and west 2.6 miles to Pico Blanco Camp. Pico Blanco is nestled along the edge of a redwood-lined gorge. Just upstream, a waterfall oasis harbors a deep emerald swimming hole.

Trip Description

See TRIP 39 Little Sur & Jackson Camps (page 161) for the first 4 miles of this route to the **Little Sur Trail junction.**

Assuming you're not headed to Jackson Camp, you'll turn right and head westbound on the **Little Sur Trail,** climbing through a dense forest dominated by tanoaks, madrones, and redwoods. Fondly referred to as "Cardiac Hill," the following steep 1350-foot ascent to the top of **Launtz Ridge** over less than a mile ends at a minor 2194-foot crest. Pause to rest and take in impressive views of the Little Sur drainage.

From here the trail forks. The faint trail to the right leads to an unofficial campsite atop a grassy knoll. Branch left on the Little Sur Trail, which descends gradually from the crest into dense woodland. You'll soon arrive at the signed **Manuel Peak Trail junction** (5.3 miles, 2090').

Branch right at this junction and continue west on the Little Sur Trail. The next 0.3 mile drops steeply into **Duveneck's Hole,** a dilapidated group of hunting huts amid a shady redwood canyon. Skirt the north edge of the canyon beyond the shacks for your first foreboding glimpse of **Pico Blanco**'s marble-strewn south face. The cool redwood and tanoak canopy abruptly changes to dry scrubby oaks and chaparral, which is replaced in turn by arid, yucca-studded grassy slopes—a stark contrast brought on by the peak's mineral composition. **Pico Blanco**'s marble and limestone slopes drain water quickly, leaving only plants adapted to such dry conditions.

The trail switchbacks three times across the lower slopes before turning southwest for a quarter-mile descent. Consider wearing long pants for this stretch, as the narrow trail is choked with poison oak, coyote brush, and yucca. Stop every few hundred feet and check for ticks, a factor in all but the driest months.

The trail forks again at the **Pico Blanco Camp Trail junction** (7.3 miles, 1385'). The right branch leads 5.9 miles west to **Coast Road** (see TRIP 40 Coast Road to Pico Blanco Camp, page 163). Head down the left branch 0.1 mile southeast to **Pico Blanco Camp** (7.4 miles, 1300'). Just upstream from camp is a scenic waterfall oasis and swimming hole, the perfect spot for a refreshing dip. (For details about the camp and swimming hole, see TRIP 40 Coast Road to Pico Blanco Camp, page 163.)

Trip 42

MANUEL PEAK & PFEIFFER BIG SUR STATE PARK

LENGTH AND TYPE: 25.4-mile out-and-back (Manuel Peak)

RATING: Challenging

TRAIL CONDITION: Passable to Vado Camp, difficult to impassable to Pfeiffer Big Sur State Park; poison oak, trail washouts, faint tread, trail closure as of 2008 Basin Complex Fire eastbound on Mt. Manuel Trail from Pfieffer Big Sur State Park.

HIGHLIGHTS: This route follows the redwood-lined Little Sur River gorge past marble-capped Pico Blanco to the Manuel Peak summit for glorious coastal and inland views.

TO REACH THE TRAILHEAD: At Bottchers Gap the trail begins 30 feet west of the parking lot at the gated dirt Pico Blanco Road.

TRIP SUMMARY: Approach this as an out-and-back hike rather than a point-to-point trek since the Mt. Manuel Trail is closed westbound from Pfeiffer Big Sur State Park. Seriously consider curtailing your hike, however, as sections between Vado Camp and Manuel Peak

The region's native Esselen people revered Pico Blanco as a sacred mountain from which all life originated.

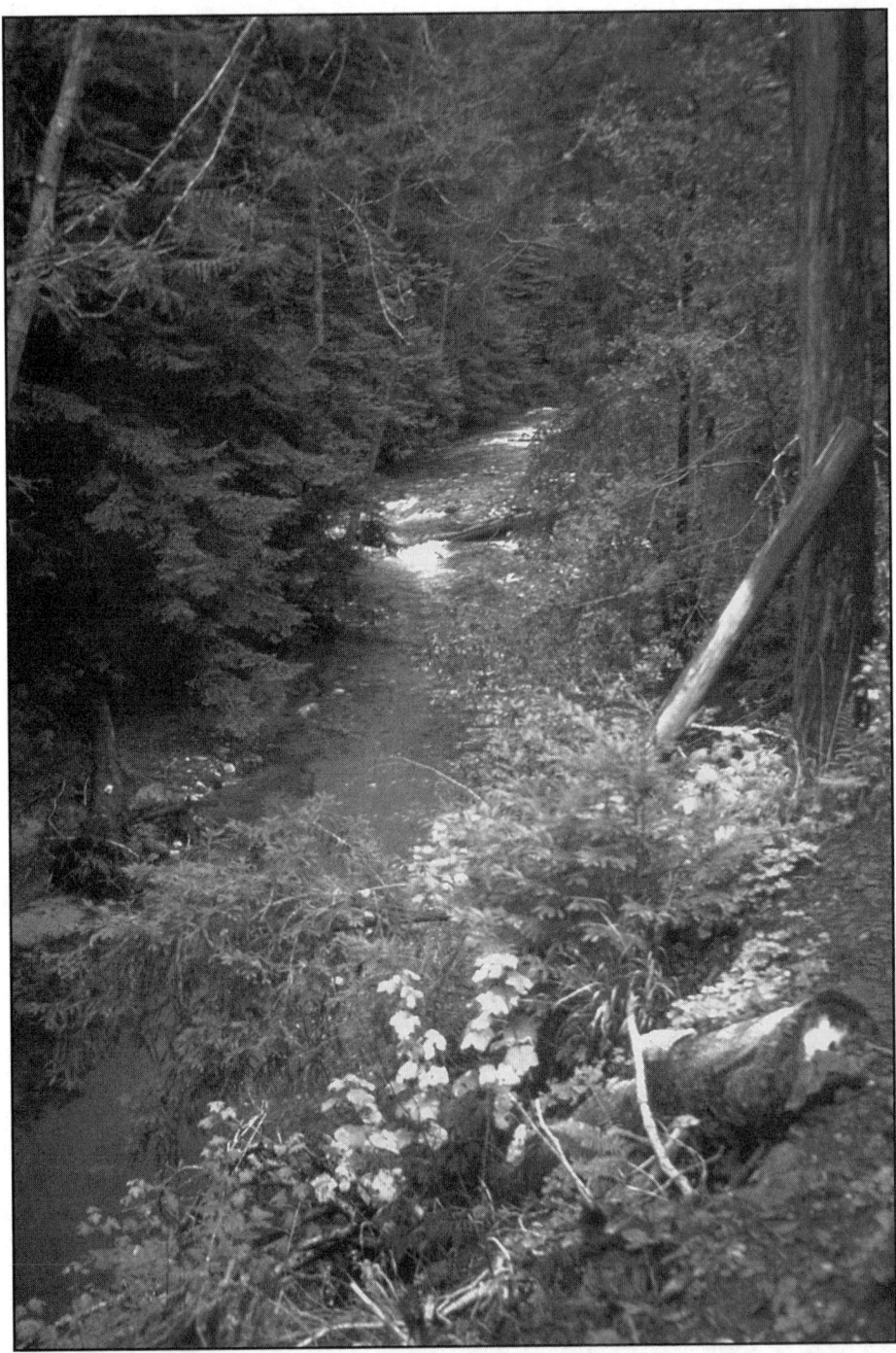

Expect solitude under the shade of towering redwoods along the South Fork Little Sur River.

are considered impassable due to trail washouts, deadfalls, and brush encroachment. From Vado Camp (ruined in 2003 by downed trees), the route switchbacks to a major ridge, where the trail practically vanishes, then summits Manuel Peak. Washouts, overgrowth, and the lack of water and trail markings make this strenuous stretch very hard to follow. In addition, during the dry season (June through November), you may not find water between Vado Camp and Pfeiffer Big Sur State Park, a grueling 11 miles on hot summer days.

Instead, plan an out-and-back overnight deep into the heart of the Little Sur drainage. Camp at Launtz Creek or Pico Blanco, then day hike the steep climb from Vado Camp to Manuel Peak. The point-to-point passage from Bottchers Gap to Pfeiffer Big Sur State Park is a two- to four-day, 18.1-mile haul along strenuous and dangerous trails due to 2008 fire damage and lack of trail restoration efforts.

As in most of the Ventana Wilderness, flies are often a nuisance, particularly in warmer months (May through October), while ticks are prevalent during the wet season (November through April). Poison oak is a year-round concern.

Trip Description

See TRIP 41 Pico Blanco (page 167) for the first 5.3 miles of this route to the **Manuel Peak Trail junction** (2090').

At the signed junction, branch left and climb past oak- and madrone-filtered views down the **South Fork Little Sur** canyon, framed by **Pico Blanco** to the west and **Post Summit** to the south. The trail crosses several minor gullies as it climbs past shady tanoak, live oak, and madrone forests into chaparral, chamise, and manzanita brush. You'll soon descend into a cool, damp redwood forest highlighted by sprawling tanoaks.

The trail drops north past a major gully, then briefly south along the north bank of **Launtz Creek** to **Launtz Creek Camp** (6.9 miles, 1920'), a favorite stop along the **Manuel Peak Trail**. Though more spacious than the recently damaged **Vado Camp,** there's only room for about three tents on its sloping creekside sites. You'll find year-round water.

Beyond camp the trail crosses the creek, turns upstream 100 yards, then climbs southwest along a few short switchbacks to the minor ridge that divides Launtz Creek and the South Fork Little Sur. You'll descend this minor ridge along a well-graded trail to the South Fork canyon floor. The trail follows the river upstream, crossing it three times over a quarter mile.

Just past the third crossing, look for several large downed trees. Provided the Forest Service or another crew has not cut or moved these trees, they mark the **Vado Camp Trail junction** (7.8 miles, 1790'). This 100-foot spur crosses the South Fork to a small east-sloping gully, the site of camp. In 2003 a major windstorm toppled several large trees directly onto the site. What remains amid the tangle would at best accommodate one or two tents along a bench on the south side of the gully. In summer and fall the South Fork often runs dry, requiring a short hike downstream for water.

Most hikers hang up their boots at Vado Camp, as the trail to **Manuel Peak** is overgrown and often difficult to follow. Between Manuel Peak and **Pfeiffer Big Sur State Park,** the trail is clearly marked, but washouts make the steep descent dangerous, especially for those lugging heavy packs. Nevertheless, as some of you have your hearts set on the summit, the trail description follows. Respect your limits and tread carefully.

From camp you'll cross the South Fork and climb west along a series of switchbacks. The trail continues its steady ascent south, dipping in and out of minor redwood-lined gullies. At the fourth **gully** (9.4 miles, 2280'), a small creeklet flows during the wet season (November through April), your last chance for water for another 8.5 miles.

Continue climbing past redwood-shaded gullies, sprawling oaks, and dense ceanothus thickets. From the first major gully, the steadily deteriorating route climbs a series of well-graded switchbacks, rising 900 feet in the next 1.1 miles on a trail that more closely resembles a deer path. Overgrown brush obscures views of **Cabezo Prieto** ridge and allows only occasional brief glimpses of Post Summit and Manuel Peak. You'll climb almost to the top of Cabezo Prieto (3554'), then battle through 0.1 mile of heavily overgrown sections to a narrow crest that offers the first of several spectacular 360-degree views.

Head south along the crest for a mile past dense stands of ceanothus, scrub oak, manzanita, and yerba santa. Check your clothing for ticks during the wet season (November through April). Also watch for poison oak. The trail crosses several bulldozed sections that make passage difficult. Just past the first saddle, the trail widens and the brush thins out somewhat.

You'll climb to a minor point, then descend to a minor saddle near a dense stand of Coulter pines, which offer welcome shade. Just past a conspicuous, yet camouflaged reflector is the spur to the **Manuel Peak viewpoint** (12.7 miles, 3379'). See TRIP 20 Manuel Peak Trail (page 105) for a description of the summit and the remaining 5.4 miles to Pfeiffer Big Sur State Park.

Los Padres Dam

■ ■ ■ ■ ■ ■ ■ ■ ■ ■ ■ ■ ■

Most of the northern Santa Lucia Range drains into the Carmel River. Above Los Padres Dam, the river flows as a small creek from the Church Creek Divide into Pine Valley, where it joins the waters from Pine Ridge, Ventana Cone, Uncle Sam Mountain, and Elephant Mountain. Before the dam was built, steelhead trout would migrate upstream from the Pacific to spawn. Landlocked rainbow trout still inhabit deep pools upstream. Two routes lead from the dam into the Carmel River watershed, each geared toward different seasons.

The Carmel River Trail offers a gentle descent south into the lush canyon, skirting the riverbanks and crossing several times. This popular route is ideal between May and October, when temperatures can soar into the 90s Fahrenheit. Sheltered beneath a shady riparian forest, the river offers drinking water and several refreshing swimming holes. In fall the colors are spectacular, low water makes for easier boulder hopping, and the fly, tick, and mosquito populations have diminished. Don't attempt this route after periods of heavy rain, as the river may be swift and dangerous to cross.

When the river is swelled, opt for the westbound Big Pines Trail, which leads to winter camps. Ambitious hikers can continue south toward Ventana Double Cone or west toward Bottchers Gap for a ridgetop circuit of the northern Ventana Wilderness. Breathtaking views abound.

DIRECTIONS: To reach the Los Padres Dam Trailhead from the north, drive 5.2 miles south of Carmel on Highway 1, then turn left and head eastbound on Carmel Valley Road (County Road G16). In 11.7 miles you'll reach the heart of Carmel Valley Village, your last opportunity for gas, food, and supplies. Continue through the village another 4.3 miles to the junction with the north end of Cachagua Road. Turn right and take this narrow paved road 5.9 miles to Nason Road. Turn right and drive 0.6 mile, passing the USFS Carmel River Station on your right. Park at the lot a minute farther on the right beside a locked gate.

From Southern California and the central Salinas Valley, leave Highway 101 at Greenfield and take Elm Avenue (County Road G16) 5.8 miles southwest to Arroyo Seco Road (County Road G17). The two roads merge for the next 6.5 miles until you

reach a fork. Take the right branch onto Carmel Valley Road (County Road G16) and drive 17 miles to the south end of Cachagua Road. Turn left, drive 1.3 miles to a junction with Tassajara Road, and then continue straight 4.5 miles to Nason Road. Turn left on Nason and drive 0.6 mile to the parking lot on the right just past the USFS Carmel River Station. There is no fee. There are no facilities or water at the station.

VISITOR CENTER: Big Sur Station: (831) 667-2315. The station is on Highway 1, a half mile south of Pfeiffer Big Sur State Park. Open daily 8 a.m.–6 p.m. Memorial Day through Labor Day, 8 a.m.–4:30 p.m. the rest of the year.

NEAREST CAMPGROUNDS: White Oaks Campground (7.9 miles along Tassajara Road) and China Camp (10.7 miles along Tassajara Road) are small USFS campgrounds open year-round on a first-come, first-serve basis. Both charge a $5 parking fee. Facilities include vault toilets, fire rings, and picnic tables. For more information contact the USFS Monterey District Headquarters at (831) 385-5434.

INFORMATION: No swimming allowed in Los Padres Reservoir. Fire permits required for all stoves. Dogs permitted and allowed off leash, except in designated campgrounds, where a 6-foot or shorter leash is required.

WEBSITE: www.fs.usda.gov/lpnf

PHONE: Los Padres National Forest Headquarters: (805) 968-6640

Trip 43

DANISH CREEK CAMP

LENGTH AND TYPE: 7.6-mile out-and-back

RATING: Moderate

TRAIL CONDITION: Passable, with narrow tread, poison oak, brush, and deadfalls

HIGHLIGHTS: Outstanding views of the Carmel River and Danish Creek watershed

TO REACH THE TRAILHEAD: This hike begins at the Los Padres Dam Trailhead.

TRIP SUMMARY: The Big Pines Trail ascends the ridge crest above Danish Creek, offering views deep into the Carmel River watershed. Beware of profuse low-lying poison oak along this stretch. From this ridge, the Danish Creek Camp Trail descends densely forested northern slopes to the canyon floor. Sites are nestled alongside the year-round creek. This spacious plot is the most easily reached camp from Los Padres Dam.

Trip Description

Pass through the gate at the end of the parking lot (1050'), where a trail sign points the way southwest toward **Los Padres Dam.** You'll hike a half mile along the one-lane dirt road, passing through an open grove of impressive lichen-draped valley and live oaks.

On a gentle ascent southeast, the trail reaches open ground with views west toward prominent **Blue Rock Ridge,** which parallels the **Big Pines Trail** above the reservoir. As the spillway and dam come into view (0.4 mile, 1180'), the trail branches left across the spillway, then leads toward the dam along the main road.

Pause atop **Los Padres Dam** (0.5 mile, 1120') to gaze south across the reservoir toward the **Carmel River** watershed. Skirting the lake, the road heads south, crossing a steep-walled gully lined with sycamore trees, easily identified by mottled cream-and-white bark that resembles a jigsaw puzzle. For 0.3 mile you'll climb steadily above the reservoir.

Equestrians should note the steep, narrow **spur road** (1.3 miles, 1090') that branches right from the main road and rejoins the Big Pines Trail. Used primarily as a horse trail, this 1.2-mile road does lead toward **Big Pines Camp** and cuts 0.7 mile off your route, but it presents a much steeper and more strenuous gradient.

A quarter mile farther you'll pass a road that branches left toward the reservoir and loops back to the main road. Continue straight ahead to a fork and veer right. The road soon narrows, becoming the **Carmel River Trail.** Keep watch for abundant poison oak along this narrow path. You'll climb 100 yards to the signed **Big Pines Trail junction** (1.8 miles, 1170').

Those bound for **Danish Creek, Rattlesnake Creek,** or **Big Pines/Bottchers Gap/Ventana Double Cone** will branch right (see TRIP 47 Ventana Double Cone via Big Pines Trail, page 187). While the tread is clear, the trail is severely overgrown with poison oak as it climbs switchbacks high above the western half of the reservoir to a chaparral-cloaked **ridge** (2.8 miles, 1920').

The Los Padres Dam prevents steelhead from migrating farther upstream.

Atop the open ridge, you'll arrive at a marked junction with the **Danish Creek Trail** (3 miles, 2050'). Here the trail branches left and descends toward **Danish Creek**. Though it's been a dry hike to this point, take heart, as the creek flows year-round.

Your descent begins on a gentle grade west through scrubby thickets, then turns south down a steep gully. In winter and early spring, a seasonal stream tumbles alongside the trail toward Danish Creek. After a 0.8-mile descent you'll reach **Danish Creek Camp** (3.8 miles, 1430'), set in a broad meadow amid creekside granite boulders.

Boasting colorful spring wildflowers and a canopy of oaks, madrones, and sycamores, the meadow is large enough to hold groups of up to a dozen tents. You'll find a timeworn table and cooking grate beneath a sprawling live oak, whose bark seems to be engulfing a granite boulder at its base. Be forewarned that mosquitoes and flies are thick in summer.

In colder months the south-facing campsites get a fair amount of sun. Watch for lizards and snakes, which slither amid the leaf litter to bask in the warm rays. Frequenting the creek's sunny banks are juvenile western skinks that flash bright blue tails, an adaptation that fools predators into attacking the detachable tail, allowing the skink to escape.

A few yards upstream a faint trail traces the creek's north bank. This unmaintained, heavily overgrown trail follows the creek, then scales the northwest walls of **Rattlesnake Creek** canyon on a nearly impassable route to **Rattlesnake Camp**.

DAM FIGHT ■

In 1995, California American Water, which owns the Los Padres Dam, reservoir, and adjacent lands, proposed construction of a new concrete dam to replace the current earthen dam. Critics argued that the $127 million project would mar the picturesque Carmel River Valley.

The proposed 28-story dam would drown 266 acres of habitat along Danish Creek and the Carmel River (including 24 acres in Ventana Wilderness), as well as 27 cultural and historic sites, many of which are sacred to the native Esselen tribe. It would also impact the migration of steelhead trout and destroy an estimated 90,000 trees and shrubs.

Fortunately, the Monterey Peninsula electorate voted down the project, though the fight will likely continue, as water—or the lack of it—has always driven state and local governments to quench the thirst of an ever-growing population.

■ ■

Trip 44

BLUFF & CARMEL RIVER CAMPS

LENGTH AND TYPE: 9.8-mile out-and-back

RATING: Easy to moderate

TRAIL CONDITION: Clear, poison oak, good for kids

HIGHLIGHTS: Experience wilderness solitude amid brilliant autumn colors, the gurgling Carmel River, and crystal clear wading pools.

TO REACH THE TRAILHEAD: This hike begins at the Los Padres Dam Trailhead.

TRIP SUMMARY: This route meanders through Carmel River canyon, lush with ferns and shaded by colorful deciduous trees. Those on day hikes or short weekend trips visit the riverside Bluff Camp, only 4.1 miles from the trailhead and big enough to hold a large group. Just 0.8 mile farther along the trail, the smaller Carmel River Camp lies at the confluence of Miller Creek and the Carmel River.

While summer temperatures and accompanying low water levels are best for hiking and swimming, flies are a constant annoyance, often swarming your eyes and ears. The wet season (November through April) brings an onslaught of ticks, which exploit the overgrown trail to hitchhike on unsuspecting hikers. Wet months also mean high water, which may end your hike at Bluff Camp, where a waist- to chest-high wade could be dangerous. Heavy storms can also rapidly swell the Carmel River and its tributaries, making the fords impassable.

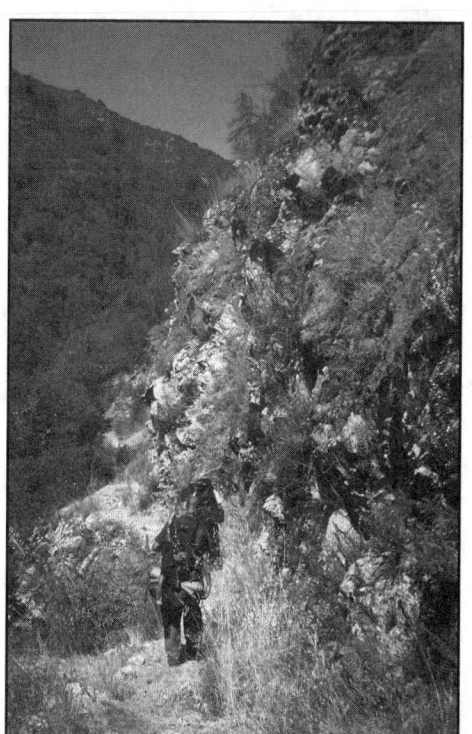

Trip Description

See TRIP 43 Danish Creek Camp (page 176) for the first 1.8 miles of this route to the signed **Big Pines Trail junction** (1170'). Those bound for **Danish Creek Camp, Rattlesnake Creek,** or **Big Pines/Bottchers Gap/Ventana Double Cone** will branch

Poison oak is common on the narrow spurs off the Carmel River Trail.

right here (see TRIP 43 Danish Creek Camp and TRIP 47 Ventana Double Cone via Big Pines Trail, page 187).

Instead, continue on the **Carmel River Trail,** which climbs high above the south end of the reservoir, emerging from dense forest dominated by live oak into drier brushy cover. A short descent on switchbacks leads down to **Danish Creek** (2.8 miles, 1050'), which flows east into the reservoir. In wet season you'll face a risky ford through high water. Although California American Water prohibits camping along the creek, there is an unofficial site along the south bank.

Crossing the creek, you'll soon reach a smaller perennial creek that cascades over a small granite-faced waterfall. One hundred yards past this creek a trail sign points south, 1 mile to **Bluff Camp** and 2 miles to **Miller Canyon** and **Carmel River Camp.** You'll climb above the river to a sharp turn cleared of vegetation, offering impressive views up the canyon to **Miller Mountain,** origin of the Carmel River's Bruce Fork.

The final 0.1 mile to Bluff Camp is entirely downhill. Less than 100 feet from camp you'll reach a junction. Though both paths descend into camp, the one that plunges straight ahead is steeper and only saves a few extra steps. The path on your left is a better choice, especially in late summer and fall when slippery dry leaves blanket the ground.

Bluff Camp (4.1 miles, 1150') is the only legal option on California American Water's private land. This delightful camp on the Carmel River offers three sites and a convenient swimming hole for a refreshing dunk. The first site lies along the west bank, adjacent to large granite boulders that border the swimming hole (3 to 4 feet deep in late spring and summer). Across the river lie the other two sites, which share a spacious bench on the east bank, large enough to accommodate a half dozen tents. An open canopy of alders and sycamores filters the sun.

Crossing the river can be a challenge. In summer and fall you can simply boulder-hop a small rock dam upstream. But in wetter months a wade is inevitable. During or after a rainstorm, crossing could involve a risky 2- to 5-foot ford across a swiftly rising river. Don't attempt to cross in such conditions.

Across the river, the trail climbs the narrow canyon to a minor ridge, leaving private land for the **Ventana Wilderness** (4.4 miles, 1430'). As you traverse the canyon's steep granite walls, the trail narrows due to washouts and erosion, requiring careful footing.

You'll soon wind back down to the signed **Miller Canyon Trail junction** (4.8 miles, 1220'), at the confluence of Miller Creek and the Carmel River. (For a description of the Miller Canyon Trail, see TRIP 48 Miller Canyon & Pine Valley Loop, page 195). Turn right at the junction and continue on the Carmel River Trail across the river to beautiful **Carmel River Camp** (4.5 miles, 1220').

Many hikers prefer this idyllic riverside camp over Sulphur Springs Camp and Buckskin Camp, farther along the Carmel River Trail. Depending on the season, you'll find a waist- to head-high swimming hole, especially welcome on hot summer days. The first two sites lie along the south bank beneath live oaks just past the confluence with Miller Creek. Each can accommodate two to three tents. Across the river lies the camp's main site, marked by a table, fire ring, and cooking grate. Just upstream from the main camp, the trail crosses the river again and follows a bend west to a smaller site beneath a filtering canopy of maples, sycamores, and alders.

Few people venture farther than Carmel River Camp, and poison oak encroaches on the little-used trail beyond. If you're continuing farther, refer to the following trip description.

ANGLER'S DELIGHT ■

Fishing season along the Carmel River centers on two species: steelhead in the lower sections in winter, and trout in the upper sections from spring through fall. From the last Saturday in April to November 15, only trout fishing is allowed from Los Padres Dam upstream. Resident rainbow and brown trout thrive at the confluence at Carmel River Camp. Your odds will improve the farther upstream you're willing to go.

You are restricted to artificial lures and barbless hooks. Anglers can keep up to five trout, though only two of those may be rainbows more than 10 inches in total length. There is no size restriction for brown trout. Visit the California Department of Fish & Game website for details: dfg.ca.gov.

■ ■

Trip 45

HIDING CANYON & ROUND ROCK CAMPS

LENGTH AND TYPE: 20.4-mile out-and-back, loop, or point-to-point

RATING: Strenuous

TRAIL CONDITION: Potentially impassable due to high water crossing along the Carmel River during the wet season, abundant poison oak, trail washouts, and faint tread

HIGHLIGHTS: Hike backcountry trails through narrow gorges, past waterfalls and deep swimming holes, to remote, peaceful camps.

TO REACH THE TRAILHEAD: This hike begins at the Los Padres Dam Trailhead.

TRIP SUMMARY: The Carmel River Trail offers numerous day-hiking and backpacking opportunities. Highlights along this 15.2-mile trail include Bluff, Carmel River, and Hiding

Canyon Camps, the gorge below Round Rock Camp, Pine Valley, and Pine Falls. (For a description of the upper Carmel River Trail, see TRIP 49 Pine Valley, page 199.)

The well-established yet overgrown trail meanders through the Carmel River canyon, carpeted with ferns and shaded by deciduous trees. The best time to hike this route is in fall, as temperatures are mild, water levels are low, ticks and flies have diminished, and autumn colors burst forth from mature sycamores, maples, oaks, and alders that line the river. Heavy rainfall may end your hike at Bluff Camp, as the Carmel River and its tributaries can rise a few feet, making passage hazardous. Be aware of changing weather conditions before entering the narrow canyon. If you're headed to Hiding Canyon Camp, regardless of the season, expect to forge or boulder-hop the river more than two dozen times. Walking sticks and river shoes are a big help.

Trip Description

See TRIP 44 Bluff & Carmel River Camps (page 179) for the first 4.5 miles of this route to **Carmel River Camp.**

Just upstream from the main site at Carmel River Camp (1220') the trail crosses the river and follows a bend west beneath a filtering canopy of maples, sycamores, and alders. Few people venture beyond the camp, and poison oak encroaches on the little-used trail beyond. At times, you may find yourself waist high in this highly toxic plant. Watch for the plant's distinctive three-leaf cluster. Hungry ticks also lay in wait for unsuspecting hikers. Wear long pants and check every few minutes for hitchhiking pests.

One of the most dramatic gorges in the wilderness is found just below Round Rock Camp.

For the most part, the tread is well established and easy to follow, except at a few of the numerous river fords. If you find yourself on anything other than an obvious trail, you've likely wandered off course. Simply backtrack until you rejoin the official trail.

After two more river crossings, you may catch whiffs of sulfur (similar to the smell of rotten eggs), your pungent introduction to **Sulphur Springs Camp** (5.8 miles, 1350'). Unfortunately, these hot springs rich in hydrogen sulfide are not large enough to soak in. One site is equipped with a table and cooking grate. This camp and Buckskin Flat Camp are the smallest and least attractive of the camps along the **Carmel River**. You're better off staying at Carmel River Camp or venturing farther to idyllic **Hiding Canyon Camp**. The latter lies just 3.4 miles from the trailhead but requires more than two dozen river crossings, which, depending on water levels, poison oak, flies, and ticks, can be an arduous trek.

From Sulphur Springs, the trail crosses a year-round creek that originates from the east slope of **Elephant Mountain,** which forms the granite southwest wall of the Carmel River drainage 4020 feet above. Upstream, you'll cross five more times amid riparian woodlands dominated by bigleaf maples, black oaks, sycamores, and alders before arriving in **Buckskin Flat Camp** (7.4 miles, 1580'). Marked by a sign, the riverside site sits atop a grassy flat. There is no table or cooking grate.

In fall, leaves bearing deep hues of yellow, orange, and red blanket the forest floor and surface pools. It's the perfect season to hike the river, as water levels remain low and you can boulder-hop its course with ease.

AUTUMN COLORS EXPLAINED ■ ■ ■ ■ ■ ■ ■ ■ ■ ■ ■ ■ ■ ■

Every autumn, brilliant hues paint the canyon floor along the Carmel River. Many changes occur in the leaf of a deciduous tree before it falls from the branch. The process begins in the abscission layer, where the leaf and stem connect.

In fall, plant hormones respond to diminished daylight, swelling the cells of the abscission layer and forming a cork-like material that gradually cuts off flow between the leaf and the tree. Deprived of water and nutrients, the leaves stop producing green-hued chlorophyll and other colors become visible. Oranges come from carotene, yellows from xanthophyll, bright reds and purples from anthocyanin, and browns from tannins. As the abscission layer continues to swell, the cells disintegrate until the leaf either falls or is blown from the tree.

The process is an energy-saving strategy. Without their leaves, trees are able to go dormant in the winter. Other than limited root growth, their biological processes come to a temporary halt.

SIDE TRIP ■

Although Round Rock Camp is not the most ideal backcountry camp, the gorge in which it rests is among the most beautiful in the Santa Lucia Range. The 0.6-mile Round Rock Camp Trail leads to the canyon floor, where the swift river plunges from pool to pool, carving its deep path between massive smooth granite walls.

From the junction, descend 0.2 mile to the river and make your way downstream 50 feet. Be mindful of slippery boulders and poison oak, which recoils in the fissures. The sounds of cascading water echo up from the gorge below. Enjoy the solitude as you take a bracing dip in the headwaters of the Carmel River.

You'll cross the river to a small grassy terrace and unofficial campsite—actually, more picturesque than camp proper. The trail climbs 0.2 mile, then descends south past riverside tangles of blackberry and poison oak. The overgrown yet established trail crosses the river just downstream from an enormous boulder, perhaps Round Rock itself, which looms over a shallow wading pool. A couple hundred feet later you'll reach Round Rock Camp (10.2 miles, 1920'), with a table and room enough for up to a dozen small tents atop a grassy terrace.

■ ■

Past Buckskin Flat Camp, you'll climb 0.3 mile to a small ridge, then return to the river's edge for a gradual ascent that at times feels more like a continual wade. The trail launches into another series of river fords, crisscrossing through mats of blackberries, thimbleberries, and ubiquitous poison oak. Head-high chain ferns shade still pools, while horsetail rushes and mosses grow in spongy clumps between granite boulders.

Past the tenth ford, the trail passes a significant canyon and tributary that stem from **Uncle Sam Mountain,** the massive granite ridge looming more than 4750 feet overhead. Swift runoff from this major peak follows the **Church Creek Fault,** among the largest fault systems in the **Ventana Wilderness,** whose shattered course provides a natural channel. If you're on your way to **Round Rock Camp,** you'll observe this northwest-trending fault in deep channels and waterfall basins along the Carmel River.

The twelfth crossing skirts a moss-covered granite wall—be aware that both the USGS and USFS maps inaccurately label this the site of Hiding Canyon Camp, which lies 0.2 mile farther upstream. Expect to get your feet wet in all but the driest months, as the trail is often submerged by high water.

True to its name, **Hiding Canyon Camp** (9.2 miles, 1740') is easy to miss. You'll reach the turnoff just as the trail leaves the river's edge to climb the canyon. Just across the river, the camp offers two large sites, each with a table and cooking grate. The first site sits atop a narrow terrace along the west bank. The larger, preferred site is just a few feet upstream near an enormous ponderosa pine with a 6-foot-plus diameter. You'll recognize ponderosas by their golden puzzle-piece bark and pine needles bunched in threes.

If you're willing to hike upriver off trail for 0.4 mile, you'll pass through a narrow sandstone gorge and arrive at **Ventana Mesa Creek Falls,** which tumbles into a swimming hole. Farther upriver, the canyon widens and turns south, entering a second gorge at the confluence with **Ventana Mesa Creek.** A few feet farther upstream the creek cascades into a deep granite-lined pool. If the water level is low enough in late summer and fall, you can press on for 200 feet to a larger swimming hole and waterfall within a mossy, fern-lined grotto. The refreshingly cold water is a welcome escape on a hot summer day.

From Hiding Canyon Camp, the Carmel River Trail continues across the river and ascends the east-facing canyon wall. Climb 0.1 mile to a stunning overlook of the narrow river gorge. The trail leads up a minor ridge to the easily missed unmarked **Round Rock Camp Trail junction** (9.6 miles, 2030'). If you're continuing on the Carmel River Trail, refer to TRIP 50 Hiding Canyon & Round Rock Camps (page 202) and follow that trail description in reverse.

Trip 46

VENTANA DOUBLE CONE VIA CARMEL RIVER TRAIL

LENGTH AND TYPE: 31-mile out-and-back, loop, or point-to-point

RATING: Challenging

TRAIL CONDITION: Potentially impassable due to high water crossing along the Carmel River Trail during the wet season, with abundant poison oak. Passable yet difficult with deadfalls, washouts, and brush encroachment along Ventana Double Cone Trail.

HIGHLIGHTS: Find solitude atop 4853-foot Ventana Double Cone as you soak up panoramic views of the furrowed Santa Lucia Range and broad Pacific.

TO REACH THE TRAILHEAD: This hike begins at the Los Padres Dam Trailhead.

TRIP SUMMARY: This book describes several routes to the remote summit of Ventana Double Cone, in the heart of Ventana Wilderness. For general information on the Ventana Trail, see the summary for TRIP 38 Ventana Double Cone via Ventana Trail (page 155).

From Los Padres Dam, this route ascends the cool Carmel River canyon along year-round sections of the river to Hiding Canyon Camp, where it begins a steep 3113-foot climb over 6.3 miles to the summit. Watch for poison oak.

As at most peaks along this dramatic coast, the best times to hike are between mid-November and April, taking advantage of cooler temperatures, fogless days, and fewer pesky mosquitoes and flies. This route is also a good choice in summer heat and fall drought, as from Hiding Canyon Camp you can reach the summit with a daypack and plenty of water.

Be prepared for rain and snow if you hike in winter, when snow levels can drop to 2000 feet and the river may be impassable.

Trip Description

See TRIP 44 Bluff & Carmel River Camps (page 179) for the first 4.9 miles of this route to **Carmel River Camp.**

Just upstream from the main site at Carmel River Camp (1220') the trail crosses the river and follows a bend west beneath a filtering canopy of maples, sycamores, and alders. Few people venture beyond the camp, and poison oak encroaches on the little-used trail beyond. Hungry ticks also lay in wait—wear long pants and check every few minutes for hitchhikers.

After two more river crossings, you'll reach **Sulphur Springs Camp** (5.8 miles, 1350'). This and Buckskin Flat Camp are the smallest and least attractive of the camps along the **Carmel River.** Instead, stay at Carmel River Camp or **Hiding Canyon Camp.** The latter lies just 3.4 miles from the trailhead but requires more than two dozen river crossings, which, depending on the season, can be an arduous trek.

From Sulphur Springs, the trail crosses a year-round creek that originates from the east slope of **Elephant Mountain.** Heading upstream, you'll cross five more times before arriving in **Buckskin Flat Camp** (7.4 miles, 1580'), atop a grassy flat. There is no table or cooking grate.

Past camp, you'll climb 0.3 mile to a small ridge, then return to the river's edge for a gradual ascent. The trail launches into another series of river fords, crisscrossing through mats of blackberries, thimbleberries, and ubiquitous poison oak. Past the tenth ford, the trail passes a significant canyon and tributary that stem from **Uncle Sam Mountain,** the massive granite ridge towering more than 4750 feet overhead.

The twelfth crossing skirts a moss-covered granite wall—be aware that both the USGS and USFS maps inaccurately label this the site of Hiding Canyon Camp, which lies 0.2 mile farther upstream. Expect to get your feet wet in all but the driest months, as the trail is often submerged by high water.

The spur to Hiding Canyon Camp (9.2 miles, 1740') is easy to miss. You'll reach the turnoff just as the trail leaves the river's edge to climb the canyon. Just across the river, you'll find two large sites with a table and cooking grate. The first site sits atop a narrow terrace along the west bank, while the second, larger site is just a few feet upstream near an enormous ponderosa pine.

If you're willing to hike upriver off trail for 0.4 mile, you'll pass through a narrow sandstone gorge and arrive at **Ventana Mesa Creek Falls,** which tumbles into a swimming hole. Farther upriver, the canyon widens and turns south, entering a second gorge at the confluence with **Ventana Mesa Creek.** A few feet farther upstream the creek cascades into a deep granite-lined pool. If the water level is low enough in late summer and fall, you can press on for 200 feet to a larger swimming hole and waterfall within a mossy, fern-lined grotto.

The **Puerto Suelo Trail** (9.2 miles, 1740') begins atop a flat bench on the west bank just downstream from Hiding Canyon Camp. Those bound for **Ventana Double Cone** or **Bottchers Gap** will climb this trail to the **Ventana Trail junction.** In drought years it's best to fill water bottles here.

You'll begin a steep climb west through a minor gully and across a small creek, then wander through several other minor gullies, dry practically year-round. In half a mile the trail begins a series of switchbacks, ascending a brushy slope to a minor saddle. Continue past fragrant stands of bays and tanoaks and across small tributaries to **Uncle Sam Creek.** The trail crosses and then recrosses the creek, which may be your last opportunity for water between here and the summit.

Continue climbing northwest through overgrown ceanothus thickets. The last 0.3 mile of the Puerto Suelo Trail ascends very steep, short switchbacks. Just 0.1 mile from the saddle, clear water bubbles up from two neighboring springs, reliable in all but the driest months.

Climb the final 200 feet to the Puerto Suelo saddle and Ventana Trail junction (11.8 miles, 3530'). See TRIP 38 Ventana Double Cone via Ventana Trail (page 155) for the final 3.7 miles to the summit (15.5 miles, 4853').

Trip 47

VENTANA DOUBLE CONE VIA BIG PINES TRAIL

LENGTH AND TYPE: 35.4-mile out-and-back, loop, or point-to-point

RATING: Strenuous to challenging

TRAIL CONDITION: Difficult with deadfalls, washouts, and brush encroachment

HIGHLIGHTS: Find serenity atop this summit with breathtaking views of a vast wilderness.

TO REACH THE TRAILHEAD: This hike begins at the Los Padres Dam Trailhead.

TRIP SUMMARY: This book describes several routes to the remote 4853-foot summit of Ventana Double Cone, in the heart of Ventana Wilderness. For general information on the Ventana Trail, see the summary for TRIP 38 Ventana Double Cone via Ventana Trail.

This route offers a consistent grade and spectacular views, particularly in winter and spring. Be aware that the first 4 miles are overrun with poison oak, and developed trails along the fire break make the trail difficult and confusing to follow.

Although Ventana Wilderness offers hundreds of dog-friendly hiking trails, be aware that poison oak can also be carried on animals' fur.

As at most peaks along this dramatic coast, the best times to hike are between mid-November and April, taking advantage of cooler temperatures, fogless days, and fewer pesky mosquitoes and flies. Be prepared for rain and snow if you hike in winter, when snow levels can drop to 2000 feet and the river may be impassable.

During the driest months (August through November), you may not find water until Big Pines Camp (upper Danish Creek) or Pat Spring. In drought years there's even a chance these two water sources could run dry. In such conditions, consider one of the alternative routes.

Trip Description

See TRIP 43 Danish Creek Camp (page 176) for the first 3 miles of this route to the signed **Danish Creek Trail junction** (2050').

From this junction, the **Danish Creek Trail** branches left and descends to **Danish Creek Camp** (3.8 miles, 1430'), set in a broad meadow beside year-round **Danish Creek** (see TRIP 43 Danish Creek Camp). You'll continue straight through this junction on the **Big Pines Trail,** skirt a minor summit, and follow the ridgeline on a narrow overgrown trail for the next 0.3 mile.

You'll soon cross a steep overgrown **jeep road** (3.3 miles, 2110'), more commonly used as a horse trail, which angles right and descends 2.6 miles to **Los Padres Dam.** A few paces past the road you'll reach an oak-rimmed grassy ridge. In spring the black oaks sprout vibrant foliage amid a brilliant blanket of flowering poppies, lupines, shooting stars, and deer vetches.

The trail widens and follows an old road that climbs the Danish Creek watershed from saddle to ridge. For the most part, you'll have to scrape past encroaching chamise, sage, and broom, so check often for ticks, particularly during the wet season.

You'll quickly pass another old **jeep road junction** (3.4 miles, 2500') on your left. Also used as a horse trail, this road leads southwest to Danish Creek, 0.3 mile upstream from Danish Creek Camp. Onward 0.3 mile, you'll reach a third **spur road** (3.7 miles, 2650'), which doglegs right and heads first north-northeast through dense madrone and oak forests, then northwest on a gravel road to **Blue Rock Ridge.**

Bypassing these spurs, the Big Pines Trail continues west across forested slopes and exposed brush-covered ridges. After a moderate climb that almost tops a 2778-foot ridge, the trail switchbacks and descends to a minor **saddle** (4.9 miles, 2640') capped by a bare outcrop of pale-green serpentine, California's state rock. The unobstructed views from this open ridge are outstanding, stretching northwest across **Monterey Bay** and the **Santa Lucia Range,** which rise abruptly from the wave-washed Pacific. A short climb from the saddle you'll reach the signed **Ventana Wilderness Boundary** (5 miles, 2680').

CALIFORNIA'S STATE ROCK ■ ■ ■ ■ ■ ■ ■ ■ ■ ■ ■ ■ ■ ■ ■ ■

Rare elsewhere on Earth, serpentine is common in California, scattered across some 2200 square miles. Originally part of the ocean floor, serpentine was thrust to the surface during ancient shifts in the Earth's crust. Intense heat and pressure metamorphosed the rock into a smooth, sometimes soapy green stone.

Due to its unique chemical composition, serpentine supports equally unusual plant species. In addition to a low water-holding capacity, soil derived from serpentine is low in calcium, phosphorous, and nitrogen and high in such toxic heavy metals as magnesium, chromium, and nickel. Most plants simply cannot tolerate these conditions.

Regardless, certain "serpentine endemics" have adapted to this soil and thrive on these shallow rocky outcrops. The rare vegetation in turn attracts birds, reptiles, amphibians, and mammals that may otherwise not be in the area. Slowly stroll across these barrens for glimpses of a rare ecosystem.

■ ■

Following the ridge up a gentle grade, you'll soon begin a steep half-mile descent south to a minor **saddle** (5.8 miles, 2250'). The route crosses forested slopes of oaks, pines, and madrones, the latter distinguished by deep red flaky bark that peels back to expose a smooth orange trunk. Past the saddle, the trail skirts waist-high brush, ascends 0.2 mile west to a 2525-foot ridge summit, then quickly descends to a saddle within earshot of Danish Creek.

From here you'll begin the second largest climb on the Big Pines Trail, first across dry slopes covered in thickets of manzanita, ceanothus, and chamise and then beneath dense madrone canopies. Again, watch for profuse amounts of poison oak—thankfully, the last concentration of this toxic trailside companion en route to **Ventana Double Cone.** The steep ascent ends after a few switchbacks, emerging amid chaparral brush atop a 3097-foot **ridge summit** (7.2 miles).

From the summit, the trail begins a gentle descent that branches away from the roadbed within 0.1 mile (7.3 miles, 3020'). While orange flagging marked this turn on my hike, it remains an easily overlooked left turn through a narrow stretch of scrub oak, bay, and ceanothus thickets. If you miss the turn and continue along the roadbed 50 feet, you'll reach a maze of narrow overgrown deer trails that lack the packed tread of the well-established Big Pines Trail.

From the turnoff, you'll descend south past steep slopes with numerous deadfalls and encroaching brush to a minor saddle, then descend farther to another minor saddle (7.8 miles, 2980'). From here the trail ascends through shady hardwood forests past scattered young pines a few hundred yards above Danish Creek's gurgling headwaters.

Over the next 0.2 mile the trail narrows between fire-scarred pine snags, a target of industrious woodpeckers, which excavate their nests in spring in large snags. You'll follow the contour to a nearby **gully** (8 miles, 3220'), home to a small granite-lined creek between December and March. A few yards farther you'll cross another seasonal tributary and clamber across a tangle of downed debris. The trail passes a third seasonal creek (8.1 miles, 3260'), climbs beneath the remnants of a pre–Basin Complex pine forest, crosses a grassy bowl, and in 50 yards reaches the **Big Pines Camp Trail junction** (8.8 miles, 3350'). After the 2008 Basin Complex Fire, little remains of the camp, and the trail is deemed challenging at best. From this junction, the main trail continues straight and contours southwest 0.1 mile to another junction (8.9 miles, 3340'). Here you'll find a shortcut spur toward **Pat Spring Camp.** Fire destroyed trail signage, but with a watchful eye you can spot carved into the sign assurance of Pat Spring and the Ventana Trail.

If you skip the recommended shortcut, you'll continue west on the Big Pines Trail, climb briefly, then cross a seasonal tributary, the nearest water source to **Spaghetti Camp** (expect water from first rains through March). After a moderate 0.1-mile ascent beneath shady oaks, madrones, and pines, you'll arrive in camp.

Spaghetti Camp (9.1 miles, 3620') also marks the junction with the **Skinner Ridge Trail** (which leads west 6.3 miles to **Bottchers Gap**) and the Ventana Trail (which leads south 8.4 miles to Ventana Double Cone). Camp is flat and can easily accommodate two tents. The nearest reliable water source between December and March is upper Danish Creek, 0.1 mile along the Big Pines Trail, while during dry months (May through November) you may have to hike as far as Pat Spring, a mile along the Ventana Trail.

From camp the Ventana Trail crosses oak- and pine-clad slopes, skirting mounds of fallen snags and woody debris. You may surprise quail, woodpeckers, and band-tailed pigeons along this little-used trail. Half a mile later you'll reach an unmarked junction with the previously described shortcut spur from the Big Pines Trail.

Continue half a mile farther past the unofficial camp to a major saddle and four-way **junction** (10.1 miles, 3770') with the westbound Pat Spring Camp Trail and eastbound Pat Spring Trail.

See TRIP 38 Ventana Double Cone via Ventana Trail (page 155) for a description of the remaining 7.6 miles from this junction to the summit of Ventana Double Cone.

SIDE TRIP ■

You can save yourself time and energy by taking the shortcut toward **Pat Spring Camp** (8.9 miles, 3340'), which leads 0.4 mile to the **Pat Spring Trail**. The shortcut spur is on your left, 20 feet from the Big Pines Trail sign. It begins as a narrow trail that descends southwest 0.1 mile across the creek's upper headwaters (9 miles, 3290'). Fifty feet farther the trail climbs from the gully to the **Ventana Trail junction**. Look for the inconspicuous VENTANA LOOKOUT TRAIL sign posted on a tree trunk and turn left.

One hundred yards eastbound on the **Ventana Trail**, you'll reach an **unofficial camp,** just off the trail on your left. Shaded by large pines and madrones, the first site is perched alongside the south branch of Danish Creek, though it's often dry by late spring. The second site lies just above the creek on the opposite bank. Together the sites can accommodate a half dozen tents. If this stretch is dry, you can either head back to the last creek crossing or continue on the Ventana Trail and camp closer to **Pat Spring.**

Onward, you'll make a gentle 0.1-mile-ascent to a minor saddle and the easily missed four-way junction with westbound **Pat Spring Camp Trail** and eastbound Pat Spring Trail (9.7 miles, 3770').

■ ■

China Camp

■ ■ ■ ■ ■ ■ ■ ■ ■ ■ ■ ■ ■

NESTLED AT 4270 FEET in a prominent saddle beneath a dense canopy of oaks and madrones, China Camp offers one of the easiest access points to Ventana's high country. This chapter also describes lower-elevation routes off Tassajara Road, along the Church Creek, Horse Pasture, and Tony Trails. Tassajara Road may be closed during storms due to fallen trees or small mudslides. Two routes extend from China Camp: the westbound Pine Ridge Trail and the northwest-bound Miller Canyon Trail.

Although the Pine Ridge Trail is the most heavily used path in the backcountry, most people begin from Big Sur and never reach Pine Ridge. This eastern section of the trail is remote, challenging, and strenuous, offering a trek across diverse terrain with sweeping panoramas of the vast wilderness. The route from China Camp suffers from encroaching brush, and few people hike farther than Pine Valley, whose dramatic sandstone cliffs shelter a spectacular waterfall and pine-studded meadow. This is the most direct route to the Black Cone Trail, but be prepared for a heavily overgrown path from Divide Camp to the north end of the Black Cone Trail atop Pine Ridge. Much of this terrain is intolerable in summer, when nagging flies swarm and temperatures soar into the upper 90s Fahrenheit.

From spring through fall, the Carmel River and Miller Canyon Trails offer pleasant routes downriver, though both trails are cloaked with poison oak. The trailhead for the Church Creek Trail lies in the heart of the wilderness, 5 miles beyond China Camp along Tassajara Road. The only trail that ascends the Church Creek drainage, it takes in some of Ventana's most dramatic sandstone outcrops.

DIRECTIONS: Heading south on Highway 1 from Monterey, turn left on Carmel Valley Road (County Road G16) in Carmel and head eastbound. In 11.7 miles you'll reach Carmel Valley Village, your last opportunity for gas, food, and supplies. Drive through the village and continue another 11.3 miles to the Tassajara Road junction.

Heading north on Highway 101 from Southern California, turn off on Route 101 Business, Greenfield's southernmost exit. In half a mile you'll turn left on Elm Avenue (County Road G16) and head southwest 5.8 miles to Arroyo Seco Road (County Road

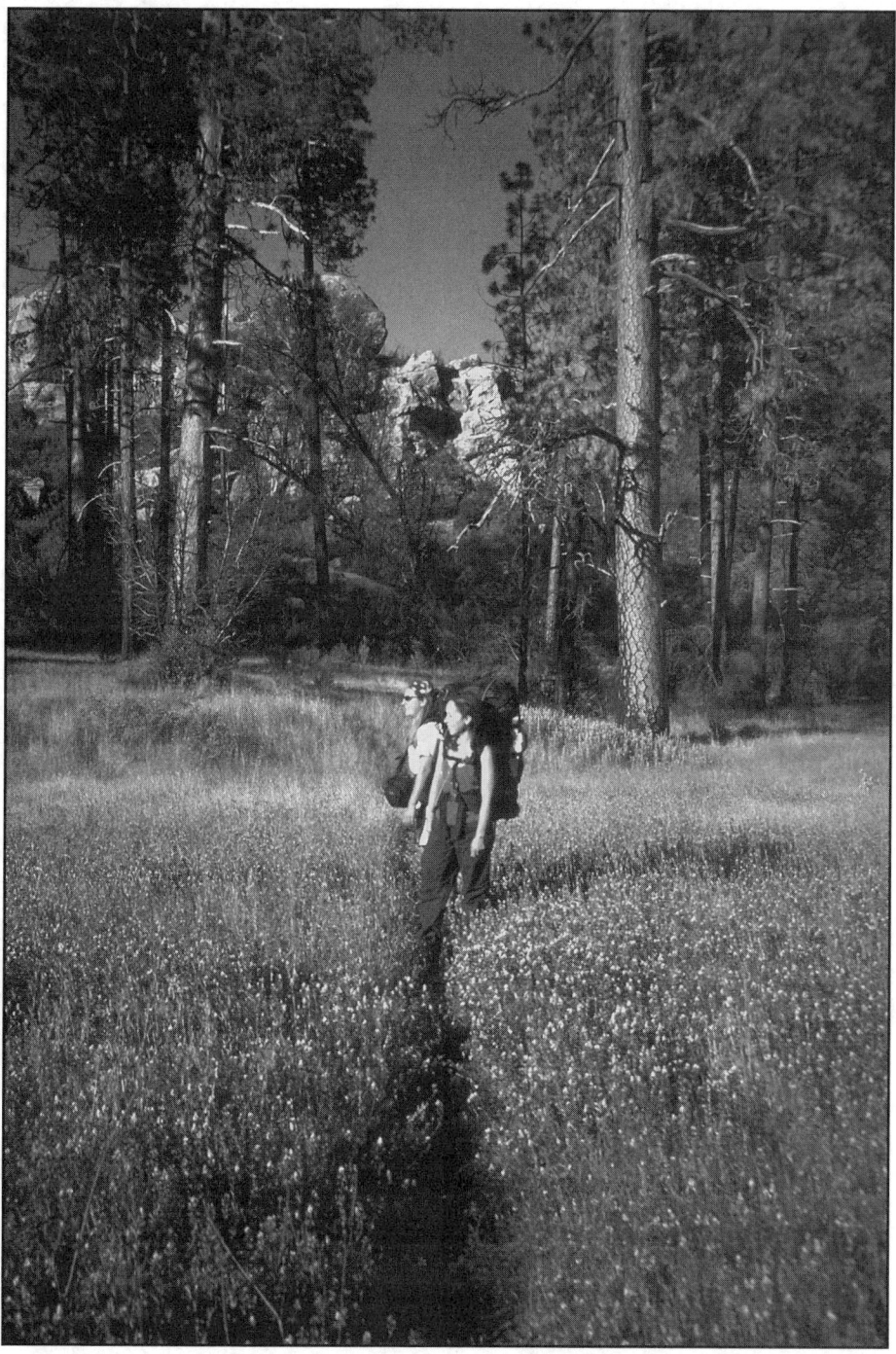

Towering ponderosa pines in the open meadow of Pine Valley.

G17). The two roads merge for 6.5 miles and then fork. Take the right branch and continue 17 miles northwest on Carmel Valley Road to the Tassajara Road junction.

From the Tassajara Road junction, turn southwest and drive 1.3 miles to a fork with Cachagua Road. Take the left branch and continue 10.7 miles along Tassajara Road to the China Camp entrance. The pavement ends 1.8 miles from the junction, and 7.6 miles farther you'll pass White Oaks Campground (for details see Nearest Campground below). From there it's 1.3 miles to the entrance road at China Camp.

To reach the campground, hang a sharp right off Tassajara Road and drive 200 feet. If you're not camping, park in the small lot across Tassajara Road from the camp entrance.

VISITOR CENTER: Big Sur Station: (831) 667-2315. The station is on Highway 1, 4.2 miles south of Andrew Molera State Park and just south of Pfeiffer Big Sur State Park. Open daily 8 a.m.–6 p.m. Memorial Day through Labor Day, 8 a.m.–4:30 p.m. the rest of the year. USFS Monterey District Headquarters, King City: (831) 385-5434.

NEAREST CAMPGROUNDS: Two small USFS campgrounds, White Oaks Campground (7.9 miles along Tassajara Road) and China Camp (10.7 miles along Tassajara Road), are open year-round on a first-come, first-serve basis (6 sites; free). Facilities include vault toilets, fire rings, and picnic tables. There is no water available at the campgrounds.

INFORMATION: There's no fee if you park at the turnout on Tassajara Road directly across from the China Camp entrance. Fire permits are required for all stoves. Dogs are permitted and allowed off leash, except in designated campgrounds, where a 6-foot or shorter leash is required.

WEBSITE: www.fs.usda.gov/lpnf

PHONE: Los Padres National Forest Headquarters: (805) 968-6640

Trip 48

MILLER CANYON & PINE VALLEY LOOP

LENGTH AND TYPE: 24.1-mile loop

RATING: Strenuous

TRAIL CONDITION: Difficult to impassable, poison oak, faint tread, trail washouts

HIGHLIGHTS: This loop takes in deep narrow river gorges rich in ferns and lined with colorful hardwoods where you'll find waterfall oases and pristine swimming holes.

TO REACH THE TRAILHEAD: Park at the large turnout on Tassajara Road across from China Camp, then stroll to the end of the entrance road. The trailhead is at the junction with gated Jeffery Road. There is no water at the trailhead.

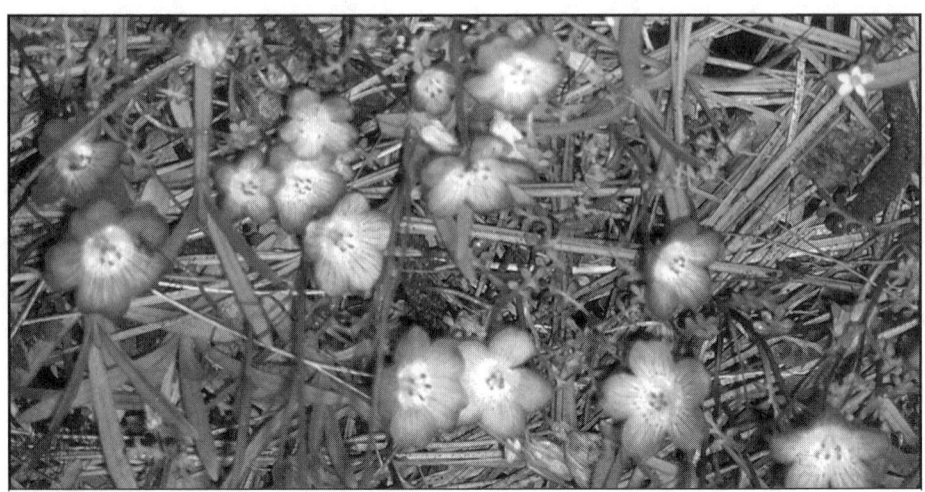

The recently charred landscape within Miller Canyon brought nutrients back into the soil to allow forest succession to begin anew.

TRIP SUMMARY: This route offers several loop, out-and-back, and point-to-point options. The following description comprises a loop through Miller Canyon to the Carmel River confluence, up Pine Valley to the river's headwaters at Church Creek Divide, then back to China Camp via the Pine Ridge Trail. This order assumes hikers will spend the final night in scenic Pine Valley, followed by a 2000-foot climb over the remaining 5.3 miles. Taking the reverse route would mean spending the last night at less scenic Miller Canyon Camp, followed by a nearly 3000-foot climb over the final 7.1 miles to the trailhead.

If you can arrange a shuttle vehicle, an excellent 15-mile point-to-point hike leads from China Camp along Miller Canyon and the Carmel River to Los Padres Dam. Highlights include scenic views from golden oak savannas and stays at the riverside Carmel River and Bluff Camps.

Miller and Carmel River Canyons are most pleasant in fall, when the lush hardwood forests turn brilliant hues of yellow, orange, and crimson. In late summer and fall, ticks, flies, and mosquitoes have diminished and temperatures are ideal for wading the creeks and rivers. After heavy winter storms, easy boulder-hopping crossings can turn swift and dangerous. In spring the broad meadows and open savannas are blanketed in wildflowers and vibrant new growth. Unfortunately, regardless of the season, the bottomland trails are heavily overgrown with poison oak.

Trip Description

Head northwest along gated **Jeffery Road** (4270') past sprawling oaks, peeling red madrones, and towering Coulter pines. The latter boast the world's heaviest cones. After a moderate mile-long descent, the road reaches a seasonal stretch of the **Miller Fork,** usually dry from May until the first winter rains. In a quarter mile you'll enter private property, posted by the Tanoak homeowners association. Follow the road past several private driveways, another seasonal branch of the Miller Fork, and the Tamarack homes' pond, then descend 0.1 mile to a second gate (1.8 miles, 3400'). Beyond this gate the route enters the **Ventana Wilderness**.

Continue 0.1 mile along the road until it doglegs sharply right and begins a steep climb east. The trail begins at this sharp turn, leading 0.1 mile to a junction with another road. Fifty feet down this road, you'll reach a fork. Take the left branch. The road ends at the **Miller Canyon Trail junction** (2 miles, 3360').

Miller Canyon Trail branches right 150 feet to another gate. Pass through the gate for a gentle descent toward a minor gorge that parallels **Miller Canyon.** The trail closely follows the Miller Canyon Fault northwest. Contouring above the minor canyon, the trail returns to private property along the banks of an alder-lined creek (3 miles, 2880'), where you'll find a few unofficial camps. Don't expect to find water during the dry season (May through October).

From the creek, the trail climbs to a series of minor saddles offering fine views. Atop the third saddle, the trail descends 0.3 mile to a more dependable creek that usually flows through early summer. Here you'll find the **Nason Cabin site** (4.3 miles, 3090'), featuring scattered homestead relics along a small creekside clearing. The site also hosts an unofficial camp. Beyond this point the already narrow trail suffers from overgrown brush and destructive washouts. In wet season, hitchhiking ticks are prolific.

The trail climbs to a fourth saddle for oak-filtered views along the **Carmel River** and Miller Fork, featuring fire-scarred ridges and cleft gullies that shelter rare Santa Lucia firs. A range of textures and hues distinguish the distinct plant communities. Along the canyon floors, lush deciduous forests flash vibrant green in the spring and deep orange, red, and yellow in the fall.

From the fourth saddle (4.9 miles, 3070'), the trail steadily descends 2.2 miles to **Miller Canyon Camp,** leading past a sixth saddle and through a minor gully. In wet months the trail crosses a nettle-lined seasonal creek beneath a small waterfall. Continue 150 feet to the **Hennickson Trail junction** (6.4 miles, 2420').

Although the US Forest Service has abandoned the **Hennickson Trail** to the elements, hikers still pass this way. The route rockets up 900 feet in 2 miles along a brushy waterless trail to the **Tin House** on **Hennickson Ridge.**

Past the junction, the Miller Canyon Trail continues past endemic stands of Santa Lucia firs, easily identified by densely foliated crowns that extend from the base of the tree and lower branches that nearly touch the ground. The trail descends 0.4 mile past talus slopes to a small seasonal tributary and a 20-foot waterfall that flows from the first winter rains until summer.

The trail follows this small tributary through its narrow gorge, crossing it a second time through shoulder-high thickets of stinging nettles. This invasive nonnative plant features clusters of small white flowers that bloom from the base of stinging pubescent leaves.

A few hundred yards past the stinging nettles, the trail approaches the Miller Fork for the first of 20 crossings. After heavy winter storms, these fords become increasingly swift and dangerous downstream. In all other seasons it's an easy boulder-hop across to **Miller Canyon Camp** (7.1 miles, 2000').

This is the larger of two official camps along the Miller Canyon Trail. The first site is perched atop the east end of a creekside bench a few yards from the crossing, marked by a dilapidated LOS PADRES NATIONAL FOREST sign, a table, and a fire ring. A hundred feet farther, the second site sits atop the west end of the bench and is large enough to accommodate up to two tents.

Beyond camp the trail leads 0.1 mile to the first major river bend and your second boulder-hop across the Miller Fork. You'll follow an old roadbed heavily overgrown with poison oak and cross the river three more times before arriving in **Clover Basin Camp** (7.7 miles, 1870').

This camp occupies a large meadow amid a marshy basin near the banks of the Miller Fork. Equipped with a fire ring and tree stump seating, the camp can accommodate up to four tents. Mosquitoes and flies can be a nuisance in all but the driest months. American Indians roamed this watershed for thousands of years, as evidenced by mortar holes in rocks adjacent to camp. Here the Esselen tribe hunted a wide variety of birds, fish, and mammals and gathered a variety of acorns to leach and grind into flour.

Past camp, you'll closely follow the Miller Fork, occasionally picking your way through unavoidable thickets of poison oak. The trail meanders along the deep, narrow river gorge blanketed in ferns, mugwort, and blackberries, as well as colorful alders, maples, buckeyes, and bays. You'll cross the river 16 more times before reaching the **Carmel River Trail junction** (10.2 miles, 1220').

From this junction, the trail crosses the Miller Fork just above its confluence and returns upstream to China Camp along the **Carmel River** and **Pine Ridge Trails**. See TRIP 45 Hiding Canyon & Round Rock Camps (page 181) for the route description to **Hiding Canyon Camp** and TRIP 50 Hiding Canyon & Round Rock Camps (page 202) for the route from Hiding Canyon to China Camp (follow the latter in reverse). If you're on a point-to-point trip from China Camp to **Los Padres Dam**, continue downstream along the Carmel River Trail 4.8 miles below the confluence to the Los Padres Dam Trailhead. Refer to TRIP 44 Bluff & Carmel River Camps (page 179) and follow that trail description in reverse.

Trip 49

PINE VALLEY

LENGTH AND TYPE: 12-mile out-and-back

RATING: Moderate

TRAIL CONDITION: Passable to difficult, poison oak

HIGHLIGHTS: Tall ponderosas amid an open meadow, ancient sandstone cliffs, buttes, and boulders, and Pine Falls, which cascades 50 feet into an emerald swimming hole

TO REACH THE TRAILHEAD: Park at the large turnout on Tassajara Road across from China Camp. The trailhead is on the camp side of the road, 100 feet south of the parking lot and 150 feet south of the camp entrance. The trail begins on a saddle above China Camp. It is marked, though encroaching brush often obscures the sign. There's no water at the trailhead.

TRIP SUMMARY: This trail leads past old-growth pine forests, waterfall oases that shelter deep swimming holes, and wildflower-strewn meadows that remind one of the Sierras. Naturally, this is a popular year-round day hike, so it's best to avoid it during major holidays. Though the valley lies within day-hike range, allow at least six hours for the round-trip to enjoy the scenery or visit Pine Falls for a refreshing swim. The route is ideal in spring and fall,

as temperatures are moderate and storms infrequent. Summer temps can reach the upper 90s Fahrenheit, and flies and mosquitoes pose a nuisance. Winter temps can dip below freezing, and snow is common above 4000 feet. If your timing is perfect, however, between winter storms the valley can hit the upper 60s Fahrenheit, and you'll likely have the valley all to yourself.

Trip Description

The route begins at a marked trailhead on a major saddle above **China Camp** (4350'), 6 miles from **Pine Valley** and 24 from **Big Sur.** Like most trails in the **Ventana Wilderness,** this one is not regularly maintained.

Pine Falls cascades 50 feet into an emerald swimming hole below Pine Valley.

In 1999 fire scorched the area, allowing fire-adapted species to thrive. As a result, trail sections over the first 1.2 miles are heavily overgrown. You'll gradually climb 400 feet, then descend the same elevation through shoulder-high brush dominated by ceanothus and tanoak.

In 0.6 mile you'll emerge from the worst of the overgrown sections at the route's high point (4750'). Views stretch south to the **Black Cone Trail** ridgelines and the **Church Creek** and **Tassajara Creek** drainages, west along the **Coast Ridge,** and southeast toward **Cone and Junipero Serra Peaks.** Rising nearly a mile above the Pacific, Cone Peak is perched atop the farthest visible ridge, 17 miles south. Dominating the horizon, 5862-foot Junipero Serra rises high above the unseen **Salinas Valley.**

The trail gradually descends a scenic ridge across golden grasslands and past thickets of new growth sprouting from the remains of a charred forest. The ridge separates the **Miller Creek** drainage and the Church Creek drainage. You'll continue through oak woodlands and grasslands speckled with stalks of Our Lord's candle, top a minor saddle, and climb the ridge to a prominent saddle. Views vanish briefly as the trail switchbacks southwest and then climbs north to the second highest point along the route (2.1 miles, 4740'). From here the route is all downhill to Pine Valley.

Pause for glimpses through the bare branches of burned snags. Look west to spot the sandstone formation that parallels Church Creek Fault. The trail turns southwest on a steep grade, dropping 850 feet through open oak woodlands carpeted with vibrant wildflowers in spring. After 1.5 miles the trail switchbacks down to **Church Creek Divide** (3.6 miles, 3650'). This divide marks the four-way junction of the westbound **Pine Ridge Trail,** the southeast-bound **Church Creek Trail,** and the northwest-bound **Carmel River Trail** to Pine Valley.

Forming a deep saddle between two west-trending ridges, the divide sits atop the 29-mile east-west **Church Creek Fault.** For millions of years the North American and Pacific plates have ground past one another, here creating Church Creek canyon. From the divide, the fault continues northwest, following the Carmel River Trail to **Hiding Canyon Camp,** ascending the **Puerto Suelo Trail** to the prominent **Puerto Suelo** saddle, and emerging at the Pacific near **Kaslar Point.** To the northwest lie the headwaters of the **Carmel River,** while to the southeast lie the headwaters of the **Salinas River** along Church Creek. Oddly enough, the latter winds some 80 miles north of the Carmel River before finding its way to sea.

From the divide, the Carmel River Trail turns right and leads 1.7 miles to the wildflower-strewn meadows and tall pines of Pine Valley. Over the first 0.3 mile you'll cross the typically dry headwaters of the Carmel River. As the grade levels off (4.5 miles, 3160'), you'll notice sandstone cliffs to your right and hear trickling water off to your left. The scene is reminiscent of the Sierras, with ponderosa pines rising from an open meadow beside steep sandstone cliffs.

You'll continue through mixed evergreen and riparian forests, highlighted by rare endemic Santa Lucia firs at the valley's east end. A large gate marks the official **Pine Valley entrance** (5.3 miles, 3140'), at a junction with the Pine Valley–Pine Ridge Trail and the cross-country trail to Pine Falls. The main trail leads to a year-round stretch of the Carmel River. If you have time, don't miss the side trip to the falls.

SIDE TRIP ■

The 0.7-mile trail to **Pine Falls** is narrow, overgrown, and washed out in a few precarious places. Your payoff is a scenic waterfall oasis and swimming hole, among Ventana's most spectacular sights.

From the Pine Valley–Pine Ridge Trail junction (5.3 miles, 3140'), turn left and cross the river, heading downstream a few yards before recrossing past the first of three small unofficial campsites. The trail closely follows the river, crisscrossing it multiple times on the way downstream past riparian forests and endemic Santa Lucia firs.

You'll emerge at an overlook directly above 50-foot Pine Falls (6 miles, 2700'). The descent to its base is hazardous, as you must clamber across slick boulders. Use the conveniently placed rope to negotiate the final 20 feet through a minor gully. The crystal clear pool is wide and deep enough for swimming, but as temperatures only reach the high 50s Fahrenheit at best, your swim will be a quick one. Enjoy the brisk plunge and return the way you came.

■ ■

If you're bound for the more spacious upper meadow, turn right at this junction onto the Carmel River Trail, following a decrepit sign marked BEAR BASIN. You'll pass through a gate toward a small cabin on private land. A longtime Pine Valley resident lives and gardens on the small plot to your right.

A hundred feet past the cabin you'll ascend a minor knoll, then descend into upper Pine Valley and the official **Pine Valley Camp** (5.4 miles, 3200'), equipped with a fire ring and room for up to three tents. Six or seven unofficial campsites also lie nestled amid the pine-studded meadow, each equipped with a fire ring and room for up to three tents. These fill up quickly on holiday weekends.

Scamper up the valley walls at dawn or dusk for spectacular pine-filtered views, highlighted by grazing deer and active woodpeckers. If the valley is deserted, you may even hear the cry of a lone coyote or happen across the tracks of an elusive bobcat along the riverbanks.

PINE VALLEY NATIVES ■ ■ ■ ■ ■ ■ ■ ■ ■ ■ ■ ■ ■ ■ ■ ■ ■

For thousands of years, fertile Pine Valley was home to the Esselen people, providing them with excellent hunting, gathering, and living grounds. The Esselen may have used fire to clear underbrush and maintain the pine stands and broad meadow, where deer, rabbits, antelopes, and even bears once commonly grazed. In the adjacent forest, doves, quails, and other game birds flocked beneath the abundant canopy of oaks, bays, pines, and madrones. Wild roses grow in dense thickets on the east edge of the valley, perhaps cultivated by the Esselen for straight, strong arrow shafts. Beneath the sandstone cliffs, women took harvested acorns from the surrounding oak woodlands and ground the nutritious meat into flour. Their mortar holes still pepper sandstone outcrops just downstream from the Pine Valley–Pine Ridge Trail junction.

Today, few Esselen remain to answer the many questions one might have about their ancestors' lives in Pine Valley or elsewhere along the Santa Lucia Range. Most of their people were decimated by disease brought by Spanish missionaries. Those who survived were often captured and sent to work in the Spanish missions. Others were killed without mercy. Sadly, much of their culture, language, mythology, and religion was also lost.

■ ■

Trip 50

HIDING CANYON & ROUND ROCK CAMPS

LENGTH AND TYPE: 18.8-mile point-to-point

RATING: Strenuous

TRAIL CONDITION: Difficult to impassable, poison oak, steep faint tread

HIGHLIGHTS: This peaceful wilderness escape leads through steep, narrow gorges to cascading waterfalls, deep emerald pools, and remote camps.

TO REACH THE TRAILHEAD: Park at the large turnout on Tassajara Road across from China Camp. The trailhead is on the camp side of the road, 100 feet south of the parking lot and 150 feet south of the camp entrance. The trail begins on a saddle above China Camp. It is marked, though encroaching brush often obscures the sign. There's no water at the trailhead.

TRIP SUMMARY: This trip offers hikers overnight excursions within the rugged northern Santa Lucia Range. If you can arrange a shuttle vehicle, the 18.8-mile one-way route takes you from China Camp to Los Padres Dam past pine-studded meadows, lush forests, secluded canyons, narrow gorges, waterfalls, and swimming holes. Highlights include Pine

Valley, Pine Falls, the pools and waterfalls below Round Rock, Ventana Mesa Creek Falls above Hiding Canyon Camp, Carmel River Camp, and Bluff Camp.

You can also arrange two- to four-night out-and-back trips, spending at least one night in Pine Valley and the other night(s) at Round Rock or Hiding Canyon Camps. Or you can take the 24.1-mile loop that leaves China Camp on the Miller Canyon Trail and returns through Pine Valley (see TRIP 48 Miller Canyon & Pine Valley Loop, page 195).

These trails are ideal in spring and fall, as temperatures are moderate and storms infrequent. Summer temps can reach the upper 90s Fahrenheit, and flies and mosquitoes pose a nuisance. Winter temps can dip below freezing, and snow is common above 4000 feet. Poison oak is a year-round problem on the lower Carmel River Trail.

Trip Description

See TRIP 49 Pine Valley (page 199) for the first 5.3 miles of this route to **Pine Valley**.

The **Carmel River Trail** crosses Pine Valley's broad meadow to a four-way junction with the **Pine Falls spur** and **Pine Valley–Pine Ridge Trail** (3140'). Consult TRIP 49 Pine Valley for the route to **Pine Falls** and TRIP 52 Pine Ridge, Sykes Hot Springs, & Big Sur (page 207) for a description of the Pine Valley–Pine Ridge Trail. This route leads northwest along the Carmel River Trail.

You'll pass through a wooden gate on your right and cross private property in sight of the owner's small cabin. The trail ascends a minor knoll and enters a large open meadow. In a scene reminiscent of the Sierras, deer graze beside towering pines amid grasslands blanketed in spring wildflowers.

The Carmel River Trail leads past Jack English's cabin in the heart of Pine Valley.

Offering pine-filtered views of the surrounding sandstone cliffs, the trail ascends northwest 200 feet in half a mile to a saddle (6.2 miles, 3414') that divides the **Carmel River and Hiding Canyon Creek drainages.** From this saddle, the route drops past four shallow gullies, then switchbacks across the seasonal headwaters of **Hiding Canyon Creek** (6.7 miles, 2950'). Continue downslope, following the path of the Church Creek Fault.

Crossing the headwaters eight more times, the route passes from exposed south-facing slopes to a shady creekside route past sycamores, bays, alders, and oaks. Expect to find year-round water by the eighth crossing (8.1 miles, 2140').

Past this crossing you'll leave the creek and ascend through dense overgrowth. During the wet season (November through April), ticks lie in wait amid the chamise- and broom-clad slopes. Wear light-colored pants to protect your legs and easily spot these hitchhikers. The trail switchbacks high above Hiding Canyon Creek for far-reaching vistas of the Carmel River drainage.

Leaving the canyon behind, you'll cross a minor ridge, switchback, and descend 0.1 mile southwest to the **Round Rock Camp Trail junction** (9.2 miles, 2030'). This easily missed unmarked junction leads to a spectacular overhanging gorge.

SIDE TRIP ■

From the **Round Rock Camp Trail junction,** hike 0.2 mile downslope to the headwaters of the **Carmel River,** then meander downstream 50 feet cross-country. The swift river plunges from pool to pool, carving a deep path through smooth massive granite walls. Be mindful of slick boulders and poison oak that shelters in the crevices. Pause for a refreshing dip in the brisk water.

Cross the river on the main trail past an unofficial campsite atop a small grassy terrace. The trail gradually ascends the canyon for 0.2 mile, then descends south along the riverbanks amid thickets of blackberry and poison oak. Make your way through this tangle and cross the river just downstream from an enormous boulder—perhaps Round Rock—which overlooks a shallow swimming hole.

Follow the trail 200 feet farther to **Round Rock Camp** (10.2 miles, 1920'), set atop a small grassy terrace. Marked by a table and a sign, the camp is roomy enough for up to a dozen small tents.

■ ■

From the Round Rock Camp Trail junction, the Carmel River Trail steeply descends the east-facing canyon wall. Pause to enjoy views on the way down. In a few minutes you'll reach the Carmel River's east bank. Expect to get your feet wet in all but the driest months—during heavy rainfall the river actually floods the trail.

Just across the river lies **Hiding Canyon Camp** (9.2 miles, 1740') and the nearby **Puerto Suelo Trail junction.** True to its name, the camp is easy to miss. The turnoff lies just downstream from the first crossing. You'll find two large sites, each with a table and cooking grate. The first site sits atop a narrow terrace along the west bank, while the larger, preferred site lies a few feet upstream near an enormous ponderosa pine with a 6-foot-plus diameter. You'll recognize ponderosas by their golden puzzle-piece bark and pine needles bunched in threes.

SIDE TRIP ■

If you're willing to hike upriver off trail for 0.4 mile, you'll pass through a narrow sandstone gorge and arrive at **Ventana Mesa Creek Falls,** which tumbles into a swimming hole. Farther upriver, the canyon widens and turns south, entering a second gorge at the confluence with **Ventana Mesa Creek.** A few feet farther upstream the creek cascades into a deep granite-lined pool. If the water level is low enough in late summer and fall, you can press on for 200 feet to a larger swimming hole and waterfall within a mossy, fern-lined grotto. The refreshingly cold water is a welcome escape on a hot summer day.

■ ■

Refer to TRIP 45 Hiding Canyon & Round Rock Camps (page 181) and reverse that description for the remaining 9.2 miles of this route to the Los Padres Dam Trailhead.

Trip 51

VENTANA DOUBLE CONE VIA PINE VALLEY

LENGTH AND TYPE: 31.8-mile out-and-back

RATING: Challenging, faint tread and overgrown along Puerto Suello Trail

TRAIL CONDITION: Passable to difficult, poison oak

HIGHLIGHTS: Stop at secluded waterfall oases on your way to 4853-foot Ventana Double Cone, which boasts panoramic views of the Santa Lucia Range.

TO REACH THE TRAILHEAD: Park at the large turnout on Tassajara Road across from China Camp. The trailhead is on the camp side of the road, 100 feet south of the parking lot and 150 feet south of the camp entrance. The trail begins on a saddle above China Camp. It is marked, though encroaching brush often obscures the sign. There's no water at the trailhead.

TRIP SUMMARY: This book describes several routes to the remote 4853-foot summit of Ventana Double Cone, in the heart of Ventana Wilderness. For general information on the Ventana Trail, see the summary for TRIP 38 Ventana Double Cone via Ventana Trail (page 155).

This route from 4270-foot China Camp leads 15.9 miles to the summit (4853'). Although the trailhead lies more than 2000 feet higher than the Bottchers Gap Trailhead and nearly 3400 feet above Los Padres Dam, it descends 2530 feet to Hiding Canyon Camp, then climbs 3113 feet in 6.3 miles to Ventana Double Cone. Highlights include the scenic waterfalls at Pine Falls, Round Rock, and Ventana Mesa Creek (see TRIPS 49 and 52). These short detours are well worth the extra mile, especially in summer, as the bracing water will revive you after a sweaty toil to the summit.

As at most peaks along this dramatic coast, the best times to hike are between mid-November and April, taking advantage of cooler temperatures, fogless days, and fewer pesky mosquitoes and flies. This route is also a good choice in summer heat and fall drought, as from Hiding Canyon Camp you can reach the summit with a daypack and plenty of water. Be prepared for rain and snow if you hike in winter, when snow levels can drop to 2000 feet and the river may be impassable. Also watch for poison oak.

If you can arrange a shuttle vehicle, consider combining trips for an excellent point-to-point backcountry excursion. From China Camp, you'll summit Ventana Double Cone, then descend the Carmel River Trail to Los Padres Dam (see TRIP 46 Ventana Double Cone via Carmel River Trail, page 185) for a 31.4-mile grand tour of the wilderness.

Trip Description

See TRIP 50 Hiding Canyon & Round Rock Camps (page 202) for the first 9.2 miles of this route to **Hiding Canyon Camp**.

The **Puerto Suelo Trail** (9.6 miles, 1740') begins atop a flat bench on the west bank just downstream from camp. Those bound for **Ventana Double Cone** will climb this trail toward the **Puerto Suelo** saddle and the **Ventana Trail junction**. In drought years it's best to fill water bottles here.

You'll begin a steep climb west through a minor gully and across a small creek, then wander through several other minor gullies, dry practically year-round. In half a mile the trail begins a series of

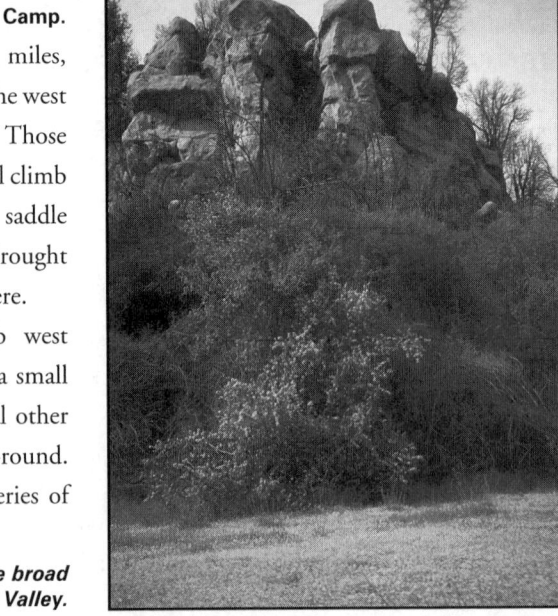

Sandstone cliffs rise above the broad pine-studded meadow at Pine Valley.

switchbacks, ascending a brushy slope to a minor saddle. Continue past fragrant stands of bays and tanoaks and across small tributaries to **Uncle Sam Creek**. The trail crosses and then recrosses the creek, which may be your last opportunity for water between here and the summit.

Continue climbing northwest through overgrown ceanothus thickets. The last 0.3 mile of the Puerto Suelo Trail ascends very steep, short switchbacks. Just 0.1 mile from the saddle, clear water bubbles up from two neighboring springs, reliable in all but the driest months.

Climb the final 200 feet to the Puerto Suelo saddle and **Ventana Trail junction** (12.2 miles, 3530'). The Ventana Trail branches left at this junction and climbs above the saddle toward Ventana Double Cone.

See TRIP 38 Ventana Double Cone via Ventana Trail (page 155) for the final 3.7 miles to the summit (15.9 miles, 4853').

WINDOW ON THE WILDERNESS ■ ■ ■ ■ ■ ■ ■ ■ ■ ■ ■ ■ ■ ■

Ventana Wilderness owes its name to the rugged twin peaks of 4853-foot Ventana Double Cone. Legend relates that a rock arch once spanned the deep cleft between the peak's sister spires, forming a natural window on the wilderness. Arriving in the area in the late 1700s, early Spanish inhabitants named the double summit *Ventana* (Spanish for window).

Descendents of the native Esselen people believe the legendary arch served as a gateway for the souls of all native people as they left their earthly existence. Others claim it was the portal through which the Great Spirit heard humankind's collective prayers.

The magnificent double summit still dominates the Ventana Wilderness skyline, inspiring newfound reverence among modern-day visitors.

■ ■

Trip 52

PINE RIDGE, SYKES HOT SPRINGS, & BIG SUR

LENGTH AND TYPE: 23.1-mile point-to-point

RATING: Challenging

TRAIL CONDITION: Passable to difficult, poison oak

HIGHLIGHTS: This arduous hike takes in rugged ridges, steep canyons, and exposed hillsides, rewarding the faithful with waterfalls, hot springs, and swimming holes.

China Camp (Trip 52, East)

TO REACH THE TRAILHEAD: Park at the large turnout on Tassajara Road across from China Camp. The trailhead is on the camp side of the road, 100 feet south of the parking lot and 150 feet south of the camp entrance. The trail begins on a saddle above China Camp. It is marked, though encroaching brush often obscures the sign. There's no water at the trailhead. The first 1.2 miles of the trail are heavily overgrown yet passable.

TRIP SUMMARY: This trip offers hikers several overnight itineraries within the rugged northern Santa Lucia Range. If you can arrange a shuttle vehicle, consider two point-to-point routes that cross the Ventana Wilderness: (1) the Pine Ridge Trail from China Camp to Big Sur, and (2) the Pine Ridge Trail, Black Cone Trail, and Marble Peak Trail from China Camp to Arroyo Seco. Highlights on the route to Big Sur include massive ponderosa pines atop ridges and large meadows, ancient redwood groves along the Big Sur River, and oak-dotted golden hillsides blanketed in spring wildflowers.

If you can't arrange a shuttle, consider the following out-and-back destinations:

Accessed via China Camp, Pine Valley is well worth a 1.7-mile detour along the Carmel River Trail. From there a 0.7-mile downstream trek leads to Pine Falls, a 50-foot cascade that fills a deep swimming hole.

Past Pine Valley, the Pine Ridge Trail leads to spectacular views atop Pine Ridge, reminiscent of a Sierra crest. Expect snow above 4000 feet in the winter and profuse wildflowers in spring. The trail is lightly traveled between Pine Ridge and Sykes Camp. Several sections between the ridge and the Big Sur headwaters are heavily overgrown, and heavy winter rains spawn dangerous trail washouts. Trekking poles are a good idea.

Redwood Camp offers solitude deep within a redwood-lined canyon, while Sykes Camp is well-known for its three small 100°F hot springs, which are often crowded during spring break and on summer weekends.

Trip Description

See TRIP 49 Pine Valley (page 199) for the first 3.6 miles along the **Pine Ridge Trail** to **Church Creek Divide** (3.6 miles, 3650').

This divide marks the four-way junction of the westbound Pine Ridge Trail, the southeast-bound **Church Creek Trail,** and the northwest-bound **Carmel River Trail** to **Pine Valley.** If you plan to spend a night in Pine Valley, expect an easy 1.7-mile detour.

If you're not bound for Pine Valley, the route from Church Creek Divide continues straight, west along the Pine Ridge Trail. Immediately past the saddle the trail climbs past heavily overgrown madrones, manzanitas, and ceanothus, fire-adapted species that thrive on this fire-scarred hillside. You'll cross two small gullies laden with blackberries, horsetails, and fragrant hedge nettles. These seasonal creeks run dry by summer.

SIDE TRIP ■

If you do stay in Pine Valley and are westbound, consider taking the **Pine Valley–Pine Ridge Trail** onward to the Pine Ridge Trail instead of hiking back through Church Creek Divide. The 1.5-mile Pine Valley–Pine Ridge Trail leads onward to the Pine Ridge Trail, saving you 2.4 miles overall, though requiring an additional 500 feet of climbing through heavy overgrowth. You'll find the trailhead at the official **Pine Valley entrance** (5.3 miles, 3140'), at a junction with the Carmel River Trail and the cross-country trail to **Pine Falls**.

From this junction, the trail (marked BEAR BASIN) crosses the **Carmel River** past a campsite that can accommodate up to four tents. Passing the site, you'll climb steeply above Pine Valley. A passage through live oaks, tanoaks, and ceanothus gives way to views northwest toward flat-topped 4766-foot **Uncle Sam Mountain**, **Puerto Suelo** (the deep saddle left of Uncle Sam's base), and the rocky twin peaks of 4853-foot **Ventana Double Cone**.

You'll climb 800 feet in the first mile to a shallow saddle (6.3 miles, 3950'), at a junction with an abandoned spur to **Bear Basin**. This spur leads right 1.1 miles to spacious **Bear Basin Camp,** alongside reliable, spring-fed **Bear Basin Creek**. Directly upslope from camp another spur ascends southwest half a mile through dense overgrowth to the Pine Ridge Trail, though poor trail conditions make for extremely slow going.

If you intend to head west along the Pine Ridge Trail, continue from the shallow saddle (6.3 miles, 3950') on the Pine Valley–Pine Ridge Trail another half mile to the Pine Ridge Trail, although this section is also overgrown.

■ ■

Cool crystalline waters offer a respite from the brush-choked, sun-drenched slopes leading into the Big Sur River basin.

After half a mile past head-high brush and scattered black oaks, madrones, and ponderosa pines, you'll round a minor ridge and reach the **Divide Camp Trail junction** (4.1 miles, 3800'). The spur leads 200 feet to the first of two sites in the shade of large pines, oaks, and alders. Each can accommodate up to two tents. A hundred feet west of camp is a small spring that dwindles to a muddy seep by midsummer and early fall.

Past the spur junction, the Pine Ridge Trail climbs above camp, meanders southwest past two small seeps, and leads 100 feet farther to a larger spring-fed creeklet lined with enormous chain ferns. A large fallen oak blocks the trail, requiring careful footing, especially if you're carrying a heavy pack. Past the creeklet, trail conditions worsen, and you must forge through overhead thickets of ceanothus. Fortunately, there's very little poison oak, and the trail is well graded. In spots the brush clears, offering glimpses of Ventana's high peaks. Flat-topped Uncle Sam Mountain lies 6 miles northwest, rising above the Puerto Suelo saddle. A long ridge leads left from the saddle up to Ventana Double Cone.

Ascending toward Pine Ridge, you'll cross a small spring-fed creek (4.7 miles, 4000'), the most reliable water source in the 3.6 miles between Divide Camp and **Pine Ridge Camp**. The route contours past an unnamed 4751-foot peak to the south, then reaches the **Pine Valley–Pine Ridge Trail junction** (5.8 miles, 4230'). Westbound hikers who spend the night in Pine Valley rejoin the Pine Ridge Trail here (see side trip on the previous page for details).

Past the junction, the trail becomes increasingly overgrown with bay laurel, ceanothus, manzanita, and scrub oak, species that are thriving in the wake of numerous fires, particularly the 1999 Kirk Complex Fires. Press on through the encroaching brush to ascend a minor saddle (6.5 miles, 4410'). Pause here for views southeast along **Tassajara Creek** canyon to the highest point in the **Santa Lucia Range**, 5862-foot **Junipero Serra Peak**.

FIRE AS A SHAPING FORCE ■ ■ ■ ■ ■ ■ ■ ■ ■ ■ ■ ■ ■ ■ ■

Over just two days in fall 1999, the Ventana Wilderness was hit by some 1200 lightning strikes as a subtropical system from the Gulf of California unexpectedly formed into a massive electrical storm over the Santa Lucia Range. This awe-inspiring display ignited the Kirk Complex Fires, a series of 47 wildfires that swept across more than 90,000 acres of the wilderness over three months, sparing only the most protected canyons and barren ridges.

The region is no stranger to fire. Every acre of the wilderness has been scorched at least twice this century. As a result, many plants are well adapted to fire. Since the Kirk Complex Fires, aggressive brush has overrun the eastern section of the Pine Ridge Trail, rendering it impassable to many hikers' standards. Without maintenance, this section may be completely overgrown within the next couple of years.

From the saddle, the trail gently ascends 200 feet, then quickly descends to Pine Ridge (7.3 miles, 4550'). Listen for woodpeckers at work on the enormous charred pine snags that stand like sentinels atop the ridge. This ridge separates the three major drainages of the northern Santa Lucia Range. The Carmel River headwaters of **Blue Creek** lie just north of the ridge, the **Big Sur River** headwaters of **Cienega Creek** flow southwest, and Tassajara Creek runs southeast into the **Arroyo Seco,** then north to the **Salinas River** and out to sea. From Pine Ridge, your major climbing is behind you. Unfortunately, your major bushwhacking is not.

A few minutes along the ridge you may notice a metal plaque nailed to a burnt snag with flagging tied around its base. This unofficial sign marks the north end of the **Black Cone Trail** (7.4 miles, 4540'). Though the trail has been officially abandoned, volunteers recently cleared its entire length (see TRIP 53 Black Cone Trail to Arroyo Seco, page 215). It offers an incredibly scenic, well-graded southeast passage across Ventana's major ridges.

From this junction, another abandoned spur strikes through the encroaching brush—easily overlooked were it not for an unofficial marking flag. If you're willing to tear through brush, this spur descends to Bear Basin Camp and then climbs 0.8 mile to a south-climbing ridge and a junction with the Pine Valley–Pine Ridge Trail.

Continue on the Pine Ridge Trail. As you leave the ridge, look southeast toward the Black Cone Trail, which crosses the flanks of 4965-foot **South Ventana Cone.** The 2800-foot descent into the Big Sur River canyon begins moderately at first, along a narrow gravel path that veers west and crosses three minor gullies. The vegetation changes and retreats somewhat from the trail. Thickets of chamise, yucca, manzanita, and wartleaf are only knee- to waist-high, allowing ocean views on clear days.

You'll pass large pine snags as you descend 300 feet in 0.3 mile to the signed **Pine Ridge Camp Trail junction** (7.7 miles, 4260').

SIDE TRIP ■

Pine Ridge Camp Trail descends 0.1 mile to a flat-topped ridge with incredible westward views. **Pine Ridge Camp** (7.8 miles, 4170') offers one large site in the sparse shade of madrones, pines, and tanoaks that survived 1999's ravaging fires. The site can accommodate up to five tents. Beyond camp, past a large burned madrone, a narrow trail leads northwest a few feet to a reliable spring-fed creeklet. Campers enjoy unparalleled views of the deep Big Sur drainage as it rises from the Pacific. This is also a spectacular place to watch a sunset and enjoy the solitude.

■ ■

From the junction, the Pine Ridge Trail descends past scorched ponderosa snags. Pause to admire views southeast toward the Black Cone Trail, which slices a nearly level route from South Ventana Cone toward Black Cone. Continue your descent on a steep grade for the remaining 2500 vertical feet to the Big Sur River canyon. Although encroaching brush is less of a problem along this narrow section, the tread is loose and washed out in places. Use caution when carrying a large pack.

You will pass thickets of chamise, ceanothus, fragrant black sage, scattered yuccas, and sticky monkeyflowers, the latter bearing bright orange blossoms and predictably sticky leaves. The route reaches a long saddle with views northwest toward Ventana Double Cone, which rises some 2500 feet from **Redwood Creek** below. You will descend past a hillside covered in invasive broom to a small gully just below a major saddle. Cross the gully to the **Big Sur Trail junction** (10.3 miles, 2320').

The Pine Ridge Trail veers right at the junction for the final 500 vertical feet to Redwood Creek. After 0.3 mile the thick brush finally gives way to redwoods nestled along the steep ravines and canyon bottoms. The spectacular views are behind you, but so are the worst trail conditions, and poison oak makes its reappearance. After a series of switchbacks, temperatures dramatically drop, as the trail enters the cool, damp redwood microclimate.

On a level grade the trail crosses Redwood Creek and passes the first of four official sites at **Redwood Camp** (11.2 miles, 1800'). The first small site along the west bank can accommodate up to two tents. To reach the other sites, you will have to hike farther downstream along a spur.

SIDE TRIP ■

Ten feet past the first site in **Redwood Camp**, you'll reach a 0.1-mile spur to the other sites. Cross the creek on the large redwood log and hike 100 feet downstream to the second site. Though there's only room for one tent, the sloping site does include a fire ring. The third site lies 50 feet farther downstream, amid large boulders and old-growth redwoods along the east bank. This small, shady site can accommodate up to two tents. The fourth and largest site sits atop an open bench 100 feet farther along the east bank, 70 feet past a small seep. Redwoods, tanoaks, and bays ring the perimeter, while starflowers and wild strawberries carpet the forest floor. This site can accommodate up to 10 tents.

■ ■

From camp the Pine Ridge Trail heads south and climbs above the west bank of Redwood Creek. To continue westbound along the Pine Ridge Trail, refer to TRIP 59 Sykes & Redwood Camps (page 246) and follow that trail description in reverse.

Trip 53

BLACK CONE TRAIL TO ARROYO SECO

LENGTH AND TYPE: 26.2-mile point-to-point, 30.2-mile out-and-back, or 31.6-mile loop

RATING: Challenging

TRAIL CONDITION: Passable to difficult, poison oak, overgrown brush, faint tread

HIGHLIGHTS: Epic views from the flanks of mountains along the recently restored Black Cone Trail

TO REACH THE TRAILHEAD: Park at the large turnout on Tassajara Road across from China Camp. The trailhead is on the camp side of the road, 100 feet south of the parking lot and 150 feet south of the camp entrance. The trail begins on a saddle above China Camp. It is marked, though encroaching brush often obscures the sign. There's no water at the trailhead.

TRIP SUMMARY: Following the 1977 Marble-Cone Fire, the US Forest Service abandoned the Black Cone Trail, which was quickly reclaimed by dense thickets of chaparral. The 1999 Kirk Complex Fires raged along most of the trail, exposing its residual tread. Soon volunteers from the Ventana Wilderness Alliance hiked the area to see whether it would be feasible to reestablish the trail. In cooperation with the USFS, volunteers removed brush and debris and regraded the trail.

As is the case with most wilderness trails, it still suffers from overgrowth, washouts, and annoying ticks, flies, and mosquitoes. Fortunately, there's little poison oak above 3500 feet on the northern section of the trail, though it fills in again near Strawberry Camp. Bring a walking stick to counteract the slope and navigate slippery sections.

Santa Lucia fir, a rare species endemic to the Santa Lucia Mountains, inhabits the steep, rocky slopes along the Black Cone Trail.

In summer, temperatures can reach the upper 90s Fahrenheit along this exposed 8.6-mile trail, and coastal fog obscures your views. In spring, ticks are a nuisance, but onshore winds promise far-reaching views east to the Arroyo Seco and west to the Big Sur watershed and broad Pacific. Fragrant wildflowers blanket the ridgelines, gullies, and steep ravines. In winter the possibility of snow keeps nighttime temps below freezing as howling winds funnel up the canyons. The fog rolls well offshore in fall, ushering in wonderful views, comfortable temps, and diminished tick, fly, and mosquito populations. However, water can be scarce along much of the route. Fill up at Mosquito Springs, White Cone Springs (0.4–0.8 mile past Venturi Camp), the headwaters of the North Fork Big Sur (not reliable by late summer), Black Cone Camp, and Strawberry Creek.

This trail serves as an important link between the northern and southern Ventana Wilderness, connecting the trails of the Carmel, Little Sur, and Big Sur watersheds with those of the Arroyo Seco watershed. The route from China Camp offers at least three point-to-point trips. If you can arrange a shuttle vehicle, destinations include: (1) Arroyo Seco Campground (26.2 miles); (2) Church Creek Trailhead (24.1 miles); and (3) Horse Pasture Trailhead (27.6 miles). The latter two trips can also be loop trips if you're willing to hike several steep miles up Tassajara Road (5.4 miles from the Church Creek Trailhead and 5.2 miles from the Horse Pasture Trailhead). Or your loop can begin and end at the Church Creek Trailhead via the Church Creek, Pine Ridge, Black Cone, Marble Peak, and Horse Pasture Trails (see TRIP 54 Church Creek to Pine Valley Camp, page 221). The Black Cone Trail descends (albeit gently) more than 1700 feet in the 7.8 miles between Pine Ridge and Strawberry Camp—if you're willing to return along the trail and regain this elevation, several point-to-point trips lead through the heart of the wilderness.

Out-and-back destinations from China Camp include: (1) Mosquito Springs Camp (17.2 miles round-trip); (2) South Fork Camp (36 miles round-trip); (3) Strawberry Camp (30.2 miles round-trip); and (4) Willow Springs Camp (38.4 miles round-trip).

Trip Description

See TRIP 52 Pine Ridge, Sykes Hot Springs, & Big Sur (page 207) for the first 7.3 miles of this route to the **Black Cone Trail junction** atop **Pine Ridge** (4540').

If you're in desperate need of water, you can either descend 0.3 mile farther along the **Pine Ridge Trail** to **Pine Ridge Camp** (a spring runs year-round in all but the driest years) or hike 0.8 mile along the **Black Cone Trail** to the **Mosquito Springs Trail junction** (a half-mile spur leads to year-round water at **Mosquito Springs Camp**).

At the Black Cone Trail junction, a metal plaque nailed to a charred snag points the way. Veer left and head south along the western flanks of 4965-foot **South Ventana Cone.**

Over 0.8 mile the loose-packed trail passes low-lying thickets of manzanita, scrub oak, ceanothus, yerba santa, and a few yuccas. The first prominent saddle marks the **Mosquito Springs Camp Trail junction** (8.1 miles, 4470').

SIDE TRIP ■

Mosquito Springs Camp Trail leads east, dropping 500 feet in half a mile. This can be a slippery descent over loose tread obscured by overgrowth. Fortunately, someone has placed yellow flagging at the major switchbacks. As the trail levels off, you'll reach **Mosquito Springs Camp** (8.6 miles, 3940'), which offers a few flat tent sites nestled between granite talus and aggressive growth stemming from the 1999 Kirk Complex Fires. Be aware that the one or two decent sites lie along the runoff path for winter storms. True to the camp name, mosquitoes thrive here in spring and early summer, diminishing again by fall. While water is available before camp during the wet season (November through April), it's reliable year-round at camp in all but the driest years.

■ ■

From the junction, the Black Cone Trail contours just west of the ridgelines that separate the **Big Sur** and **Arroyo Seco** drainages. You'll meander on and off the spine, eventually arriving at a saddle atop a steep, narrow canyon that holds the western headwaters of **Tassajara Creek,** just below point 4135 feet on the USFS map. The saddle hosts **Venturi Camp** (10.7 miles, 4100'), littered by such random artifacts as a pair of pliers and a rusty rake. There's enough room for two tents, but the nearest water is 0.4 mile farther along the trail at **White Cone Springs.** The sheer topography exposes the camp to strong, cold winds that funnel up from the canyon.

Beyond camp the trail skirts the western flanks of an enormous white granite peak known locally as **White Cone.** Over the next 0.3 mile you'll pass two impressive peaks marked as 4721 feet and 4719 feet on the USFS map (the trail doesn't thread the peaks as drawn on the USFS map, but remains well below them on the contour). You'll soon reach the first of three reliable springs (11.1 miles, 4240'), though this one may run dry in drought years. White Cone Springs is 0.1 mile farther, gushing over moss-covered white granite cliffs. Head east 0.4 mile toward a massive granite face to find the **third spring** (11.5 miles, 4100').

Beyond the springs, the trail descends toward a prominent forked **ridge** (12.1 miles, 4100'), offering views northwest to the Big Sur watershed and Pacific. From this vantage point, you can see most of the remaining 3 miles of the Black Cone Trail as it winds past the western flanks of **Black Cone** before dropping into **Strawberry Valley.**

Pine Valley Camp

54

Divide Camp

53

VENTANA

53

Pine Ridge Trail

PB 46

China Camp

Bear Basin Camp

Pine Ridge Trail

54

Church Creek/
Divide

WILDERNESS

14

Church Creek Trail

Church Creek Road

To Pine Ridge Camp (0.3 mile)

South Ventana Cone

The Caves

TRACT 38

Mosquito Springs Camp

53

22

22

23

PB 50

The Mesa

54

19

Black Cone Trail

Los Padres National Forest

PB 51

28

27

26

PB 59

30

28

27

Venturi Camp

26

Ventana Wilderness

PB 56

PB 57

PB 57

PB 58

PB 59

36° 14' 00"

53

BIG SUR

Big

South Fork Camp

WILD AND SCENIC RIVER

Black Cone

Black Cone Camp

Strawberry Camp

ES

53

OS

True North

Magnetic North

14.5°

0   .5   1 mile

0   1   2 kilometers

After a strenuous 25 miles, reward yourself with a refreshing dip along the Arroyo Seco.

Onward, the trail dips through a small canyon that channels a headwater of the **North Fork Big Sur River** (12.6 miles, 3670'). Across the canyon, the trail ascends to **Shotgun Ridge** (12.9 miles, 3700'), which overlooks the dozens of creeks, creeklets, springs, ravines, gullies, and broad valleys of the Big Sur drainage below. The ridge was named for a rusty 20-gauge shotgun that was left in the brush with other debris by the crew that forged this trail in the 1960s.

Beyond the ridge, the mostly waterless route reaches another small seep trickling from the mountainside (13.3 miles, 3610'). Fifty yards farther you'll reach the 200-yard spur down to comfortable **Black Cone Camp**. A year-round spring issues forth from the hillside in camp, which can accommodate up to four tents with room to spare. Nearby, look for an ice-mold stove that the Forest Service installed when the camp was established in the 1960s.

Beyond the spur, the trail leads 0.3 mile toward a large reliable **creek** (13.6 miles, 3600'), another headwater of the North Fork Big Sur. The creek lies along the northeastern flanks of Black Cone, which dominates the eastern skyline less than half a mile from the trail. From here you'll contour past three minor ridges to the divide (14.3 miles, 3690') between **Strawberry Creek,** the **Salinas River** headwaters, and the North Fork Big Sur. The trail gradually descends an old bulldozed firebreak. Although the trail widens, poison oak makes a comeback along the remaining 0.8 mile to **Strawberry Camp.**

As you descend into Strawberry Valley, you'll cross two small seasonal creeklets (usually dry by midsummer), following the second creeklet 0.1 mile to **Strawberry Camp.** The Black Cone Trail ends here at the **South Fork Trail junction** (15.1 miles, 2840'). Though perched in a small valley, the camp lies on sloping ground. The site can accommodate up to four tents in the shade of a sprawling oak. While the creek may run dry by late summer, a 0.3-mile jaunt downslope to the **Marble Peak Trail junction** will lead to water.

For a description of the remaining 12.1 miles to **Arroyo Seco Campground,** refer to TRIP 56 Willow Springs & Strawberry Camps (page 234) and follow that trail description in reverse.

Trip 54

CHURCH CREEK TO PINE VALLEY CAMP

LENGTH AND TYPE: 17-mile out-and-back, 34.2-mile loop, 22.3-mile point-to-point (Los Padres Dam), or 32.5-mile point-to-point (Arroyo Seco)

RATING: Strenuous to challenging

TRAIL CONDITION: Passable to difficult, poison oak

HIGHLIGHTS: This route leads past ancient sandstone formations deep within Church Creek canyon, highlighted by vast oaks and ponderosa pines amid grassy slopes and spring wildflowers.

TO REACH THE TRAILHEAD: To reach the Church Creek Trailhead, drive 5.4 miles past the China Camp entrance along Tassajara Road. At 5.2 miles you'll pass the Horse Pasture Trailhead on your left. Continue 0.2 mile farther to a sharp left bend through a conspicuous gully. Park in the small lot on your right and walk 50 feet back up the road to the crossing at the Church Creek Trailhead. There are no facilities or water at the trailhead.

If you miss the trailhead and continue down Tassajara Road, you'll reach another parking area in 1.1 miles. There, 17.2 miles from the Carmel Valley Road junction, a dirt road leads to a Zen Buddhist monastery that contains Tassajara Hot Springs.

TRIP SUMMARY: From the Church Creek Trailhead, hikers can choose from at least four route options, each featuring a stay at beautiful Pine Valley. Destinations include: (1) Pine Valley (17 miles out-and-back) via the Church Creek and Carmel River Trails; (2) Los Padres Dam Trailhead (22.3 miles point-to-point) via Pine Valley, Hiding Canyon, and the Carmel River; (3) Arroyo Seco Campground (32.5 miles point-to-point) through Church Creek with a detour to Pine Valley via the Pine Ridge, Carmel River, Black Cone, and Marble Peak Trails; or (4) the Church Creek Trailhead (34.2 miles out-and-back) with a detour to Pine Valley via the Pine Ridge, Black Cone, Marble Peak, and Horse Pasture Trails and Tassajara Road. While the last two routes could bypass the detour to Pine Valley, that 1.7-mile trail leads to one of Ventana's premier camps. As is the case with most wilderness trails, these routes suffer from overgrown brush and poison oak, faint tread, fallen snags, and other obstacles.

The out-and-back route along the Church Creek Trail ascends 2070 feet in 6.8 miles to Church Creek Divide, at the junction with the Carmel River Trail to Pine Valley. Though this route to the divide is 3.2 miles longer and gains 670 feet more elevation than the Pine Ridge Trail, it offers your only chance to take in Church Creek canyon's incredible sandstone formations. Remnants of a seafloor formed millions of years ago, these ancient beds jut from the canyon walls along the downthrown side of the Church Creek Fault. Native Esselen tribes once used these outcrops as shelters. Many of their pictographs remain on cave walls.

Trip Description

A sign at the trailhead (2180') states that Pine Ridge Trail is 7 miles away and Pine Valley 8 miles. You'll quickly cross a small stream and enter the **Ventana Wilderness**. The trail parallels the creek in the shade of bigleaf maples, live oaks, Coulter pines, and ceanothus thickets. For the next half mile the well-defined yet slightly overgrown trail recrosses the creek three times and ascends minor ridges and gullies to the **first of seven divides** (0.8 mile, 2770').

Pause at the saddle to take in views southwest to the **Church Creek** and **Tassajara Creek** confluence, northwest to massive sandstone beds along the canyon bottom, and west along

"The Caves" is named after the sandstone formations that form primitive shelters along the ancient canyon walls above Church Creek.

the spine of the ridge that separates the **Big Sur** and **Arroyo Seco** watersheds. The **Black Cone Trail** closely follows this distant ridge.

Beyond the saddle, you'll meander past tilted sandstone layers and descend into **Wildcat Camp** (1.1 miles, 2750'). This small camp is limited to one tent site along a narrow bench shaded by bays, elderberries, alders, and sycamores. The reliable creek dwindles to a trickle in summer and fall.

Past camp, you'll cross the creek and begin a moderate climb past chaparral, chamise, sage, and bush poppies. Over the next 0.6 mile the trail wriggles across two divides, crosses a seasonal creek (dry by late summer), and reaches the **third divide** (1.7 miles, 3240'), offering a view southeast toward **Junipero Serra Peak,** which lords 5862 feet over the **Santa Lucia Range.**

You'll continue between sandstone outcrops featuring smooth overhanging rims and convex floors and walls. A honeycomb pattern along the sandstone faces is the result of weathering, which forms deep cavities known as **tafoni.** Archaeological evidence proves the Esselen used larger tafoni caves for shelter from the sun, wind, and rain.

The trail briefly strays from the formations and descends half a mile past brushy slopes, crossing a small reliable **creek** (2.2 miles, 2760'). Past the gully, the trail steepens for a 0.2-mile descent to a large arroyo, or dry boulder-strewn creek bed, lined with yuccas, Coulter pines, sycamores, sage, and poison oak. Onward, the trail climbs 200 feet to the fourth divide along broad grassy slopes, radiant in spring with blooming owl's clover, lupines, poppies, and popcorn flowers. From this divide, you can see the trail along the east canyon wall past the fifth divide to **Church Ranch Road.**

At points over the next 0.3 mile the tread grows faint and confusing, particularly where a large fallen live oak blocks the trail. Clear deer trails lead down to the creek, while the less distinct main trail contours northwest above the creek. You'll cross a shallow gully and small seasonal creek, then ascend a minor ridge past oak- and pine-clad slopes to the fifth divide.

Labeled THE MESA on the USFS map, this broad, flat-topped divide lies just below the junction with Church Ranch Road. Climb the steep, oak-studded grassy slopes past a dilapidated sign a few feet from the junction (3.4 miles, 2690'). The trail joins this private road and contours past **The Mesa** 0.8 mile to **Church Ranch Bridge**. Cross the bridge for views across the canyon of sprawling black oaks, Coulter pines and their massive cones, and recently charred Santa Lucia firs.

You'll soon enter **Bruce Church Ranch** through an open wooden gate posted PRIVATE PROPERTY (4.2 miles, 2580'). For the next 1.5 miles the trail crosses the ranch past grazing horses, wooden barns, and fences. From the entrance gate, the road abruptly turns after 0.2 mile, crosses the creek, and leads to private homes. At this turn, the Church Creek Trail continues straight along a vague trail (4.4 miles, 2590').

Beyond the ranch, the trail closely follows Church Creek for the next 0.3 mile before beginning a moderate ascent of the east bank toward a minor ridge. Pause here for views of the sloping sandstone beds that parallel **Church Creek Fault,** as well as the open ridges and oak savannas back along the trail. Past an often-dry creek bed (4.7 miles, 2630'), the trail reenters the Ventana Wilderness and climbs 0.2 mile, skirting prime wildlife habitat. These oak savannas teem with grazing deer, moles, rabbits, mice, stealthy bobcats, and scavenging coyotes. Acorn woodpeckers hammer away noisily at the thick bark of oaks and pines, building caches for their favorite nut.

As the trail again strays from the creek, it climbs past scattered oaks to the **sixth divide** (5.3 miles, 3130'). Notice the striking differences in plant communities amid the sandstone outcrops, with chaparral on higher slopes, small clusters of Santa Lucia firs and ponderosa pines nestled along the canyon, and open oak woodlands below. Past two small seasonal creeks, the trail wraps along steep slopes through dense thickets of ceanothus, manzanita, scrub oak, and poison oak.

Fire-scarred madrones, ponderosas, black oaks, and manzanitas have made an impressive comeback since the 1999 Kirk Complex Fires ravaged these slopes. Unfortunately, these aggressive, fire-adapted species are quickly overtaking the trail. Someone has managed to slash back much of the encroaching vegetation, but regular maintenance is needed to keep the trail clear. Beyond these densely overgrown sections, the trail crosses several gullies past the often-dry headwaters of Church Creek to the seventh and final divide, **Church Creek Divide** (6.8 miles, 3651').

PICTURES FROM THE PAST ■ ■ ■ ■ ■ ■ ■ ■ ■ ■ ■ ■ ■ ■ ■ ■

On Bruce Church Ranch, amid arching overhangs and rock shelters labeled THE CAVES on the USFS map, visitors will find a series of ancient pictographs. The many handprints on these rock walls offer proof of the practically vanished Esselen people, whose homeland once encompassed the Ventana Wilderness. A 1972 excavation of the rock shelters along Church Creek recovered artifacts that prove the Esselen survived in this canyon for many years following the arrival of Spanish missionaries in 1770, perhaps remaining in remote areas of the Santa Lucia Range through the mid-1800s.

Hostility toward American Indians was commonplace in California during this period. Most Esselen either assimilated, succumbed to disease, or were killed in warfare. Tragically, much of their culture, trading systems, religion, and language were also lost. No one knows why the Esselen left this rock art, but in 1929, poet Robinson Jeffers wrote the following verse to commemorate the pictographs:

Hands

Inside a cave in a narrow canyon near Tassajara
The vault of rock is painted with hands,
A multitude of hands in the twilight, a cloud of men's palms, no more,
No other picture, There's no one to say
Whether the brown shy quiet people who are dead intended
Religion or magic, or made their tracings
In the idleness of art; but over the division of years these careful
Signs-manual are now like a sealed message
Saying "Look: we also were human; we had hands, not paws. All hail
You people with the cleverer hands, our supplanters
In the beautiful country; enjoy her a season, her beauty, and come down
And be supplanted; for you also are human."

— Reprinted by permission of Jeffers Literary Properties

■ ■

The divide marks the junction with the **Pine Ridge** and **Carmel River Trails**. If you're bound for **Pine Valley**, see TRIP 49 Pine Valley (page 199) for a description of camp and the 1.7-mile route into the valley via the Carmel River Trail. If you're bound for **Arroyo Seco Campground** or a grand wilderness loop along the **Black Cone Trail**, see TRIP 53 Black Cone Trail to Arroyo Seco (page 215) for details.

CHAPTER seventeen

Arroyo Seco

■ ■ ■ ■ ■ ■ ■ ■ ■ ■ ■ ■ ■

N EAR ITS SOURCE, the Arroyo Seco is anything but a dry wash, as its Spanish name might suggest. Only as it approaches the Salinas River does it dwindle into a desiccated sandy riverbed. This relatively unknown river originates in the eastern Ventana Wilderness amid some of Big Sur's most spectacular backcountry. Its fanlike drainage encompasses numerous tributaries. The Arroyo Seco is fed from the north by Paloma and Piney Creeks; from the west by Tassajara, Church, and Willow Creeks; and from the southwest by Lost Valley Creek. To the south its headwaters descend off the east face of Coast Ridge and the north face of Cone Peak, and to the southeast it flows from Junipero Serra Peak into Roosevelt and Santa Lucia Creeks. Together these tributaries slice through diverse mountainous terrain, carving narrow gorges that shelter deep emerald pools.

As with most of the Ventana Wilderness, the best time to visit the Arroyo Seco is in spring or fall. Be aware that ticks and mosquitoes flourish in spring and summer, and in fall many small tributaries run dry. During heavy winter storms, the small creeklets, creeks, and rivers swell rapidly and can be difficult or dangerous to cross. Summer is an excellent time to enjoy the river's numerous swimming holes, though air temperatures are often uncomfortably hot, and flies can be a nuisance.

The narrow, winding 18-mile Arroyo Seco Road—or Arroyo Seco–Indians Road, as labeled on the USFS map—threads through the wilderness, connecting Santa Lucia Memorial Park Campground near Jolon with the Arroyo Seco resort area, west of the Salinas Valley town of Greenfield. The road has been permanently closed to public vehicles since its seasonal closure in late fall 1994. The stretch between the Arroyo Seco Campground and Escondido Campground remains closed to all vehicles, due to landslides. The road is open to hikers, equestrians, and bicyclists year-round, if they can get past the landslides. The stretch between Escondido and Memorial Park campgrounds is closed seasonally, starting with the first rains of the season through approximately April. Contact Monterey County Public Works for current road conditions: (831) 755-4800, www.co.monterey.ca.us/publicworks.

The road's fate is uncertain. Los Padres National Forest officials proposed to remove landslide debris and perform road maintenance to reopen the road. Opposition from

Calm pools along Willow Creek are densely shaded by alders above Tassajara Camp.

environmental organizations, including the Ventana Wilderness Alliance and the Center for Biological Diversity, sought to have the problematic road either closed to vehicle traffic entirely or restored with less impact to the Arroyo Seco watershed.

DIRECTIONS: From the north, drive south on U.S. Highway 101 to Salinas and exit at Arroyo Seco Road/Mission la Soledad in the town of Soledad. Drive 1.1 miles west on Arroyo Seco Road to a sharp bend left, where it meets Fort Romie Road (County Road G17). From this junction, Arroyo Seco Road merges with County Road G17 for 8.5 miles south to a junction with Elm Avenue (County Road G16). Turn right on Elm and drive 5.8 miles southwest to the junction with Arroyo Seco. Bear left (west) on Arroyo Seco.

Arroyo Seco

From the south, drive north on U.S. Highway 101 and take the Route 101 Business exit in Greenfield, 15 miles north of King City. Half a mile from the exit, you'll reach Elm Avenue. Turn left on Elm and drive 5.8 miles southwest to the junction with Arroyo Seco Road. Bear left (west) on Arroyo Seco.

Arroyo Seco Road merges with Carmel Valley Road (County Road G16) for 6.5 miles until you reach a fork. Bear left along Arroyo Seco Road, which leads 4.4 miles to a bridge over the Arroyo Seco. Onward half a mile, the road enters the self-service pay station at popular Arroyo Seco Campground (see below for campground details).

If you're not camping, continue along the road 0.4 mile beyond the entrance to a large parking lot and a gate where the pavement ends. From here you must traverse the narrow, winding road on foot, bike, or horse. The Marble Peak Trailhead lies 2.4 miles farther along Arroyo Seco Road.

VISITOR CENTER: Big Sur Station: (831) 667-2315. The station is on Highway 1, 4.2 miles south of Andrew Molera State Park and just south of Pfeiffer Big Sur State Park. Open daily 8 a.m.–6 p.m. Memorial Day through Labor Day, 8 a.m.–4:30 p.m. the rest of the year. USFS Monterey District Headquarters, King City: (831) 385-5434.

NEAREST CAMPGROUND: The northern section of Arroyo Seco Road ends at Arroyo Seco Campground (39 sites, $15–30/night for primitive sites and $20–40/night for car camping), along the lower Arroyo Seco. Facilities at the year-round campground include flush toilets, hot showers, and RV sites.

INFORMATION: There's a $5/night parking fee at the campground. Fire permits are required for all stoves in the backcountry. Dogs are permitted and allowed off leash, except in designated campgrounds, where a 6-foot or shorter leash is required.

WEBSITE: www.fs.usda.gov/lpnf

PHONE: Los Padres National Forest Headquarters: (805) 968-6640

Trip 55

TASSAJARA HOT SPRINGS

LENGTH AND TYPE: 19.2-mile out-and-back, 15.3-mile loop, or 11.5-mile point-to-point

RATING: Moderate to strenuous

TRAIL CONDITION: Passable to difficult, poison oak

HIGHLIGHTS: Hikers follow Tassajara Creek through narrow gorges that shelter hidden pools, while guests of the Tassajara Zen Mountain Center can enjoy the mineral-rich hot springs.

TO REACH THE TRAILHEAD: This hike begins where the pavement ends on Arroyo Seco Road.

TRIP SUMMARY: This route along Arroyo Seco Road and the Marble Peak Trail to the Tony Trail or the Horse Pasture and Tassajara Cutoff Trails accesses rugged, steep-walled Tassajara Creek canyon and its invigorating hot springs and swimming holes.

Only take this route when the Tassajara Zen Mountain Center is open. The center is open only to guests with reservations from late April to early September: (831) 659-2229 or (415) 865-1899 for reservations, sfzc.org/tassajara. From late September to early April, Tassajara is closed to the public while the resident community immerses itself in Zen training. The public does have right-of-way through the grounds year-round, but the monks would prefer not to have unregistered guests. Without reservations you cannot use the hot springs or bathhouses.

The climb from Willow Creek canyon to Tassajara can be arduous. The trail is overgrown, and along steeper sections the narrow tread suffers from slides and washouts. Expect flies, ticks, and lots of poison oak. Nevertheless, these routes via the Tony, Horse Pasture, and Tassajara Cutoff Trails lead into one of Ventana's most beautiful canyons.

The route from Arroyo Seco offers several out-and-back, loop, and point-to-point options, including: (1) Arroyo Seco to Tassajara Zen Mountain Center to the Church Creek Trailhead via the Tony Trail and Tassajara Road (11.5 miles point-to-point, if you can arrange a shuttle vehicle); (2) Arroyo Seco to Tassajara Zen Mountain Center via the Horse Pasture and Tassajara Cutoff Trails, returning via the Tony Trail (15.3-mile loop); and (3) Arroyo Seco to Tassajara Zen Mountain Center via the Tony Trail (out-and-back 19.2 miles). Choose this last route if you're unable to arrange a shuttle vehicle. The Horse Pasture Trail is overgrown with waistdeep poison oak, ruling it out for those highly allergic to this plant. The Tony Trail is steeper and considered abandoned by the US Forest Service, though as of this writing it was passable.

PROTECTING THE STEELHEAD ■ ■ ■ ■ ■ ■ ■ ■ ■ ■ ■ ■ ■ ■ ■

Steelhead trout have thrived in coastal waters and freshwater rivers for millions of years. Now these fish are endangered. The Arroyo Seco is one of the few tributaries of the Salinas River that supports a small population of the threatened trout. Unfortunately, loss and damage of their freshwater habitat is a leading reason for their population decline.

Fortunately, wilderness advocates have launched a campaign to permanently preserve the wild and free Arroyo Seco from dams, diversions, and new development by adding it to the National Wild & Scenic River System. This designation is part of the Wild & Scenic Rivers Act of 1968. As of 2010, a bill was introduced to protect about 19 miles of the Arroyo Seco.

Wilderness advocates urge the public to voice support for permanent protection of the Arroyo Seco. For more information contact the Ventana Wilderness Alliance: (831) 423-3191 or ventanawild.org.

■ ■

Trip Description

Arroyo Seco Road continues from a locked gate directly above the parking lot (1540'). The road beyond winds high above the **Arroyo Seco.** Listen for the swift river below as it cascades past smooth outcrops and plunges into deep pools. You'll be tempted to take one of the many short spurs to the banks of these refreshing pools to escape the heat and sun along the exposed road.

After 2.4 exposed miles, the road widens at a turnout where cars once parked for the **Marble Peak Trailhead** (1340'). Set out from the signed junction on your right, descending narrow, steep **Marble Peak Trail.** You'll brush past manzanita brush and poison oak in the shade of sprawling coast live and black oaks. The steep trail drops to a sturdy **bridge** (2.7 miles, 960') across a narrow stretch of the Arroyo Seco, 150 yards above the river's confluence with **Willow Creek,** fed by **Tassajara** and **Church Creeks.** You'll find a refreshing swimming hole just below the bridge.

Beyond the bridge, you'll follow an old roadbed, then veer west on a broad path to a steep bluff. This bluff overlooks the Arroyo Seco, Willow Creek, and the **Horse Pasture Trail,** which slices through dry chaparral along Tassajara Creek canyon. Onward, the trail parallels Willow Creek Fault and ducks through two gullies to the **Horse Pasture Trail junction** (3.6 miles, 1070').

To reach Tassajara Creek canyon, you'll either take the Horse Pasture Trail 2.1 miles to the **Tassajara Cutoff Trail,** which leads a mile to the monastery, or continue on the Marble Peak Trail to the **Tony Trail,** which climbs 3.1 miles of steep switchbacks to the monastery. Both routes are laborious and suffer from encroaching brush. Though it offers an easier grade through the canyon, the Horse Pasture Trail is overgrown with waist-high poison oak, and there are no campsites along the trail. Neither route is suitable if you're toting a heavy pack.

Although the Forest Service doesn't make trail maintenance or construction a priority, it would be valuable to build a trail along Tassajara Creek to the Tassajara Cutoff Trail. This new route would connect to Tassajara Road and eliminate the need to maintain the Horse Pasture and Tony Trails, not to mention lead through one of the backcountry's most spectacular canyons.

In the meantime, you're better off staying at one of the camps along **Willow Creek** (**Willow Springs** is a favorite) and dayhiking to the hot springs. Remember, reservations are required at the **Tassajara Zen Mountain Center,** and it's closed to the public between late September and early April.

SIDE TRIP ■

The 4.8-mile **Horse Pasture Trail** (3.6 miles, 1070') crosses brush-choked slopes high above Tassajara Creek on its 1300-foot ascent to **Tassajara Road.** It's a hot, exposed route in summer and a tick-infested trek in spring. Regardless, it's useful if you're headed to the **Church Creek Trailhead,** Tassajara Cutoff Trail, or the Zen Mountain Center.

After 2.1 miles, you'll reach the **Tassajara Cutoff Trail junction.** This trail leads a mile to Tassajara Creek and 0.3 mile farther to the monastery. Gorgeous pools line the narrow canyon, offering welcome opportunities to swim and lounge about on smooth, sun-warmed rocks.

The Horse Pasture Trail continues another 2.1 miles to Tassajara Road, where a left turn leads 0.2 mile to the Church Creek Trailhead and 1.3 miles to the monastery.

■ ■

A few feet past the Horse Pasture Trail junction, amid open stands of oaks and pines, a 70-foot spur leads from the Marble Peak Trail to the well-established though unofficial **Horse Pasture Camp** (3.7 miles, 1070'). Equestrians frequent this idyllic camp amid a small rock-studded meadow, which in spring is blanketed in colorful wildflowers. Camp can accommodate

A refreshing swimming hole entices backpackers just below Horse Bridge.

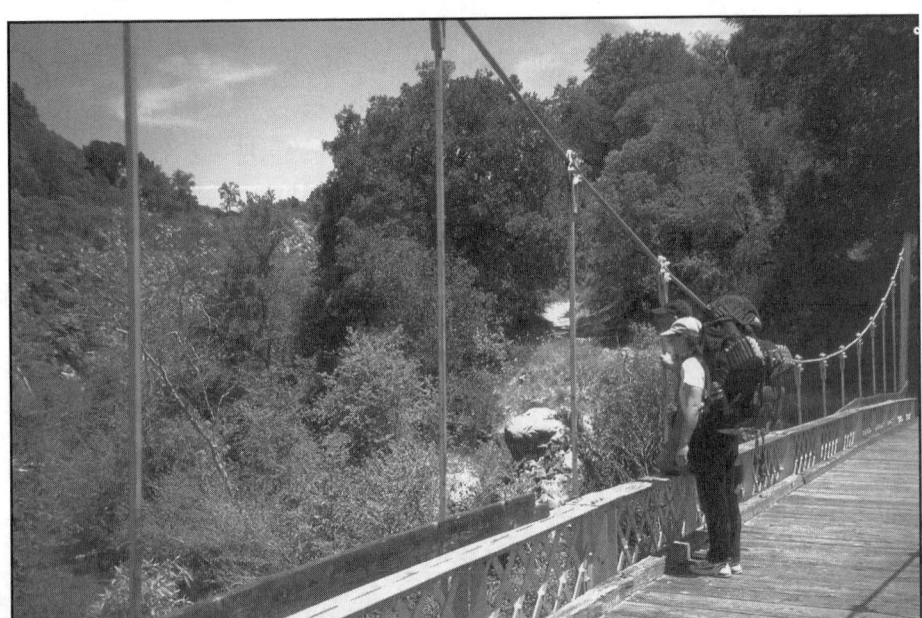

up to two tents in the shade of live oaks and maples. Two small cascades gurgle away not 50 feet from camp, but the route to Willow Creek is heavily overgrown with poison oak.

Beyond the spur to camp, the Marble Peak Trail widens along an abandoned road. You'll climb high above the creek past two small gullies with reliable springs, enter a side canyon lined with poison oak, then descend to **Tassajara Creek Camp** (4.7 miles, 1150'). Two sites lie along the south bank. To reach the first site, descend from the main trail to a flat bench downstream from the confluence of Willow and Tassajara Creeks. Overlooking the confluence a minute farther along the main trail, the second site can accommodate up to three tents in the shade of maples and live and valley oaks. Campers can also take a dip in small pools along the alder-lined creek.

A few hundred yards past camp, you'll reach the first of 15 boulder-hops across Willow Creek. The first 11 occur in fairly rapid succession over the next mile as the trail closely follows the river's course. The 12th crossing is 0.2 mile farther, the next 0.4 mile farther, and the 14th a half mile beyond that. From late spring until the first winter rains, you should make it without wetting a toe. Along the south bank 150 feet past the last crossing, you'll reach the **Tony Trail junction** (6.5 miles, 1800').

Here you'll find an unofficial primitive camp with two small sites, each with a fire ring and room for up to two tents. The camp lies under a dense canopy of alders, maples, and sycamores with a lush understory of ferns, poison oak, and thimbleberries, which produce edible berries in early summer.

The Tony Trail leads 3.1 miles to Tassajara Creek and the Zen Mountain Center. The public has legal right-of-way across the monastery grounds to Tassajara Road, though the monks prefer to not have unannounced guests (reservations must be made in advance). The monastery is closed to visitors from fall to spring. In summer, visitors with reservations may enjoy the creekside hot springs, waterfalls, and swimming holes. Visitors may stay overnight in private or communal rooms. Day-use fees ($30/adults, $12/children) include soaks in the bathhouses. A vegetarian lunch is also available by reservation and costs $13/adults and $9/children.

From the Tony Trail junction, you'll cross Willow Creek and an adjacent **creeklet** (your only source of water until Tassajara Creek) and ascend a steep, unstable slope on a moderately overgrown trail. Though the trail is marked ABANDONED on USFS maps, it shows signs of recent maintenance, unlike many "maintained" trails within the wilderness. Check for hitchhiking ticks in spring. You'll ascend 16 switchbacks to precarious slopes above Willow Creek, climbing 1150-foot ridge in 1.5 miles. Pause atop this ridge for views of the Willow Creek drainage to the south and Tassajara Creek drainage to the north.

From this point, the trail is virtually all downhill the 1.6 miles to Tassajara Creek and the monastery. A small unofficial trail leads half a mile upstream to a **waterfall**—impressive in winter, though a mere trickle by late summer. The trail crosses the creek and leads 0.4 mile downstream past meditation grounds, bathhouses, small rooms, and residences to the parking lot and Tassajara Road. The steep, unpaved road continues 1.5 miles farther to the Church Creek Trailhead (11.5 miles, 2180'). Heavy rains may close this stretch.

PARADISE FOUND ■ ■ ■ ■ ■ ■ ■ ■ ■ ■ ■ ■ ■ ■ ■ ■ ■ ■ ■

The Tassajara Zen Mountain Center is nestled in rugged, mineral-rich Tassajara Creek canyon. Humans have used these healing grounds for centuries. The native Esselen people used the hot springs as traditional ceremonial grounds, as depicted in surviving pictographs on cave walls in Church Creek canyon.

In the 1860s, crews forged Tassajara Road and built the original resort cabins and pools along the banks of Tassajara Creek. Today the site is home to *Zenshin-ji* (Zen Mind Temple), a Soto Zen Buddhist monastery established in 1966. From May through August, Tassajara welcomes guests to workshops, retreats, and work-study programs in this remote wilderness valley. For more information visit sfzc.org/tassajara.

Trip 56

WILLOW SPRINGS & STRAWBERRY CAMPS

LENGTH AND TYPE: 24.2-mile out-and-back, loop, or point-to-point

RATING: Strenuous

TRAIL CONDITION: Passable to Willow Springs; dense poison oak, brush, and faint tread to Strawberry Camp

HIGHLIGHTS: Wind your way through narrow gorges and verdant canyon bottoms past crystal-clear tributaries and cool, dark pools.

TO REACH THE TRAILHEAD: This hike begins where the pavement ends on Arroyo Seco Road.

TRIP SUMMARY: This route from Arroyo Seco Road along the Marble Peak and South Fork Trails to Strawberry Camp and beyond offers multiple out-and-back and point-to-point destinations, including: (1) Willow Springs Camp (13.8 miles out-and-back); (2) Pine Ridge Trail junction via Black Cone Trail (14.6 miles one way, with option to continue 15.8 miles to Pfeiffer Big Sur State Park or 5.4 miles to Pine Valley); (3) Tassajara Hot Springs (11.5 miles point-to-point to the Church Creek Trailhead); and (4) Tassajara Hot Springs via Tony Trail (19.2 miles out-and-back).

From Arroyo Seco Campground, you'll climb steep Arroyo Seco Road for 2.4 miles above the lower Arroyo Seco. Short spurs from the road drop to the banks of the river, where you can roam the canyon floor, swimming, sunning, climbing, and boulder-hopping around each bend.

Trip Description

See TRIP 55 Tassajara Hot Springs (page 229) for the first 6.5 miles of this route to the **Tony Trail junction.**

Past the Tony Trail junction (1800') on the **Marble Peak Trail,** you'll make three boulder-hops across **Willow Creek** in fairly rapid succession over the next 0.4 mile, emerging at **Willow Springs Camp** (6.9 miles, 1970') amid a magnificent grove of live oaks. One of the most charming camps along the Marble Peak Trail, Willow Springs is large enough to accommodate up to 12 tents, depending on one's willingness to camp on slightly sloping ground. In early morning, even the soundest sleepers will wake to the chorus of numerous birds marking their territories and finding mates along the fertile canyon ripe with insects, acorns, seeds, and fruit.

Past camp the trail ascends through shaded gullies, then climbs a series of switchbacks more than 800 feet in 1.3 miles to the first of two saddles. Pause for views down Willow Creek canyon and beyond to the **Salinas Valley.** From here you'll head south 0.1 mile to the second, more prominent saddle (8.2 miles, 2770') at the head of Willow Creek canyon, overlooking the headwaters of Willow and **Zigzag Creeks.**

Ahead, the Marble Peak Trail descends one of the most level, well-graded routes in the Ventana's chaparral landscape. The trail traverses two major side canyons and contours past numerous smaller gullies before crossing reliable **Camp Creek** (10.4 miles, 2760'). You'll climb from this canyon to the fourth saddle, then descend to less reliable **Shovel Handle Creek** (11.3 miles, 2720'). After a steep climb 200 feet across a minor ridge, you'll pass a fairly reliable small spring and reach the second saddle. From here the trail descends 0.2 mile to the **South Fork Trail junction** (11.8 miles, 2750').

At the junction, turn right onto the 5.2-mile **South Fork Trail,** which quickly crosses **Strawberry Creek** and climbs gently upstream 0.3 mile into **Strawberry Valley** and **Strawberry Camp** (12.1 miles, 2840'). The sole site lies on slightly sloping ground and is big enough for up to three tents. This is a popular camp among equestrians due to the small open valley and it's proximity to water through late summer. In fall the creek may seem more like a seep, though you can usually find water a few feet downstream.

Directly above camp lies the **Black Cone Trail junction** (12.1 miles, 2840'). This incredibly scenic 7.8-mile route traverses some of Ventana's highest ridges and mountains, connecting the trails of the Arroyo Seco drainage with the trails of the **Big Sur River** and **Carmel River** drainages. If you're bound for the coast, the Black Cone Trail links up with the **Pine Ridge Trail** at **Pine Ridge** (see TRIP 53 Black Cone Trail to Arroyo Seco, page 215). For a broader wilderness tour, the Pine Ridge Trail leads west 15.8 miles to **Pfeiffer Big Sur State Park** and east 5.4 miles to **Pine Valley** (see TRIP 52 Pine Ridge, Sykes Hot Springs, & Big Sur, page 207).

Trip 57

JUNIPERO SERRA PEAK

LENGTH AND TYPE: 12.4-mile out-and-back

RATING: Strenuous to challenging

TRAIL CONDITION: Passable to difficult, poison oak

HIGHLIGHTS: Epic panoramas from the highest peak in the Santa Lucia Range

TO REACH THE TRAILHEAD: If you're driving north or south on Highway 101, take the Jolon Road exit, 10 miles south of Greenfield and a mile north of the Salinas River crossing. Take Jolon Road (County Road G14) 17.8 miles south to the Mission Road junction. Turn onto Mission Road and drive 0.2 mile to the Hunter Liggett Military Reservation gate (expect to show your driver's license and vehicle registration to enter). In 4.9 miles you'll reach a four-way junction with Del Ventura Road. Turn left and in 0.8 mile bear right along the paved road. Del Ventura turns into Milpitas Road at an unspecified spot. Travel 12 miles from the intersection, cross Rattlesnake Creek, and enter US Forest Service land. Just 5 miles farther you'll reach a spur road on your right, which leads 250 feet to the gated trailhead for Junipero Serra Peak via the Santa Lucia Trail. Just before the gate you'll find a turnout that can accommodate 10 cars.

If you're bound for Memorial Park and the Arroyo Seco Trailhead, continue on Milpitas Road 0.1 mile past a spur road on your left that leads to the USFS Indian Station. A tenth of a mile past this spur, you'll reach Santa Lucia Memorial Park Campground on the right. Here the pavement ends and the road continues 0.1 mile to the end of Milpitas Road. At this junction, take the left fork and travel a few yards, then fork left again. The road dead-ends at the gated trailhead. Park on the shoulder without blocking the gate.

If you're bound for the Lost Valley Trailhead at Escondido Camp, take the right fork from the end of Milpitas Road and drive along Arroyo Seco Road 2.6 miles to Escondido. This road closes from the first heavy rains until spring, when weather and road conditions improve. Contact Los Padres National Forest Headquarters for current road conditions: (805) 968-6640, www.fs.usda.gov/lpnf.

TRIP SUMMARY: This strenuous hike climbs nearly 4000 vertical feet in 6.2 miles across boulder-strewn hillsides, pine groves, and blue and valley oak woodlands to the summit. During the wet season, new growth highlights ancient exposed sandstone along the valleys, knolls, cliffs, and ridges. Vibrant wildflower displays progress upslope as spring advances. On clear days from the summit you'll catch glimpses of the Sierra Nevada across the Salinas and San Joaquin Valleys.

The best time to summit is during the wet season (November through April), when air quality is best and temperatures are moderate along this exposed route. Snow blankets the mountain at higher elevations after winter storms. Ticks thrive as temperatures rise, while summer brings an onslaught of flies, soaring temperatures, and blankets of fog that obscure coastal views.

Forged by the Forest Service in the early 1900s, the Santa Lucia Trail historically linked Indian Station to Arroyo Seco Campground with a detour to Junipero Serra Peak, formerly known as Sta'yokale among local American Indians.

The trail served as the only access through the eastern section of the Ventana Wilderness until Arroyo Seco Road was completed in 1939. Though its northern and southern trailheads remain open today, they are not regularly maintained. In places, the tread is faint and head-high brush aggressively encroaches on the trail.

Our Lord's candle, a semiarid yucca, thrives on rocky, open slopes where it blooms a candle-like stalk of creamy white flowers in late spring.

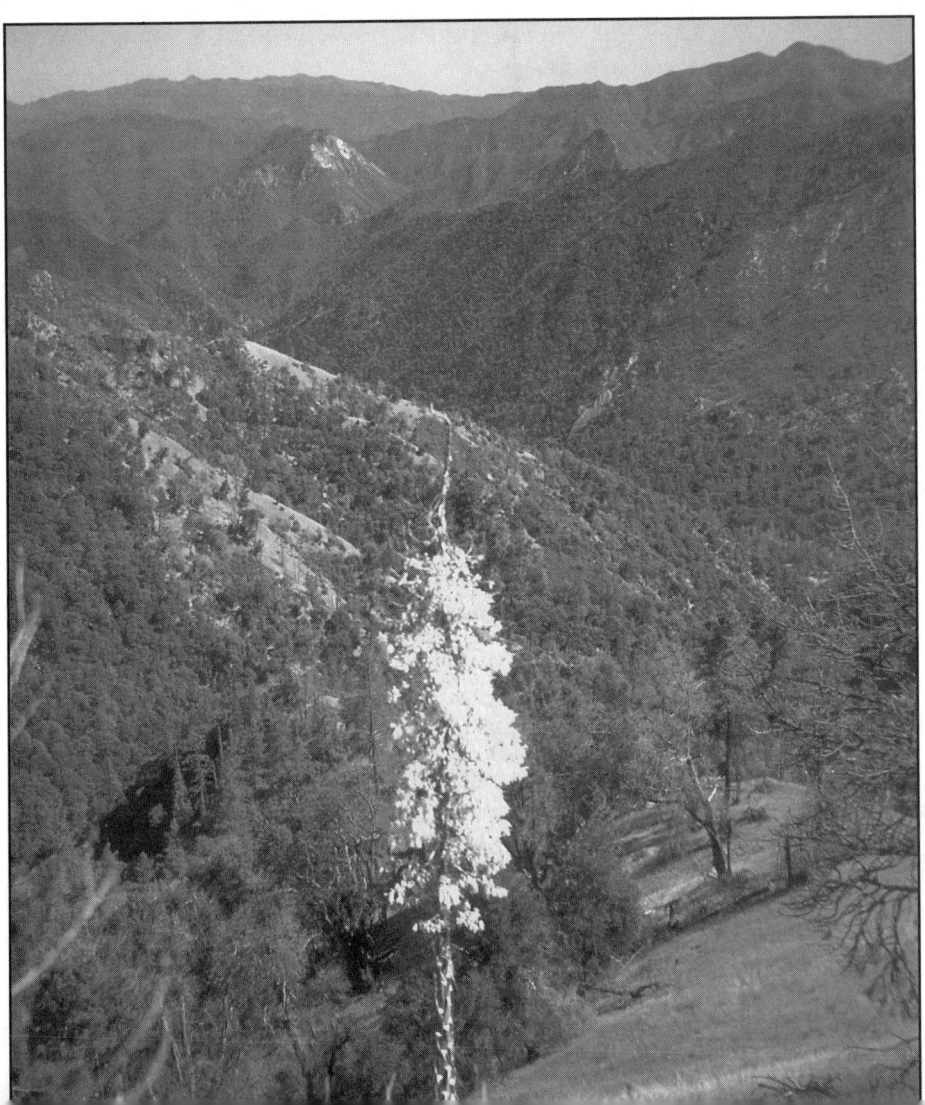

Trip Description

From the gated trailhead at road's end (2090'), the broad **Santa Lucia Trail** leads through open grassland to the east end of **Santa Lucia Memorial Park,** adjacent to steep sandstone cliffs. You'll ascend a minor ridge, climb briefly northeast, and arrive at a minor gap. Onward, the trail leads northeast past live oaks and open terrain. If you're not bound for the summit but would like to take in some of the scenery, end your climb atop the next ridge, which offers outstanding views.

Along the way you may notice the anomalous prickly pear cacti. Although **Junipero Serra Peak** does boast unusual and rare plant species, this cacti is not endemic to the **Santa Lucia Range**. Spanish missionaries brought the drought-tolerant species from Mexico as early as 1769. Modern-day specimens probably derive from stock planted by early settlers.

From the scenic ridge, you'll turn east and climb to a **saddle** (1 mile, 2350'). From this saddle, the route continues along an abandoned road to a dry creek bed lined with willows and sycamores, the latter featuring bark that resembles a jigsaw puzzle. In a few minutes you should pass a rusty **abandoned tractor** (1.4 miles, 2320'). Onward, the path narrows and gradually climbs to a junction with a **southbound trail** (1.6 miles, 2430'). Beyond this junction the trail climbs an unrelenting steep grade.

Dense brush encroaches on the trail as you enter a steep-walled arroyo canyon. In winter and spring, a small stream meanders through the wash. Lining the channel are large granite boulders, transported here during heavy floods that reshape this landscape about once every 100 years. You'll continue along a faint trail between two parallel washes before crossing the west wash (2.6 miles, 3170').

The steep route crosses a small meadow past heavy chaparral thickets to a second sloping meadow. From here you'll switchback through head-high brush to a prominent saddle and a junction with the north-trending abandoned section of the **Santa Lucia Trail** (3.7 miles, 4170'), marked by a dilapidated sign that claims you're 2 miles from the summit. You'll notice a faint trail leading east up the ridge. Fortunately, your route switchbacks toward the ridge along a more moderate grade. From this point, you're more than halfway to the summit.

Over the next 0.8 mile the trail tops a ridge, veers left past oak-clad slopes, and crosses through dense manzanita thickets to a notable saddle. Turning east, you'll skirt the north slopes and pass a junction with the heavily overgrown, abandoned **Junipero Serra Camp Trail,** which drops 600 feet in 0.4 mile to the site of the former camp. Beyond the junction you'll pass enormous Coulter and sugar pines as you climb toward a saddle between a ridge and the summit. Below the saddle, the trail leads a quarter mile to a minor ridge, where it turns south and climbs to more open terrain. The trail wanders up the western flank, then climbs south to an abandoned 40-foot **lookout tower** (6.2 miles, 5862') at the summit.

From this vantage point atop the highest peak in the Santa Lucia Range, you'll take in virtually the entire northern range, including the **Ventana and Silver Peak wildernesses, Hunter Liggett Military Reservation,** and the **Big Sur** coast. To the northwest, conspicuously flat-topped **Uncle Sam Mountain** (4766') and notched, barren **Ventana Double Cone** (4853') rise behind **Tassajara Creek** and **Church Creek** canyons. Sixty miles of visible coastline spread out beyond the **Coast Ridge.** To the west, 5155-foot **Cone Peak** rises less than 3 miles from the glistening blue **Pacific** (or perhaps engulfing fog bank). **Piñon Peak** (5264') caps a prominent ridge that extends east, masking most of the Salinas Valley, while beyond it lies the **Diablo Range,** 35 miles to the south. On extremely clear days, usually between winter storms, you may spot the high crests of the **Sierra Nevada** across the **Salinas and San Joaquin Valleys.** About 165 miles east, any visible peaks are most likely those along the east edge of Kings Canyon National Park. When ready, return the way you came.

STA'YOKALE, SACRED PEAK ■ ■ ■ ■ ■ ■ ■ ■ ■ ■ ■ ■ ■ ■ ■ ■ ■

Formerly known as Sta'yokale, Pimkolam, and Santa Lucia Peak, Junipero Serra Peak has long been of great spiritual importance to Salinian American Indians. The Salinian people continue to gather here for ceremony and prayer, trusting in the healing wisdom of this sacred mountain.

The following traditional Salinian creation story, retold by the Salinian Nation Cultural Preservation Association, explains the peak's significance:

A long time ago, waters from the ocean rose and flooded the entire world, except for the very top of Sta'yokale. Those First People who survived the deluge gathered on top with Eagle (Sa'yyo). Sa'yyo asked Kingfisher to dive down and get some mud from the bottom of the water. Kingfisher did so, but when he returned to the surface, he died. Sa'yyo scraped mud from beneath Kingfisher's nails, which he rolled into four balls. He threw one of the balls to each of the four directions. The waters receded, and the world became as it is today. And the First People who had died were brought back to life.

■ ■

CHAPTER eighteen

Big Sur

■ ■ ■ ■ ■ ■ ■ ■ ■ ■ ■ ■ ■

N ESTLED ALONG THE BASE of the rugged Santa Lucia Range, Big Sur shelters a wealth of natural treasures. From steep, redwood-lined canyons to headlands that tumble precipitously into the sea, this land is more than a string of towns or stretch of coastline. Though its attributes are many, Big Sur's beauty will elude halfhearted travelers not wanting to venture far from Highway 1.

This chapter varies from Chapter 10: Pfeiffer Big Sur State Park. While trails in that park are limited to day-use access, trails described in this chapter offer overnight treks into Los Padres National Forest and the vast Ventana Wilderness, and backcountry camps are mentioned in each route. Except for the Manuel Peak Trail, these routes do not begin at Pfeiffer Big Sur State Park, but near the town of Big Sur.

You'll hike past wildflower-strewn golden hillsides, oak woodlands, fragrant coastal scrub, and pine-studded ridges. The higher you climb, the more rewarding the views become, with glimpses east into the sheer Santa Lucias and west to the rugged coast. Hikers can access the Pine Ridge Trail at Big Sur Station, a half mile south of Pfeiffer Big Sur State Park. This is unquestionably the most popular route into the Ventana Wilderness. It leads from high above the Big Sur River to the canyon floor, linking spacious riverside camps, refreshing swimming holes, and thermal pools, including the often-crowded Sykes Camp. Other routes access portions of Big Sur from Coast Ridge Road (closed to vehicles).

DIRECTIONS: Pfeiffer Big Sur State Park is on the east side of Highway 1, 26 miles south of the Carmel Valley Road (County Road G16) junction in Carmel and 28 miles north of the Nacimiento-Fergusson Road junction near Kirk Creek Campground. Big Sur Station is also on the east side of Highway 1, a half mile south of the state park entrance. The complex serves the US Forest Service, CalTrans, and California State Parks.

VISITOR CENTER: Big Sur Station: (831) 667-2315. The station is a half mile south of the park entrance. Open daily 8 a.m.–6 p.m. Memorial Day through Labor Day, 8 a.m.–4:30 p.m. the rest of the year.

Solitude seekers must venture only a few miles from Highway 1 before being continuously rewarded the farther they climb.

NEAREST CAMPGROUND: Pfeiffer Big Sur State Park (218 sites, $35/standard site, $45/river site, $150/group site; reservations recommended). Along the Big Sur River, this 1006-acre park offers showers, Wi-Fi, and swimming. For more information call (800) 444-7275 or visit parks.ca.gov.

INFORMATION: Pfeiffer Big Sur State Park charges a day-use fee of $10. No dogs allowed on park trails. Fire permits required for all stoves and/or campfires (free and available at Big Sur Station). Campfires permitted from late November through April (fire season posted at trailhead). No wilderness permits are required in Ventana Wilderness.

WEBSITE: parks.ca.gov or www.fs.usda.gov/lpnf

PHONE: Big Sur Station: (831) 667-2315; Los Padres National Forest Headquarters: (805) 968-6640

Trip 58

VENTANA CAMP

LENGTH AND TYPE: 10.2-mile out-and-back

RATING: Moderate

TRAIL CONDITION: Well maintained to clear, poison oak

HIGHLIGHTS: Follow the Big Sur River as it cascades through steep, narrow canyon walls that shelter deep swimming holes.

TO REACH THE TRAILHEAD: At Big Sur Station the Pine Ridge Trailhead is at the end of the parking lot beyond the visitor center. Self-pay parking is $4/night for overnight guests. You'll find water, flush toilets, and maps at the visitor center.

TRIP SUMMARY: Pine Ridge is the most heavily used trail in the wilderness, as most hikers set their sights on Sykes Camp and the 100°F hot springs. Barely 4 miles into that 10-mile trek is the junction to Ventana Camp, which boasts one of Ventana's finest swimming holes. Though far from a hidden treasure, it makes a wonderful weekend trip. If you go in spring or fall, when summer crowds have diminished and temperatures are still pleasant, you'll likely have the brisk pool all to yourself.

Trip Description

The well-marked and heavily used **Pine Ridge Trail** starts from the end of the parking lot (370'). You'll briefly skirt a fenced-in pasture, then enter the cool, damp redwood- and fern-lined gullies high above **Pfeiffer Big Sur State Park Campground.** After a gradual descent and crossing of perennial **Post Creek** (0.7 mile, 280'), the trail climbs steady switchbacks to a steep ridge (0.8 mile, 850'). Pause to take in the view down canyon, where the **Big Sur River** abruptly turns from southwest to northwest on its final stretch to **Molera Beach.** Also notice the flats where the river meets the major fault of the Big Sur drainage, the **Sur Thrust Fault,** which steadily slips, compresses, and erodes rocks in its path. The river closely follows this swath of destruction to the **Pacific.**

Onward, the tread turns to loose gravel along sunny slopes with scattered views into the steep-walled river gorge. Although you'll hear cascading falls directly below, the only way to access this section of the river is along the **Gorge Trail** (see TRIP 21 Gorge Trail, page 107). Across the canyon are the exposed south-facing slopes of **Manuel Peak,** clearly marked by the **Manuel Peak Trail,** which slices through dense chaparral thickets (see TRIP 20 Manuel Peak Trail, page 105). This vegetation stands in stark contrast to this trail's forested north-facing slopes.

The trail continues through shady redwood gullies and tanoak groves devastated by sudden oak death (see sidebar, page 165, for details). Soon you'll reach a sign that marks the state park boundary and your entry into the **Ventana Wilderness** (2.3 miles, 900').

You'll climb north nearly 300 feet in the next 0.3 mile to the trail's high point, then turn east for a quick descent through two gullies. The second gully (3.3 miles, 1240') boasts a seasonal 40-foot waterfall that cascades from trailside cliffs in winter and spring, though by summer barely a trickle is heard. Onward, the trail climbs half a mile past several overlooks, then descends to a nearby ridge and the **Ventana Camp Trail junction** (3.9 miles, 1500'), marked by a dilapidated sign.

Ventana Camp Trail is a strenuous 1.2-mile spur that drops 840 feet down a series of short switchbacks to the river. From the junction, turn left down the trail and you'll quickly reach an unofficial campsite. Though waterless and not as scenic as Ventana Camp, this is where those unwilling to slog heavy gear down the steep grade choose to camp. It can hold up two tents on sloping ground. After a series of 14 switchbacks, the trail emerges at **Ventana Camp** (5.1 miles, 660'), perched atop a broad terrace on the upper Big Sur.

Shaded by oaks, madrones, and redwoods, the camp can accommodate large groups at 10 sites that flank the river. In summer, a large swimming hole in the river bend offers respite from the heat. Just past this bend, the river turns south-southwest through a steep-walled gorge, where the collective flow of the watershed's tributaries and runoff funnel through a notch less than 10 feet wide and plunge into one of Ventana's most alluring swimming holes.

If you're eastbound on the Pine Ridge Trail, refer to the following trip description for the remaining 1580-foot gain and 970-foot loss in elevation over the next 5.7 miles to **Sykes Camp**. The strenuous 900-foot vertical toil back to the Pine Ridge Trail is best done in early morning or late afternoon.

JUST WHAT THE DOCTOR ORDERED ■ ■ ■ ■ ■ ■ ■ ■ ■ ■ ■ ■

While artifacts found in the Santa Lucia Range date back 10,000 years to the Esselen, Salinian, and Ohlone-Rumsen people, Big Sur remained largely unexplored through the early 20th century. A flood of settlement and industry at the end of the 19th century emphasized the need for a direct trading route in and out of the region.

Frustrated with the time it took to reach his Big Sur patients from Monterey, Dr. John Roberts dreamed of an efficient, safe road, and even conducted early surveys. Entering the political arena as county supervisor, then state legislator, he lobbied for the construction of what would become America's most scenic roadway. Construction began in 1919, and Highway 1 opened to the public in 1938.

Trip 59

SYKES & REDWOOD CAMPS

LENGTH AND TYPE: 23.8-mile out-and-back

RATING: Moderate to strenuous

TRAIL CONDITION: Well maintained to clear, poison oak

HIGHLIGHTS: Stroll the free-flowing Big Sur past sheltered swimming holes, mineral-rich hot springs, and redwood forests to these idyllic camps.

TO REACH THE TRAILHEAD: At Big Sur Station the Pine Ridge Trailhead is at the end of the parking lot beyond the visitor center. Self-pay parking is $4/night for overnight guests. You'll find water, flush toilets, and maps at the visitor center.

TRIP SUMMARY: Winding deep into the heart of the Big Sur River drainage, the lower Pine Ridge Trail from Big Sur Station to Sykes Camp is the most popular route into the Ventana Wilderness. The total elevation gain and loss along this stretch are 2380 feet and 1490 feet, respectively. The well-maintained trail winds past three other camps in the 10 miles to Sykes Camp. Expect plenty of foot traffic in summer, while spring break brings hordes of hikers to Sykes to cluster about the 100°F hot springs, which can get crowded and, at times, rowdy.

Despite the crowds, pesky flies, and mosquitoes, summer is the best time to visit for a brisk swim (mid- to high 50s Fahrenheit) or to lounge atop the Big Sur's sunny banks and boulders. Swimming is also tolerable on warmer spring and fall days. In spring wild irises emerge from the damp forest floor, while lupines, poppies, hound's-tongues, and starflowers bloom in natural riverside bouquets, highlighted by the occasional delicate tiger lily. Temperatures remain pleasant in fall, as breezes scatter colorful autumn leaves across the canyon floor. From winter through early summer, ticks thrive amid the trailside brush. Fortunately, vegetation rarely encroaches on this well-maintained trail. If you crave solitude, hike the trail in winter. Be aware, however, that the river can rise swiftly during winter storms, making crossings deep and treacherous. The only ford along this trail is at Sykes Camp, and you can avoid this crossing to reach the hot springs.

From Sykes Camp, the Pine Ridge Trail leads 2.4 miles east to Redwood Camp, where you'll find peace beneath the trees even in busy summer months.

Trip Description

See TRIP 58 Ventana Camp (page 244) for the first 3.9 miles of this route to the **Ventana Camp Trail junction** (1500').

From this junction, the **Pine Ridge Trail** ascends 70 feet and descends 260 feet over the next 1.4 miles to **Terrace Creek Camp**. *Ventana* (Spanish for window) holds true to its name along this trail, which offers framed glimpses down the **Big Sur** drainage to the sheer peaks and ridges of the **Ventana Wilderness** and distant **Pacific**. Notched and barren **Ventana Double Cone** lords over the northeastern skyline. Legends claim a rock bridge once connected its twin peaks, framing a window-like summit nearly 5000 feet above the ocean. Whether or not that's true, the double summit served as a prominent landmark for Spanish vessels in the late 18th and 19th centuries.

Enjoy the views, as the trail soon enters shady gullies laced with ferns and moss-covered boulders amid seasonal springs. After a brief climb to a nearby ridge, you'll descend south into steep, redwood-lined **Terrace Creek** canyon. Here you'll find **Terrace Creek Camp** and the **Terrace Creek Trail junction** (5.3 miles, 1320').

The small camp flanks the creek just upstream from the junction. Don't expect solitude, as hikers stream past en route to **Sykes Camp** or back to **Big Sur Station**. You'll find one large main site for up to three tents along the east bank a few yards from the junction, just below a pit toilet. Three smaller sites lie upstream, two downstream. The steep canyon remains cool even in summer heat. In spring, carpets of redwood sorrel, mats of ferns and mosses, and delicate fairy bells line the babbling creek to its confluence with the Big Sur. If you're bound for **Coast Ridge Road** via the **Terrace Creek Trail,** see TRIP 60 Highway 1 to Terrace Creek Camp (page 251) for the trail description.

Beyond the signed camp junction, the Pine Ridge Trail ascends 510 feet and descends 210 feet in the next 1.4 miles to **Barlow Flat Camp** (see side trip on the following page). You'll skirt a ridge and head east along its marble slopes to two seasonal springs. Past the second spring, the trail enters a damp redwood glen. Microclimates vary dramatically as the trail climbs to more arid slopes and sun-drenched ridges. Across the canyon, sheer granite walls reflect the sound of roaring rapids far below in the steep canyon.

Past a second ridge, the trail switchbacks and descends into **Logwood Creek** canyon (6.5 miles, 970'). The creek is an easy boulder-hop in all but the wettest months. After crossing, you'll ascend 0.1 mile to a saddle, from which a short, steep spur climbs 200 feet in 0.1 mile to a 1290-foot summit. Detour here for far-reaching views south along the canyon. Past the spur, the trail descends 0.1 mile to the signed **Barlow Flat Camp Trail junction** (6.7 miles, 1040').

Beyond the signed camp junction, the Pine Ridge Trail ascends 900 feet and descends 690 feet in the next 2.9 miles to Sykes Camp. The trail starts out on a moderate 500-foot climb past a wall of fragile ferns, fed in wet season by a 40-foot waterfall above the trail. You may miss it entirely in summer. You'll climb through two increasingly larger redwood gullies and emerge amid arid slopes cloaked with fragile wild iris beneath oaks, madrones, and a few pine saplings. As you crest a minor ridge (8.2 miles, 1640'), the vegetation changes to a chaparral community of chamise, ceanothus, and poison oak.

SIDE TRIP ■

The **Barlow Flat Camp Trail** descends steep switchbacks 150 feet in 0.2 mile to the outskirts of **Barlow Flat Camp** (6.9 miles, 890'). This is the most spacious camp along the Pine Ridge Trail, often welcoming large groups in summer. The first three sites sit atop a flat, redwood-shaded bench above the south bank of the Big Sur. Three more open sites are nestled amid fragrant bays, maples, alders, and sycamores closer to the water's edge. Five more sites lie beneath redwoods, tanoaks, and peeling madrones along the north bank. The crossing is often wet until summer and may be impassable during or after heavy winter rains. A narrow trail leads upstream past the fifth site to an 80-foot-long swimming hole and sandy beach.

The swimming opportunities at Barlow Flat are excellent. Its sun-drenched rocky outcrops are perfect for basking in the sun and diving into some of the deeper pools. Expect water temps in the low 50s Fahrenheit in spring and fall and the low 60s on warm summer days. Temps may rise 10°F on a hot summer day.

A cross-country route leads to more alluring swimming holes downstream, though passage can be treacherous in rainy season. The first pool is adjacent to the site farthest downstream along the south bank. Onward, 150 yards downstream, cascades plunge through the narrow gorge into deep, hidden pools. From late spring through fall, it's best to wade rather than scale the sheer canyon walls. Don't even attempt passage in winter, as the frigid river can be swift and dangerous. Beyond an Olympic-sized pool, a gossamer 80-foot fall plunges from a small tributary into the Big Sur. If you're willing to swim and wade a minute farther downstream, you'll reach another emerald pool.

■ ■

Beyond this exposed ridge, you'll descend 200 feet to a cool, damp redwood gully cloaked with six-fingered ferns, which bear delicate palmate fronds. Beyond the gully, the route contours 0.2 mile along **Dolores Creek** canyon to a small knoll and dips directly above hidden **Sykes Hot Springs.** You'll continue your descent southeast, switchback northwest, then descend 150 feet to the Big Sur. The trail emerges at **Sykes Camp** and the **Sykes Hot Springs Trail junction** (9.6 miles, 1080').

Most hikers end their trek at Sykes, as the Pine Ridge Trail ascends 1760 feet and descends 1130 feet in the next 2.3 miles to **Redwood Camp.** This less-traveled stretch is predictably ill maintained. Encroaching brush poses a nuisance in wet season when hitchhiking ticks are abundant.

SIDE TRIP ■

Sprawled along a 0.1-mile stretch of the Big Sur, **Sykes Camp** offers campers their choice of 10 sites. The best lie upstream from the Pine Ridge Trail.

From the trail junction, cross the river and head upstream to a sandy beach and adjacent emerald pool. This wet ford can be swift and treacherous in winter as the river swells. You'll soon reach the first of six sites, with room for up to two tents beneath live oaks and madrones. Fifty feet farther upstream, you'll reach a pit toilet amid three large redwoods. The second and third sites lie nearby along a narrow gravel bench. Each can accommodate up to three tents.

A larger fourth site is perched above the rocky bank in the shade of fragrant bays, madrones, and live oaks, whose roots grasp riverside boulders. Secluded pools below this site are often less crowded than pools closer to the hot springs. Perch atop the sun-baked boulders and watch small trout dart between the white water cascades and calm pools.

Beyond the fourth site, the camp trail leads 60 feet upstream, crosses the river, and emerges on a sandy beach beside another attractive pool. Just above this pool lies the fifth site, which can accommodate up to two tents. Onward, 80 feet past a bend, is the similarly small sixth site, atop a sandy flat bordered by a smooth rock face and alders.

Downstream, the unmarked 0.4-mile spur to **Sykes Hot Springs** is heavily used and easy to follow—ignore erroneous descriptions of bushwhacking from camp. Those who want to keep their feet dry will have to navigate sheer rock faces laced with poison oak. The preferred route requires a few boulder-hops or wades that may be difficult or impassable in rainy season.

From where the Pine Ridge Trail crosses the Big Sur, head downstream along the south bank 25 feet to the first crossing. Onward, you'll pass a small single-tent site, recross the river, and reach two more sites, equipped with a pit toilet. Beyond the third site, the trail crosses the river twice in 100 feet and arrives at a fourth site. A third of a mile downstream, you'll catch a whiff of sulfur from the first of several small hot seeps.

The trail ascends 60 feet to the first of three small pools, each large enough for up to four adults. Directly below the pool lies a stone- and sandbag-lined hot tub, 6 feet across and 2 to 3 feet deep. Perched beside the clear, bracing waters of the Big Sur, these mineral-rich 100°F pools are among Ventana's most popular destinations. Don't expect a private soak in summer or on weekends and holidays in spring and fall.

■ ■

From Sykes Camp, you'll cross the Big Sur and climb 0.3 mile to a long, narrow saddle. Passing a rocky ledge, the trail crosses a gully and small seasonal creek. Leaving the canyon, switchbacks climb to a south-trending ridge (10.6 miles, 1680'), offering impressive views down the Big Sur's steep **North Fork** and **South Fork** drainages. The terrain and temperatures vary widely as the brushy route leads to a second exposed ridge, ducks through a small redwood-fringed gully, then returns to the dry slopes of chamise, manzanita, scrub oak, live oak, black sage, and scattered pines and yuccas. Just as suddenly, you'll reenter shady groves along Redwood Creek.

Descending 0.1 mile, you'll reach an unmarked spur on the right (11.9 miles, 1780') to Redwood Camp's larger sites. If you miss this narrow spur, just continue 150 yards farther past two small sites and cross the river. The larger sites now lie a minute downstream.

The first site on the east bank sits amid large boulders and old-growth redwoods. Seventy feet downstream past a small seep, the trail leads to the biggest site, which can accommodate up to 10 tents. This site is perched atop a flat bench carpeted in wild strawberries, starflowers and sorrel in the shade of redwoods, tanoaks, and madrones.

If you continue eastbound on the Pine Ridge Trail, expect conditions to worsen. Overgrown brush, loose tread, and exposed slopes make the 2770-foot climb over the next 3.9 miles to **Pine Ridge** a strenuous adventure.

Sykes Hot Springs is one of Big Sur's most popular backcountry destinations.

From Pine Ridge, the **Black Cone Trail** leads into the heart of the wilderness, skirting some of Ventana's highest peaks and ridges (see TRIP 53 Black Cone Trail to Arroyo Seco, page 215). If you intend to hike the entire 23.1 miles of the Pine Ridge Trail, Redwood Camp is an excellent place to rest before beginning the long climb. Better yet, start your hike from **China Camp** to avoid excessive elevation gain (see TRIP 52 Pine Ridge, Sykes Hot Springs, & Big Sur, page 207).

Trip 60

HIGHWAY 1 TO TERRACE CREEK CAMP

LENGTH AND TYPE: 11.6-mile out-and-back or 12.9-mile loop

RATING: Moderate

TRAIL CONDITION: Clear, poison oak

HIGHLIGHTS: Take in dramatic views of the furrowed Santa Lucia Range above steep coastal canyons that shelter redwood-flanked creeks.

TO REACH THE TRAILHEAD: The trailhead is on Highway 1 at gated Coast Ridge Road (North Coast Ridge Road on the USFS map) beside the Ventana Inn. The inn is on the east side of Highway 1, 2.2 miles south of Pfeiffer Big Sur State Park and 10 miles north of Julia Pfeiffer Burns State Park. Drive 0.1 mile along the inn entrance road to the public parking area on your left, for day use only. If you're planning to camp, you must park at one of the turnouts along Highway 1 adjacent to the entrance road. From the parking area, walk up the entrance road till it forks. The left branch climbs past the restaurant, while the right branch leads to the gated trailhead.

TRIP SUMMARY: This 5.8-mile route along Coast Ridge Road and Terrace Creek Trail to Terrace Creek Camp can be approached as either an out-and-back or loop trip. You could continue east along the Pine Ridge Trail to swimming holes at the riverside Barlow Flat, Sykes, and Redwood Camps or return 5.3 miles to Big Sur Station via the westbound Pine Ridge Trail (see TRIP 59 Sykes & Redwood Camps, page 246). The latter route finishes with a 1.7-mile stroll south on Highway 1 to the inn. Though a strenuous day hike, the loop makes a pleasant weekend trip. To avoid excessive elevation gain and end on a moderate downhill gradient, consider starting from Big Sur Station.

From Coast Ridge Road, you'll climb more than 1500 feet and traverse a spectacular ridge crest. The Terrace Creek Trail closely follows its namesake's banks as the creek builds to support a narrow strip of redwoods. Temperatures drop as you descend the lush canyon through an oasis of ferns, fungi, and mosses to redwood-shaded Terrace Creek Camp.

The best times to hike this route are in winter and spring, when the swollen creek cascades past verdant new growth. Spring paints the flanks of Coast Ridge with abundant poppies, lupines, baby blue eyes, and myriad other emerging wildflowers. In summer, cool Terrace Creek canyon offers respite from the sweltering heat, though views along Coast Ridge Road disappear beneath a thick blanket of fog.

Trip Description

This hike begins along the first 4.2 miles of **Coast Ridge Road,** which offers convenient mile markers. From the gate (1040'), the road skirts the prestigious **Ventana Inn** and its short guest trails. In a few minutes, you'll pass several private driveways and cross a shallow redwood-fringed gully (1 mile, 1420').

Ancient 1000-year-old redwoods form a narrow band winding through the Big Sur River canyon.

Past this creeklet, the trail crosses a smaller gully, where a creek cascades 40 feet down a sugary white **marble stalagmite** (1.2 miles, 1460'). This formation developed as marble deposits flowed downstream and accumulated at the base of the gully. Marble is one of the oldest rocks in the youthful **Santa Lucia Range,** stretching back hundreds of millions of years to a mountain range in what is now Mexico. The ancient rocks migrated north along the numerous northwest-trending faults to create some of the region's most dramatic features.

Beyond the gully, you'll continue to climb exposed **Coast Ridge.** Briefly returning to shade, the route passes through a second **locked gate** (1.5 miles, 1635'). After half a mile, the trail switchbacks and leads to impressive views northwest along the **Big Sur River** canyon to the **Pacific.** Continue 0.3 mile to a saddle, where dramatic inland views feature 4853-foot **Ventana Double Cone,** whose barren notched peak dominates the skyline just 5 miles northeast.

The road veers right from the saddle to a minor **gully** (3 miles, 2100'), passing a steep, gated private driveway on your left. Onward, the vegetation changes to rolling grasslands, highlighted in spring by spectacular wildflowers. You'll steadily climb four minor ridges, then crest a fifth, which offers the best views thus far.

From the saddle, you'll cross to an adjacent ridge and head north toward a prominent saddle. At mile 4, the road turns east past a spur road on your left. A hundred yards farther, you'll reach a second saddle and the signed **Terrace Creek Trail junction** (4.2 miles, 2590'), also on your left.

From this junction, you'll descend 1270 vertical feet along the steep 1.6-mile trail. Start out past encroaching brush that rebounded aggressively following a fire years back. Keep watch for abundant poison oak. After 0.3 mile, the trail crosses the typically dry headwaters of Terrace Creek and switchbacks down oak- and madrone-clad slopes.

You'll follow the east bank for the next quarter mile before crossing the creek to continue your descent of the steep canyon. The creek holds true to its name, as it cascades past terraces of lush ferns, emerging mushroom caps, and delicate redwood sorrel. Follow the switchbacks another mile through the primeval redwood forest to **Terrace Creek Camp** and the **Pine Ridge Trail junction** (5.8 miles, 1320').

Nestled along the creek beneath a narrow belt of redwoods, the camp offers three small sites above the trail junction (with a pit toilet) and three below the junction. The largest site, with room for up to three tents, lies along the east bank above the **Pine Ridge Trail**.

If you're continuing east or west along the Pine Ridge Trail, refer to TRIP 59 Sykes & Redwood Camps (page 246).

Trip 61

HIGHWAY 1 TO COAST RIDGE ROAD

LENGTH AND TYPE: 7-mile out-and-back

RATING: Challenging

TRAIL CONDITION: Difficult, poison oak

HIGHLIGHTS: Clear days along Coast Ridge Road reveal 50 miles of coastal views. If fog shrouds the coast, gaze east to marvel at Ventana's nearly mile-high peaks.

TO REACH THE TRAILHEAD: This route begins along a private road on the east side of Highway 1, 7.9 miles south of Pfeiffer Big Sur State Park and 3 miles north of Julia Pfeiffer Burns State Park. Turn east off Highway 1 and park along the road without blocking access. The road continues as a private driveway, restricted to vehicles but open to hikers. After 1.1 miles, the road curves right to the signed, gated DeAngulo Trailhead.

TRIP SUMMARY: The lightly used DeAngulo (day-an-GOO-low) Trail climbs to dramatic views along Coast Ridge. Be prepared to face diminished tread, fallen debris, overgrown brush, and minor slides that challenge even the most experienced backcountry hiker.

Highway 1 to Coast Ridge Road

Trip Description

Although the **DeAngulo Trail** does not officially begin along the private road, the trail description and mileage is measured from **Highway 1** (600').

The road crosses through an open gate and ascends wide switchbacks past two private driveways. You'll climb past fragrant, invasive eucalypti and dense thickets of sage, lupine, poison oak, golden yarrow, and coyote brush to dense oak woodlands, where the **road forks** (0.6 mile, 1410'). The right fork switchbacks up a private driveway 0.1 mile to a locked gate. You'll veer left through a second open gate (0.7 mile, 1450') and pass a dilapidated sign assuring hikers that the trail does eventually begin. After a few minutes, the road passes another private residence, then switchbacks past three more private driveways. Continue climbing through a hairpin right turn to the signed **DeAngulo Trail junction** (1.8 miles, 1600'), a thousand feet above Highway 1.

Fringed with poison oak, the trail heads north through open grasslands, skirting just east of a private residence. After 100 yards, you'll cross a small shady gully past scrapped cars and make your way around a large fallen tanoak. The trail crosses a second shallow

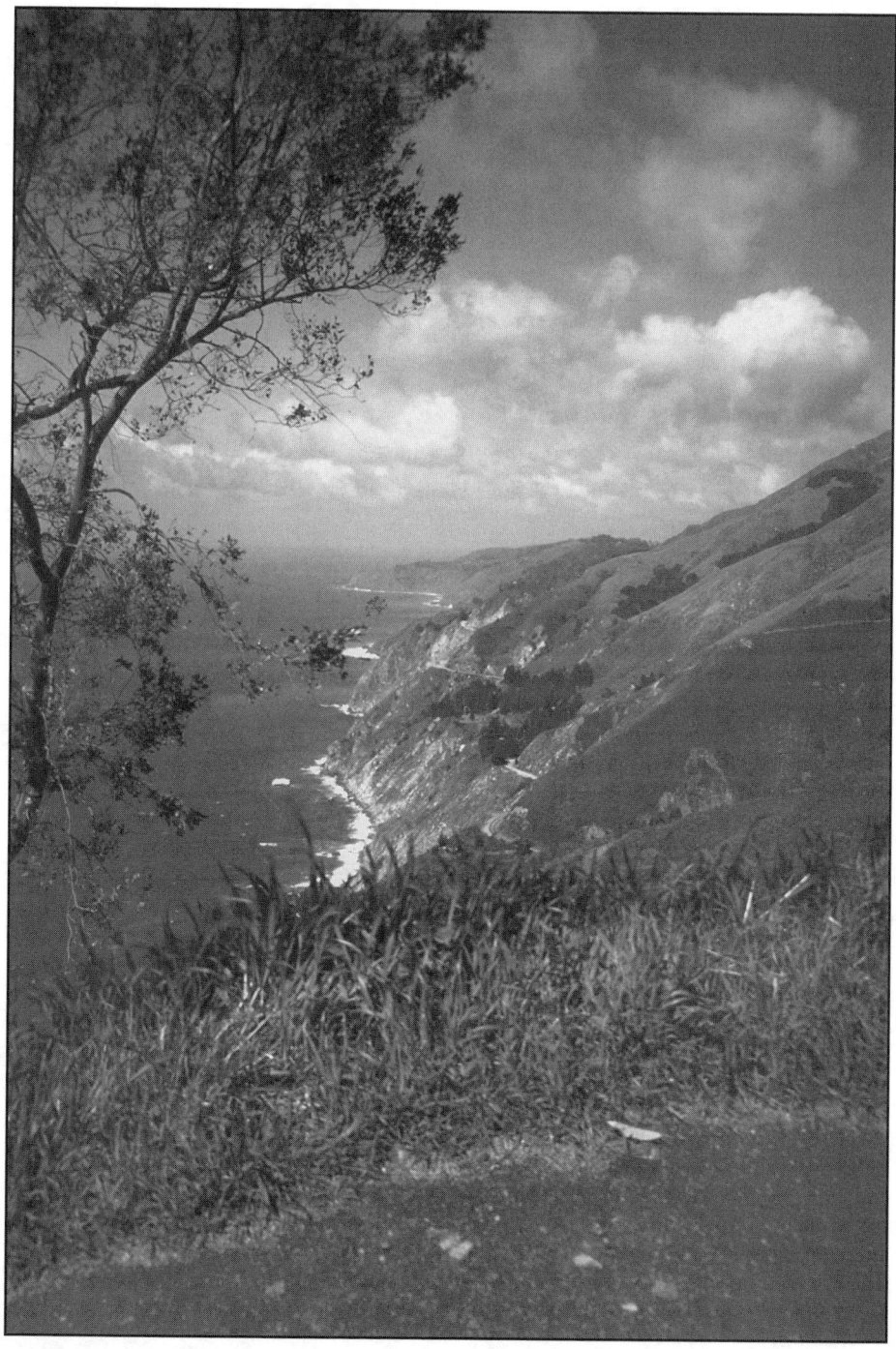

Hikers must climb a steep yet scenic private road before meeting the remote and lightly traveled DeAngulo Trail.

redwood-lined gully, briefly follows an abandoned roadbed, and skirts around a downed bay tree in another shallow gully. You'll cross several more gullies, slippery with leaves from numerous dead or dying tanoaks afflicted by sudden oak death, which has killed these trees by the thousands (see sidebar, page 165). Flags may hang from dead limbs and branches, marking the vanishing trail.

Continue climbing the steep, shady canyon to more open slopes and cross a junction with a dirt road. The trail switchbacks up a grassy ravine, climbing toward a large ponderosa pine draped with vine-like poison oak (2.3 miles, 2080'). Follow a trail sign left past a private road and stroll beneath a canopy of madrones, live oaks, bays, tanoaks, and pines to a **junction** (2.4 miles, 2170') marked by a conspicuous pine.

Avoid the abandoned road, which leads to a gully lined in poison oak. Instead, switchback right into a small grove of young pines. A minute farther the trail turns left and merges with an **old tractor path** (2.5 miles, 2240'). Head north 60 yards, then follow the next trail sign uphill to the right.

Leaving the roadbed, you'll climb past arid yuccas, which sport brilliant cream flowers on large stalks in early summer, and toyons, which produce vibrant red berries in winter. In spring, lupines, poppies, owl's clover, and baby blue eyes blanket these steep slopes. The trail climbs steadily along switchbacks to an oak-clad knoll (3 miles, 279') between **Torre** and **Partington Canyons**. Take a break and enjoy the views, as the trail continues on an extremely steep grade (about 30%) along bulldozer tracks forged during the 1985 Rat Creek Fire.

On loose rubble, you'll climb a dry wash straight up **Partington Ridge** past drought-tolerant ceanothus, scrub oaks, and yuccas. The trail passes an abandoned road (3.2 miles, 3140') on your left and continues a minute farther to a trail junction. Turn left here for a moderate, quarter-mile climb along grasslands past scattered pine and oak woodlands to **Coast Ridge Road** (3.5 miles, 3520'). If you miss the spur trail, the bulldozed wash also reaches the road along a shorter albeit more strenuous route.

From here you can either head back the way you came or continue along the road. If you turn right and hike 0.7 mile to **Cold Spring Road,** then turn left and hike 0.6 mile, you'll reach **Cold Spring Camp**. If you turn left, the road leads 8.8 miles to the **Ventana Inn** on Highway 1 (see TRIP 60 Highway 1 to Terrace Creek Camp, page 251). Whatever you decide, enjoy the solitude and spectacular views along this lonely ridgetop.

CHAPTER nineteen

Cone Peak

TOPPING OUT BELOW 6000 FEET, the Santa Lucia Range by no means approaches the lofty reaches of the Sierra Nevada, which soars more than 14,000 feet above the San Joaquin and Sacramento Valleys. But the rugged Santa Lucias certainly surpass any of the Lower 48 coastal ranges in terms of topographical relief. These peaks drop so precipitously to the rocky coves and pounding Pacific, their vertical canyon walls appear to fold in upon themselves.

No mountain illustrates this better than Cone Peak. Within 3 miles of the coast, Cone rises nearly a mile. The astonishing grade from the beach at Limekiln to the summit is the most extreme coastal slope in the contiguous United States. This abrupt change in elevation, along with a variety of soil types, supports impressive ecological diversity, including old-growth redwoods, ancient oak woodlands, endemic stands of Santa Lucia firs, and an isolated grove of sugar pines.

Despite the rugged terrain, Cone Peak and its flanks are accessible via many trails and roads. When it opens in spring, Cone Peak Road (aka Central Coast Ridge Road) enables hikers to reach the summit in less than two hours. Four trailheads start along this road: the Cone Peak Summit Trail, Vicente Flat Trail, Coast Ridge Trail, and San Antonio Trail. A network of trails also wind through Limekiln and Hare Canyons, while other trails lead to upper San Antonio Creek and Devils Canyon.

DIRECTIONS: The first four trail descriptions in this chapter start along Cone Peak Road (driving directions follow). Directions for TRIP 66 Highway 1 to Vicente Flat are listed in that route's summary information.

From the north, drive 54 miles south of Carmel on Highway 1 to the Nacimiento-Fergusson Road junction, on the east side of the highway. From the south, drive 44 miles north of Cambria and 36 miles north of San Simeon on Highway 1 to the junction. Kirk Creek Campground is on the west side of the highway, 0.1 mile north of the junction.

Head east on Nacimiento-Fergusson Road and climb 7.3 very windy miles to the signed junction with Central Coast Ridge Road (better known as Cone Peak Road). Turn left and drive north on Cone Peak Road.

Peace and solitude atop Cone Peak, the most extreme coastal slope in the lower 48

If you're driving north or south on Highway 101, take the Jolon Road exit, 10 miles south of Greenfield and a mile north of the Salinas River crossing. Take Jolon Road (County Road G14) 17.8 miles south to the Mission Road junction. Turn onto Mission Road and drive 0.2 mile to the Hunter Liggett Military Reservation gate (expect to show your driver's license and vehicle registration to enter). In 2.9 miles turn left onto paved Nacimiento-Fergusson Road, which winds 17.9 miles to the signed junction with Central Coast Ridge Road (Cone Peak Road), 300 yards past the USFS Nacimiento Station. Turn right and drive north on Cone Peak Road.

As you drive north on 6.6-mile Cone Peak Road, a saddle at Mile 3.7 marks the Vicente Flat Trailhead, while the San Antonio Trailhead is at Mile 3.9, and the Cone Peak Trailhead at Mile 5.2.

Cone Peak Road is closed from roughly November through May (specific dates vary depending on weather and road conditions). Contact Los Padres National Forest Headquarters or Big Sur Station for details (see below).

VISITOR CENTER: Pacific Valley Station: (805) 927-4211. Open daily 8 a.m.–5 p.m. The station is on the east side of Highway 1, 3 miles north of the Sand Dollar Beach Day-Use Area, 60 miles south of Carmel, and 30 miles north of Hearst San Simeon State Historical Monument (Hearst Castle).

NEAREST CAMPGROUND: Kirk Creek Campground (34 sites, $22/night; reservations recommended) is on the west side of Highway 1, 0.1 mile north of the Nacimiento-Fergusson Road junction. Kirk Creek campsites are available on a first-come, first-serve basis or by reservation. You can make reservations online at recreation.gov or by calling (877) 444-6777. This campground offers magnificent views of the Big Sur coast and a short trail to the beach.

INFORMATION: Fire permits required for all stoves. Dogs permitted and allowed off leash, except in designated campgrounds, where a 6-foot or shorter leash is required. No horses or bikes allowed on trails.

WEBSITE: www.fs.usda.gov/lpnf

PHONE: Los Padres National Forest Headquarters: (805) 968-6640; Big Sur Station: (831) 667-2315

Trip 62

CONE PEAK TRAIL

LENGTH AND TYPE: 6.4-mile out-and-back

RATING: Moderate

TRAIL CONDITION: Clear

HIGHLIGHTS: The fast track to epic views from 5155-foot Cone Peak

TO REACH THE TRAILHEAD: The signed trailhead is on the west side of Cone Peak Road at Mile 5.2 beside a small turnout for up to four cars. There are no facilities or water at the trailhead.

TRIP SUMMARY: This is the shortest trail to one of the highest peaks in the Santa Lucia Range. Trails to 5862-foot Junipero Serra, 4853-foot Ventana Double Cone, and 4417-foot Mt. Carmel require significantly more elevation gain and mileage to summit. If you're bound for this summit

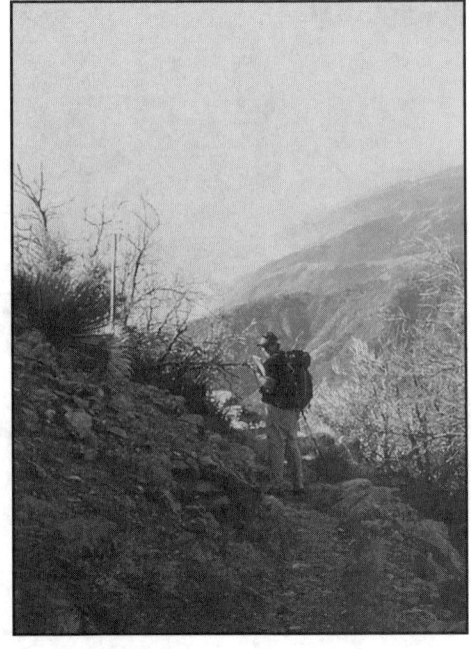

Fire-adapted species such as chamise and manzanita inhabit the flanks of Cone Peak and encroach on the trail as they vigorously grow back following a fire.

when Cone Peak Road is closed (November through May), tack on the additional 5.2 miles each way between the trailhead and junction with Nacimiento-Fergusson Road.

Lording over the southern Ventana Wilderness, Cone Peak offers boundless views along the rugged flanks of the Santa Lucias to the rocky Pacific. The hike is best enjoyed in spring and fall, when fog banks roll well offshore. In winter, snow may fall on the summit, and temperatures can drop below freezing. Bring plenty of water and extra clothing along this exposed trail, and be prepared for rapidly changing conditions.

THE HIGH ROAD ■

In 1542, Juan Cabrillo sailed past the forbidding Santa Lucia Range and wrote, "There are mountains which seem to reach the heavens, and the sea beats on them." Spanning 200,000 acres of raw wilderness, these granite and marble peaks rise more than 5000 feet above the Salinas Valley to the east and plunge west to the rugged Pacific shoreline.

If you're looking for an easy hike or drive into these mountains, think again. Few roads cross the wilderness, making it one of the largest roadless coastal tracts in the Lower 48. Fortunately, if you're reluctant to brave overgrown trails with loose tread and steep grades, there is Nacimiento–Fergusson Road, which connects the "Salad Bowl" to the surf in little more than an hour's drive.

From the east, the road crosses the oak-fringed San Antonio Valley and Hunter Liggett Military Reservation before climbing into the Santa Lucias. Three miles past the divide, you'll reach the US Forest Service's Nacimiento Station, the only structure along the route. A quarter mile farther, the road passes Old Coast Road to the south and Cone Peak Road to the north, which access most trailheads in this chapter. Where the road plummets to the Pacific, fog often engulfs the river canyons, replenishing redwoods that line these deep gullies.

■ ■

Trip Description

From the signed trailhead on the west side of **Cone Peak Road** (4000'), you'll climb past dense thickets of manzanita, wartleaf, and tree poppies, which bloom brilliant yellow by late spring. These fire-adapted species are thriving in the wake of the 1999 Kirk Complex Fires, California's 10th largest recorded wildfire, which scorched more than 90,000 acres of wilderness.

The trail climbs to a nearby saddle for your first stunning overlook of the southern **Santa Lucia Range**. Approaching a ridge, you'll turn north to a second saddle (0.5 mile,

4030'). As the trail steepens, the views encourage you onward. Watch your footing as you pass two rubble-lined gullies that continually erode onto the trail.

Skirting past a downed tree, you may notice the first instance of encroaching poison oak, a rarity at this altitude. Aggressive brush makes steady inroads, but dedicated Ventana hikers and wilderness advocates bring pruning sheers and machetes with them to keep it in check.

PRODIGIOUS CONE PEAK ■ ■ ■ ■ ■ ■ ■ ■ ■ ■ ■ ■ ■ ■ ■ ■

Remarkable in many aspects, Cone Peak has intrigued people for millennia with its varied topography, geology, botany, and cultural history. Its western slopes form the steepest coastal grade in the continental United States. Its bedrock comprises metamorphic rocks of the Salinian block, among the oldest rocks in the Santa Lucia Range. Its spectacular cliffs boast marble from an ancient seafloor that was transported here from Mexico along northwest-trending faults.

In the late 1800s, entrepreneurs found an overwhelmingly rugged peak that sheltered a wealth of natural resources. They would extract lumber, lime, tanbark, and even gold from these slopes and clefts. One company erected four enormous kilns along Limekiln Creek to purify some of the largest limestone deposits along the central California coast. The kilns still stand amid the redwoods at Limekiln State Park, along Cone Peak's western flanks.

Intrigued by the abrupt, distinct climatic zones from sea level to 5155', botanists came in search of new plant species. Habitats vary from cool, damp redwood forests to rolling oak savannas and sun-scorched chaparral, each zone hosting dramatically different flora and fauna. In the 1830s, botanists first described the area's Coulter and sugar pines and Santa Lucia firs. The latter form an extensive stand on the peak's northwest slopes. Isolated from Sierra Nevada stands, secluded stands of sugar pines are limited to the highest peaks of the Santa Lucias.

■ ■

Onward, you'll reach an unmarked junction (1.2 miles, 4380'), where a spur on your left leads 100 feet south along the ridge for encompassing views of the Santa Lucias. To your right, the main route switchbacks down a ridge with scattered views through the remains of charred trees. The trail veers northwest to the **Cone Peak Summit Trail junction** (2 miles, 4830'), atop a narrow ridge. If you're bound for **Trail Spring Camp** and the **Gamboa Trail junction,** refer to TRIP 65 Cone Peak Loop (page 266) and follow that trail description in reverse.

Cone Peak Summit Trail climbs the remaining 325 feet in 0.3 mile. Start out southeast past drought-tolerant scrub oaks, manzanitas, sticky monkeyflowers, and yuccas, which shoot forth stalks of densely clustered, edible white flowers. As the trail switchbacks to cooler north-facing slopes, the vegetation shifts to a cluster of endemic Santa Lucia firs and an isolated stand of sugar pines. The switchbacks soon lead to a dramatic **ledge** (2.2 miles, 4760') above a sheer rock face inhabited by cliff swallows, which dart skyward in search of tasty insects.

From the ledge, a final series of short switchbacks leads to the **summit** (5155'). Climb the lookout tower for more encompassing views. Breathe deeply, relax, and enjoy. Clockwise from the north are the barren peaks of 4853-foot **Ventana Double Cone** and 3709-foot **Pico Blanco**. To the northeast rises 5862-foot **Junipero Serra,** the highest peak in the Santa Lucia Range. The ancient oak savannas of the **San Antonio and Nacimiento Valleys** stretch south and southeast. From the summit, a 3.2-mile ridge drops west to the **Pacific,** comprising the steepest coastal slope in the Lower 48—even steeper than the drop from 14,494-foot Mt. Whitney to Owens Valley. On the clearest days, often after winter storms, you can see the **Sierra Nevada** peaks east across the **Salinas and San Joaquin Valleys.**

Trip 63

FRESNO CAMP

LENGTH AND TYPE: 3-mile out-and-back

RATING: Challenging

TRAIL CONDITION: Difficult to impassable, poison oak

HIGHLIGHTS: Find solitude at this camp amid the vast, remote wilderness.

Fresno Camp is primitive and difficult to access, but the solitude is worth the trek.

TO REACH THE TRAILHEAD: The trailhead is on the east side of Cone Peak Road at Mile 3.9. Trailhead parking is at Mile 3.7, just above the Vicente Flat Trailhead.

TRIP SUMMARY: You can approach this as either a 3-mile round-trip day hike or an overnight out-and-back trip with a stay at Fresno Camp, one of Ventana's largest camps. Thick brush encroaches on this lightly traveled trail.

Trip Description

From the turnout at Mile 3.7, you'll hike 0.2 mile farther along **Cone Peak Road** to the trailhead at Mile 3.9—factor this out-and-back stretch into your overall mileage. The unmarked trailhead (3290') is at an abandoned roadbed on the right-hand side of the road. Hike 200 yards along the heavily overgrown trail past chamise, broom, and wartleaf to a LOS PADRES NATIONAL FOREST sign at the **Ventana Wilderness** boundary. To the southeast lie the headwaters of the **Nacimiento River**.

After 0.2 mile, you'll reach a saddle that offers sweeping views of the **San Antonio River** canyon. Along a series of switchbacks, the trail makes an easily missed hairpin turn from east to west through head-high brush intermixed with poison oak, then veers east to north through a dry **gully** (0.8 mile, 2710'). From here you'll leave the roadbed and descend the fire-scarred slopes past thriving thickets of tanoak, madrone, and live oak.

The trail soon arrives at the usually reliable headwaters of the **San Antonio River** (1.3 miles, 2590'). You'll briefly parallel the drainage past a large fallen oak, then switchback southwest to the lush canyon floor at **Fresno Camp** (1.5 miles, 2320'). The first site sits atop a boulder-strewn flat just past the confluence of the river and the small creek your route paralleled. There's room for up to five tents in the shade of large maples and sycamores. The second site lies 120 yards upstream atop two large shady terraces.

Despite its proximity to Cone Peak Road, Fresno Camp remains one of Ventana's least-visited camps, likely due to the overgrown trail and unmarked trailhead. Judging from animal prints found along the flood plain, bears, bobcats, and cougars visit camp more often than humans. Be aware that severe winter storms may flood the camp.

Trip 64

VICENTE FLAT TRAIL

LENGTH AND TYPE: 4.8-mile out-and-back or 7.7-mile point-to-point

RATING: Moderate

TRAIL CONDITION: Clear to passable, poison oak

HIGHLIGHTS: Follow a narrow band of old-growth redwoods along sheer Hare Canyon.

TO REACH THE TRAILHEAD: The marked trailhead is on the west side of Cone Peak Road at mile 3.7 near a small turnout for up to five cars. There are no facilities or water at the trailhead.

TRIP SUMMARY: The Vicente Flat Trail descends 7.7 miles from Cone Peak Road to Highway 1. You can approach the trail as either an out-and-back or point-to-point hike. If you can arrange a shuttle vehicle, start from Cone Peak Road. This downhill route offers tremendous views of the coast, the sheer canyon, redwoods, and rolling golden savannas. The 4.8-mile out-and-back to Vicente Flat Camp is an excellent day hike or weekend trip.

Although you can hike the trail year-round, it can get quite cool and damp in the shady canyon in winter. Spring brings colorful wildflowers and new growth to the open slopes. Summer fog often obscures coastal views, while moderate fall temperatures keep fog banks well offshore.

Trip Description

From a saddle (3190') on the west side of **Cone Peak Road,** the **Vicente Flat Trail** climbs southwest toward a nearby ridge. From the ridge, you'll descend to another saddle and begin a series of short switchbacks that overlook **Hare Canyon**'s sheer north wall, composed of banded gneiss and other Salinian metamorphic rocks. Barely 3 miles long, the gorge rises from sea level to more than 3000 feet, making it one of the world's deepest canyons.

The trail descends past healthy, fire-regenerated thickets of yerba santa, chamise, and scrub oak to a small **ridge** (0.7 mile, 2500'). From here a more moderate gradient descends pine-clad slopes past the charred remains of Coulter pines that still bare their enormous cones. Onward, you'll pass large redwoods that succumbed to the 1999 Kirk Complex Fires. Some of these fire-scorched giants along upper **Hare Creek** have sprouted vibrant new shoots from their trunks, calling to mind bristled pipe cleaners.

Farther along the shady trail, gurgling water heralds your arrival on the banks of Hare Creek (1.1 miles, 2500'). You'll follow the intermittent creek for a quarter mile beneath more fire-ravaged redwoods before crossing it and a side gully. In another quarter mile, the steep trail recrosses the creek. Over the next 0.3 mile, you'll head southwest into the lush canyon, crossing the creek seven more times.

Past the fifth crossing, you'll reach **Vicente Flat Camp** (2.2 miles, 1700'). The first site is perched amid redwoods atop a flat creekside bench, with room for up to three tents. The second, more spacious site sits along the north bank and includes a table and fire ring. The third and fourth sites lie just downstream past old-growth redwoods at the extreme southern limit of their range.

Onward, the trail leads to **Vicente Flat** itself, a small meadow that hosts **two small sites** (2.4 miles, 1650'). Along the edge of the flat, two parallel paths skirt west. The upper

Ancient fire scars from large cavities inside old-growth redwoods at Vicente Flat.

trail, the main Vicente Flat Trail, climbs 0.1 mile through poison oak thickets to the **Stone Ridge Trail**. Avoid the poison oak in favor of the lower spur, which detours 70 feet to two creekside sites and rejoins the main trail only yards from the **Stone Ridge Trail junction** (2.5 miles, 1620').

If you're continuing on the scenic westbound Stone Ridge Trail, refer to TRIP 65 Cone Peak Loop. If you're bound for the coast, refer to TRIP 66 Highway 1 to Vicente Flat (page 271) and follow that trail description in reverse.

Trip 65

CONE PEAK LOOP

LENGTH AND TYPE: 15-mile out-and-back, loop, or point-to-point

RATING: Challenging

TRAIL CONDITION: Passable, poison oak

HIGHLIGHTS: Climb through coastal oak woodlands, pastoral hillsides, and thriving chaparral for tremendous views from 5155-foot Cone Peak.

TO REACH THE TRAILHEAD: The marked trailhead is on the west side of Cone Peak Road at Mile 3.7 near a small turnout for up to five cars. There are no facilities or water at the trailhead.

TRIP SUMMARY: You can approach this 15-mile loop as either an extremely strenuous day hike or a more enjoyable yet still strenuous backpacking trip, staying at one or more of the four camps along the route. Most people hike the 2.2 miles to Vicente Flat Camp, spend the night, and get a fresh start the following day. The onward route is slow going, as sections of the Stone Ridge Trail are overgrown with brush with faint, steep tread. If you do opt for a multiday trek, stay a second or third night at Goat, Ojito, or Trail Spring Camps. Regardless of your route, don't miss the 0.3-mile spur to the summit.

Instead of hiking the entire loop, consider day hiking the scenic lower section of Stone Ridge Trail. This lightly used trail offers tremendous views of surrounding peaks in the Limekiln drainage. If you're willing to descend from the Hare/Limekiln Creek divide, the trail plunges into cool redwood- and fern-lined canyons amid Limekiln's remote headwaters.

This route is best enjoyed in spring, when grassy slopes are cloaked with colorful lupines, blue-eyed grass, and California poppies. You'll climb from 1500 feet to 5155 feet through lush redwood canyons, yucca-dotted slopes, open grasslands, arid chaparral, and oak woodlands. Use caution on steep, slippery trails along the oak-clad canyon walls, and watch for hitchhiking ticks amid the encroaching brush. In summer, temperatures can be brutal and fog usually obscures coastal views, while fall brings moderate temperatures and diminished fly, tick, and mosquito populations.

CLEARING THE TRAILS ■ ■ ■ ■ ■ ■ ■ ■ ■ ■ ■ ■ ■ ■ ■ ■ ■ ■ ■

Over the past few decades, six major fires have swept through Los Padres National Forest: the 1977 Marble-Cone Fire, the 1985 Rat Creek Fire, the 1992 Cienega Fire, the 1993 Big Sur Gorge Fire, the 1999 Kirk Complex Fires, and the 2008 Basin Complex Fire. The latter scarred most of the Ventana Wilderness, burning 162,818 acres. In this era of fire suppression, enormous amounts of dead and downed trees build up, creating catastrophic damage when fires do sweep through.

Following a wildfire, charred trees and debris obscure trails and lay waste to camps. Free from the limiting shade of a forest canopy, the understory of shrubs such as ceanothus, poison oak, chamise, and manzanita aggressively sprouts new shoots, obscuring tread and sometimes choking the path altogether. Winter storms bring an onslaught of mudslides and washouts, which further erode trails, creating dangerous hiking conditions.

Fortunately, dedicated Ventana hikers and wilderness enthusiasts volunteer their time and efforts to help the US Forest Service maintain these scenic trails. If you'd like to get involved, visit the Ventana Wilderness Alliance at ventanawild.org or the Sierra Club's Ventana chapter at ventana.sierraclub.org.

Trip Description

See TRIP 64 Vicente Flat Trail (page 264) for the first 2.4 miles of this route to **Vicente Flat** (1650').

Along the edge of the flat, two parallel paths skirt west. The upper trail, the main **Vicente Flat Trail,** climbs 0.1 mile through poison oak thickets to the **Stone Ridge Trail**. Avoid the poison oak in favor of the lower spur, which detours 70 feet to two creekside sites and rejoins the main trail only yards from the **Stone Ridge Trail junction** (2.5 miles, 1620'). If you're bound for the coast on the Vicente Flat Trail, refer to TRIP 66 Highway 1 to Vicente Flat (page 271) and follow that trail description in reverse.

From the signed junction, the Stone Ridge Trail climbs northwest through dense redwoods and tanoaks into sun-dappled oak woodlands. Beyond a minor gully lined with poison oak, you'll climb to a grassy knoll that offers views up sheer-sided **Hare Canyon** toward **Cone Peak**. The trail continues past oak savannas (2.8 miles, 1830') that harbor several picnic spots, ideal for day hikers from Vicente Flat. In spring this open terrain is carpeted in vibrant wildflowers.

As you skirt a ridge composed largely of marble, the narrow trail opens on spectacular coastal views. Watch your footing along a minor washout just before you reach the saddle that divides Hare Canyon and **Limekiln Canyon** (3.8 miles, 2030'). From the saddle, a 0.2-mile spur leads west atop a ridge for views thousands of feet down-canyon to the foamy surf.

The main trail descends from the saddle along the steep north-facing slopes of the Limekiln Creek drainage. Be on your guard for poison oak along this lightly used stretch. Increasingly steeper switchbacks lead past sprawling oaks to deep redwood-lined gullies. You'll have to clamber over and around large fallen oaks and redwoods in some sections, especially difficult if you're carrying a heavy pack. The trail leads north to the **creek** (4.6 miles, 1530'), where windstorms have toppled several large redwoods.

Across the reliable headwaters, the trail leads 10 yards downstream, climbs the canyon's steep west wall, switchbacks and leads north, skirting several large fallen tanoaks. Expect to find lots of debris from dead or dying oaks afflicted by sudden oak death (see sidebar, page 165). The trail continues across a minor ridge to a shallow canyon.

Following a seasonal stream west up the canyon, you'll climb first past shady redwoods then beneath live oaks and bays to two unofficial campsites. Perched beside the stream, each offers room for up to two tents. Beyond the second site, a curious trashcan sits alongside the trail. Regular garbage pickup service is not offered in the backcountry, so please pack out all your trash.

The trail beyond climbs southwest to an obvious oak-clad **saddle** (5.4 miles, 2030'), then northwest along a nearly level ridge. A hundred feet past a minor gully lined with

Enjoy breathtaking views from pastoral coastal oak woodlands.

madrones, oaks, and bays, the trail emerges in the open (5.9 miles, 2160'). For the next half mile, you'll enjoy sweeping views of the coast, Cone Peak, and sheer Hare and Limekiln Canyons. In spring, the otherwise golden hillsides are blanketed in lupines, poppies, buttercups, blue-eyed grass, mariposa lilies, shooting stars, and blue dicks. Watch the skies for common raptors, as well as the rare and endangered California condor, which boasts a massive 9-foot wingspan.

Onward, the trail follows a gentle contour and climbs a prominent ridge to a **minor gap** (6.4 miles, 2260') for filtered views through live oaks. Continue past a cluster of ponderosa pines to the headwaters of **West Fork Limekiln Creek.** Winding 0.8 mile through several shady gullies, the trail leads to a prominent **gully** (7.2 miles, 2170') of exposed, weathered marble. In all but the heaviest downpour, it's an easy hop across.

You'll soon enter the canyon's largest eastside gully along a boulder-strewn wash beneath a dense redwood canopy. The trail continues north across two more gullies, the second hosting a reliable creek. After veering 100 yards west to a grassy slope, you'll turn northwest to the **Goat Camp junction** (8.4 miles, 2500').

A short spur trail descends southwest to **Goat Camp,** nestled in the shade of oaks and sugar pines. Offering wonderful ocean views, this remote camp can accommodate up to four tents. During wet season, the nearest water source lies only a minute farther along the Stone Ridge Trail. In dry months, you'll need to return 0.6 mile to the large gully.

Fifty yards from the Goat Camp junction, the trail contours past Limekiln's northern headwaters, which in wet season supports a small creek that sustains a few staunch redwoods. Onward 0.1 mile, the trail begins a steep climb past the charred remains of a pre-1999 forest, now overgrown with ceanothus, broom, and yerba santa. Watch your footing on the loose tread, and be alert for hitchhiking ticks in spring. Switchbacks climb 500 feet to an obvious saddle and the three-way junction with the **Gamboa** and **Ojito Camp Trails** (9.3 miles, 3450').

SIDE TRIP ■

From the junction, the unmarked **Ojito Camp Trail** heads north, dropping 600 feet in the next 0.6 mile to Devils Canyon. On my last trip, encroaching brush and large fallen snags obstructed the route, though it was flagged and remained passable.

You'll descend a gentle grade to a nearby saddle, then plunge steeply to the south bank of **South Fork Devils Creek.** A faint overgrown trail leads 200 yards downstream along the swift creek to **Ojito Camp,** which has room for up to two tents. Those willing to venture cross-country will find myriad beautiful pools and cascades.

■ ■

Back at the saddle, the Gamboa Trail begins just left of a large pine snag, 50 feet before you reach a large fallen oak across the trail. The trail follows an ancient American Indian trading route past Coulter pines and Douglas and Santa Lucia firs. Filtered views overlook the South Fork's remote swimming holes and glistening **Pacific** beyond. Trail conditions along this stretch are dramatically better than on the Stone Ridge Trail. The route is well defined with no encroaching brush. Descend the gentle grade 1.6 miles to **Trail Spring Camp** and the **Coast Ridge Trail junction** (10.9 miles, 3800').

Trail Spring Camp offers one small site on sloping ground beside the unreliable headwaters of South Fork Devils Creek. To find water in dry months, anticipate a steep 300-foot descent 0.3 mile along the boulder wash. The **Coast Ridge Trail** continues 1.5 miles across the boulder-strewn gully to the end of **Cone Peak Road.** Twenty feet above camp is the signed **Cone Peak Trail junction** (10.9 miles, 3800').

Short switchbacks climb quickly to a broad, boulder-lined creek bed, only wet during heavy rains. Here enormous sugar pines tower above an open canopy of scorched manzanitas, tanoaks, scrub oaks, and ceanothus. As you climb longer switchbacks toward the isolated summit, you'll pass rare, endemic Santa Lucia firs, Santa Lucia bedstraw, and Santa Lucia lupines.

The trail reaches a narrow ridge between Devils and Limekiln Canyons that leads west to Cone Peak's neighbor, 4843-foot **Twin Peak.** Follow this ridge east to the **Cone Peak Summit Trail junction** (12.1 miles, 4830'). The 0.3-mile spur climbs short, steep switchbacks to the 5155-foot summit (see TRIP 62 Cone Peak Trail, page 260, for details).

From here it's 2 miles east along the Cone Peak Trail to Cone Peak Road. Again, refer to TRIP 62 Cone Peak Trail and follow that trail description in reverse. At Cone Peak Road, turn right and descend 530 feet in 1.5 miles to reach the **Vicente Flat Trailhead** at Mile 3.7. For directions to **Vicente Flat Camp**, see TRIP 64 Vicente Flat Trail (page 264).

Trip 66

HIGHWAY 1 TO VICENTE FLAT

LENGTH AND TYPE: 5.3-mile out-and-back or 7.7-mile point-to-point

RATING: Strenuous

TRAIL CONDITION: Clear, poison oak

HIGHLIGHTS: Climb from golden coastal bluffs to Vicente Flat Camp, nestled beneath ancient redwoods along Hare Creek.

TO REACH THE TRAILHEAD: The trailhead is on the east side of Highway 1, across the street from Kirk Creek Campground, 36 miles north of Hearst Castle, 41 miles north of Cambria, 38 miles south of Pfeiffer Big Sur State Park, and 54 miles south of Carmel. There are no facilities or water at the trailhead. If you're bound for Cone Peak Road and plan to use a shuttle vehicle, be aware that the road is closed during the wet season (November through April). See TRIP 64 Vicente Flat Trail (page 264) for more information.

TRIP SUMMARY: You can approach this primarily uphill route as either a scenic day hike or an out-and-back overnight. Or you can use Vicente Flat as a base camp for grander tours of the wilderness via the Stone Ridge, Gamboa, and Cone Peak Trails. If you can arrange a shuttle vehicle, consider the route from Cone Peak Road to Highway 1, which is virtually all downhill (see TRIP 64 Vicente Flat Trail).

From Highway 1, this route ascends nearly 2000 feet above the wave-swept coast. Bare golden terraces allow dramatic coastal and canyon vistas as the trail climbs pastoral hilltops into redwood-lined Hare Creek. Vicente Flat offers sites amid old-growth trees and atop a sun-drenched meadow.

Spring welcomes a profusion of wildflowers to the otherwise golden slopes. Watch for the rare and fragile orchid-like chocolate lily, which blooms along the lower portion of the trail. In wet months Hare Creek abounds with life. American dippers dive for food or bob along the banks, while California newts slither slowly to the water. Red, orange, yellow, and purple fungi emerge from the damp forest floor, and lush ferns, mosses, and horsetails thrive in the verdant canyon.

Trip Description

From its marked trailhead along **Highway 1** (190'), the **Vicente Flat Trail** quickly climbs a series of switchbacks north past coastal scrub, vibrant in spring with flowering lupines, poppies, sticky monkeyflowers, and sagebrush. In 0.3 mile you'll cross a minor gully, head toward a minor saddle, then turn north across rolling grasslands and sun-drenched coastal chaparral. Crossing a gully choked with invasive blackberry and broom species, you'll hear trickling from a nearby **spring** (0.9 mile, 700').

The grade steepens as the trail passes scattered yuccas, attesting to the aridity of these exposed slopes and switchbacks. You'll soon reach a **ridge** (1.4 miles, 1000') that offers spectacular views of the vast convergence of land and sea. This is a favorite day-hiking destination.

Onward, the trail enters the **Ventana Wilderness** and after 0.3 mile reaches shade beneath a canopy of oaks, madrones, and bays. Follow the ridgeline through four gullies past a dense band of redwoods. After a steep climb to a prominent ridge (2.9 miles, 1610'), pause to rest and enjoy the views. To the east is 5155-foot **Cone Peak** and its neighbor, double-notched **Twin Peak,** which loom over **Hare and Limekiln Creeks. Hare Canyon** is one of the world's deepest gorges, while **Limekiln Canyon** boasts the steepest coastal slope in the Lower 48 on its climb to Cone Peak.

The trail descends from the ridge, veering northeast through varied microclimates that support a wide range of drought-tolerant and moisture-loving plants. Yuccas dot the open, arid slopes, while redwoods cluster in the gullies. One hundred yards past a major gully along an unreliable creek, marked by a large fallen redwood, you'll reach a spur to **Espinosa Camp.**

The spur leads 100 feet to camp (3.4 miles, 1660'), which sits atop a minor ridge in the shade of live oaks, bays, redwoods, and rare, endemic Santa Lucia firs. Two small flats can accommodate up to four tents. Rock outcrops offer unobstructed views toward the coast. This is an excellent picnic spot, though the gully nearest camp is usually dry. Just 1.8 miles farther along the main trail, the roomier **Vicente Flat Camp** is adjacent to reliable Hare Creek.

Beyond the spur, you'll round a prominent ridge and skirt a large tanoak afflicted by sudden oak death, evidenced by its large cankerous wounds (see sidebar, page 165). On a contour 0.2 mile past camp, the trail reaches the first reliable water source, a creeklet that cascades past redwoods and lush ferns. Across the creeklet and through another gully, you'll emerge on open grassy slopes with ocean views. Here the trail veers east, tops out at 1860 feet, and begins a gentle descent to Vicente Flat.

Enjoy unsurpassed views during spring and fall, when typical summer fog and winter storm fronts have passed.

Soon you'll cross three typically dry rubble-strewn **gullies** (4.1 miles, 1800'), whose confluence lies 100 feet downslope. In winter, water plunges from adjacent marble faces, misting the surrounding greenery. Beyond the next dry redwood gully, the trail contours north and enters dense forest a quarter mile from Hare Creek. Several notably large redwoods mark your arrival at Vicente Flat.

A few feet past the creek, a spur cuts upstream to Vicente Flat Camp. Poison oak is less of a concern along this well-used stretch. The main trail continues a few yards to the **Stone Ridge Trail junction** (5.2 miles, 1620') and 0.1 mile beyond to the camp's lower reaches. See TRIP 64 Vicente Flat Trail (page 264) for a description of camp.

Silver Peak
Wilderness

■ ■ ■ ■ ■ ■ ■ ■ ■ ■ ■ ■ ■

I N 1992, the Los Padres Condor Range & River Protection Act established the Silver Peak Wilderness. It originally protected 14,500 acres of this sheer region, where ridges plunge into deep V-shaped canyons and streams cascade past smooth boulders and deep pools on their way to the Pacific. An additional 17,055 acres are being added to these pristine lands within the Willow Creek and San Carpoforo drainages.

The wilderness encompasses a biologically rich landscape characterized by golden oak savannas, sun-drenched chaparral slopes, and lush riparian canyons. Northern and southern biogeographical regions converge here in a sharp dichotomy of vegetation. Redwoods push their southern limits amid verdant canyons carpeted in ferns and mosses. Watch for slithering salamanders and chatty winter wrens. Immediately adjacent, yet more typical of areas farther south, semiarid grasslands host yuccas, rufous-crowned sparrows, and scurrying alligator lizards. The wilderness also shelters such threatened and endangered species as the southern steelhead and the California condor.

Bounded on the west by the Pacific, the Silver Peak Wilderness rises thousands of feet to the crest of the Santa Lucia Range. Here, hikers can lose themselves amid river canyons, wildflower-strewn meadows, and high peaks that overlook the rugged coast.

DIRECTIONS: From San Simeon, head north on Highway 1, 1.5 miles past the Monterey County line. The Salmon Creek Trailhead is on the east side of the highway, at the heart of the Silver Peak Wilderness.

VISITOR CENTER: Pacific Valley Station: (805) 927-4211. The station is on the east side of Highway 1, a mile north of the Sand Dollar Beach Day-Use Area, 30 miles north of Hearst Castle, and 60 miles south of Carmel. Open daily 8 a.m.–5 p.m.

NEAREST CAMPGROUND: Plaskett Creek Campground (41 sites, $22/night; reservations recommended spring–fall and on holidays) is on the east side of Highway 1, 0.1 mile south of the entrance to the Sand Dollar Beach Day-Use Area, 40 miles south of Pfeiffer Big Sur State Park, and 35 miles north of San Simeon State

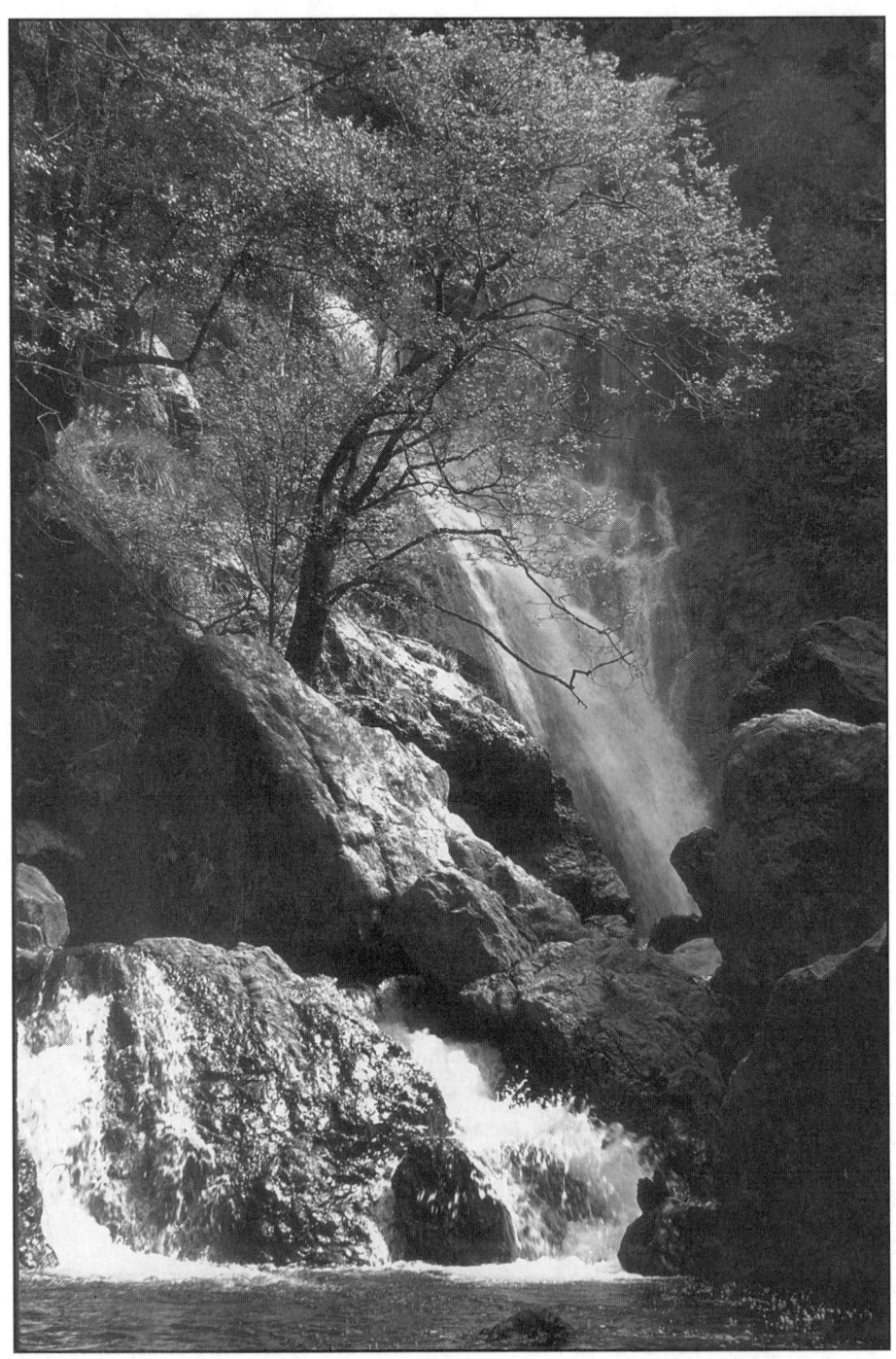

Just a short stroll from Highway 1, Salmon Falls is a wonderful stop along your coastal road trip.

Park. There's a maximum of eight people per site. Each site includes a picnic table, fire ring, and pedestal grill. Drinking water is available. For more information call Reserve America at (800) 444-7275 or visit ReserveAmerica.com.

INFORMATION: Fire permits required for all stoves. Dogs permitted and allowed off leash, except in designated campgrounds, where a 6-foot or shorter leash is required. Horses and livestock are allowed on the trail, but bikes are prohibited.

WEBSITE: www.fs.usda.gov/lpnf

PHONE: USFS Monterey District Headquarters: (831) 385-5434; USFS Pacific Valley Station: (805) 927-4211

Trip 67

PREWITT LOOP TRAIL

LENGTH AND TYPE: 12.8-mile out-and-back or loop

RATING: Strenuous

TRAIL CONDITION: Clear to difficult, poison oak

HIGHLIGHTS: Dramatic coastal views of sandy coves and jagged promontories from a remote canyon in the heart of Pacific Valley

TO REACH THE TRAILHEAD: The northern trailhead is on the east side of Highway 1, 30 miles south of Big Sur Station and 57 miles south of Carmel. The southern trailhead is on the east side of Highway 1, 0.8 mile north of the Pacific Valley Station, 2 miles north of Plaskett Creek Campground, and 17 miles north of Ragged Point. The following route description begins from the northern trailhead.

Parking for the northern trailhead is on the east side of Highway 1, at a turnout adjacent to the trailhead. There are no facilities or water at the trailhead. Parking for the southern trailhead is at the Pacific Valley Station. Parking is free at both trailheads.

TRIP SUMMARY: This hike leads past a diverse array of plant communities, from dense thickets of coastal scrub to cool redwood groves, oak and pine woodlands, and grassy savannas. The trail is best enjoyed in spring, when fields of delicate wildflowers boast profuse colors and aromas. For the best views, visit between October and April, when fog banks roll well offshore. On my last trip, the trail past Stag Camp was suffering from loose tread and active slides. Use caution.

Trip Description

From the turnout on **Highway 1,** stroll 50 feet down a single-lane dirt road to the signed **Prewitt Loop Trailhead.** According to the sign, the first backcountry camp, Stag Camp, is 4 miles from the junction (actual mileage 4.1 miles) and the entire loop trail is 12 miles (actual mileage 12.8 miles).

From the junction, turn right onto the **Prewitt Loop Trail** and head southeast past ocean views through fragrant thickets of sagebrush, coyote brush, coffeeberry, and poison oak. In 0.1 mile you'll switchback north and climb past two small seeps amid chain ferns, horsetails, and a stand of willows. At the next switchback, the trail climbs southeast past two dry **gullies** (0.4 mile, 440').

Continue on a moderate grade past a dilapidated wooden gate marking the barbwire fence line of private property. Pause for views along the open coastal slope where **Prewitt Creek** meets the **Pacific** just north of **Sand Dollar Beach**. A few minutes past the gate, you'll reach a four-way junction (0.7 mile, 630') with an unmarked private trail that leads down to the small housing development in **Pacific Valley**.

Fifty yards farther southeast, the trail crosses an abandoned, overgrown roadbed and bends east for your first glimpse of the broad Prewitt Creek watershed. Narrow belts of redwoods stretch up canyon like veins, following the moisture-bearing gullies and ravines, while

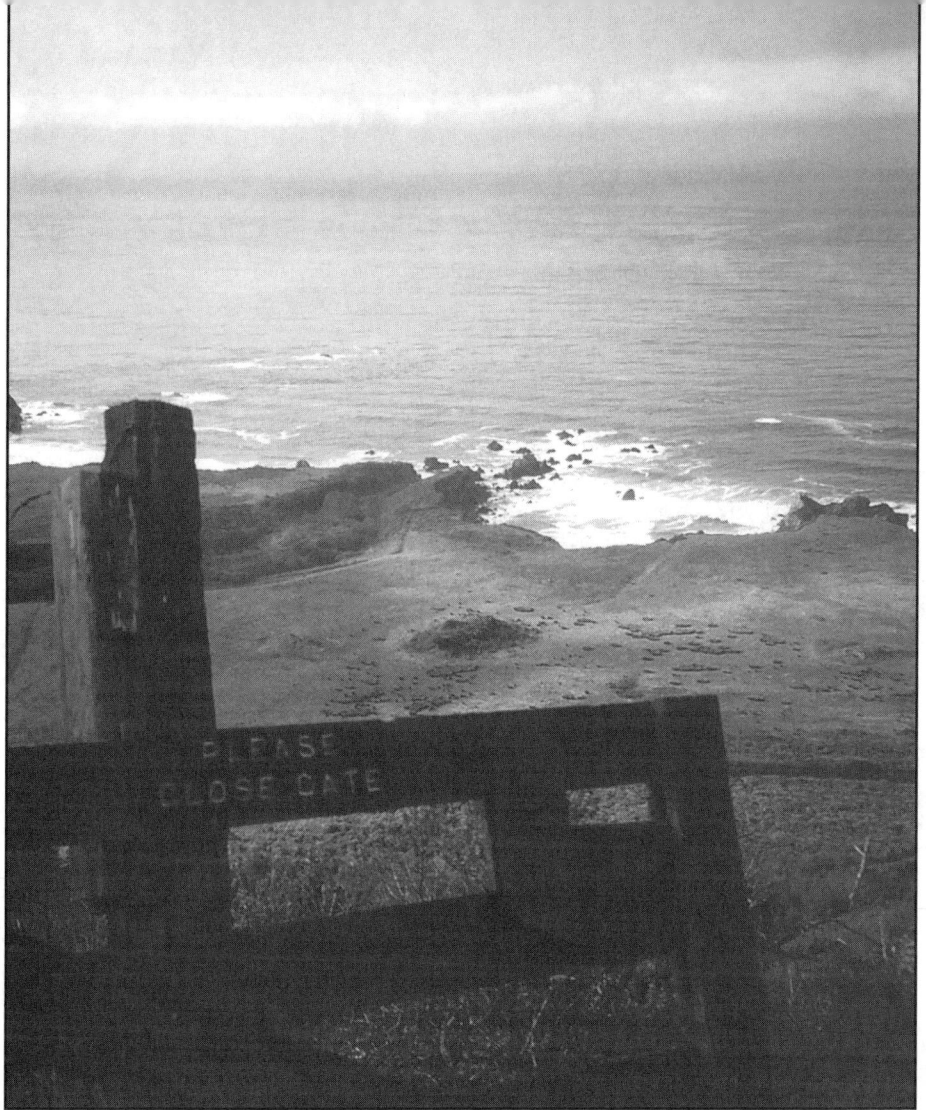

A broad marine terrace, which gave Pacific Valley its name, rises above the rocky shoreline and below the Prewitt Loop Trail.

more drought-tolerant oaks and pines stud the upper watershed. The trail contours past exposed south-facing slopes of arid chaparral and grasses, in dramatic contrast to the cooler, shadier north-facing slopes of mixed evergreens across the canyon.

The grade eases as you contour past three small dry gullies fringed with slender redwoods, live oaks, and bays. Climbing to grassy slopes studded with mature live oaks, the trail reaches the Prewitt Creek headwaters and crosses two small gullies 50 feet apart (2.6 miles, 1420'). Past the second gully, you'll switchback southeast to an easily missed spur **junction** (2.7 miles, 1530'). This spur doglegs left and climbs 150 yards to a dramatic overlook.

Past the spur, the main trail meanders through oak and pine woodlands populated by busy acorn woodpeckers, which store acorns to feed grubs they will later devour. Cross three prominent gullies (dry in all but heavy rain) to a stand of sycamores amid a fourth gully (3.8 miles, 1650'). Easily identified by mottled cream-and-white bark that resembles a jigsaw puzzle, the sycamores offer a place to picnic and enjoy canyon views. If you'd prefer a shadier spot with a picnic table, continue 0.3 mile to Stag Camp.

LUCKY COWS OR SPACE HOGS? ■ ■ ■ ■ ■ ■ ■ ■ ■ ■ ■ ■ ■ ■

Gazing across the coastal terrace and lush grasslands at Pacific Valley, you may well wonder, "How lucky can a cow be?" Local cattle ranchers also feel pretty lucky, since they pay nearly a tenth of the market rate to graze each head of cattle on public vs. private lands. In 2004, the Forest Service charged allotment holders a measly $1.43 per AUM (animal unit month) for running cattle on the public land. Market rates on private land range from $12.50 to $15 per AUM. Cheap rent and a spectacular view—something to moo about.

However, all those happy hooves inflict a toll on the land. Cows graze native flora and fauna, trample delicate riparian zones, gouge and erode unstable slopes, and disperse seeds of invasive nonnative plants. They also disturb complex ecosystems by eating blooms that sustain butterflies, insects, and birds, in turn affecting predators further up the food chain.

Burger, anyone?

■ ■

A minute past the sycamore-lined gully, the trail passes a piped spring where water spills into a manmade trough. This is the most reliable water till you reach the **South Fork** headwaters, 6.8 miles from the trailhead. Many animals use this spring. Look for the tracks and scat of such species as coyotes, bobcats, gray foxes, and the occasional mountain lion.

Continue climbing past grassy slopes that in spring burst with decadent displays of lupines, shooting stars, and California poppies. The trail dips through a minor gully past ancient oaks nearly 4 feet in diameter, then bends south and leads straight to **Stag Camp** (4.1 miles, 1760'). In the shade of sprawling tanoaks and bays, the lone site offers room for up to three small tents and includes a table and fire ring. Although the trail leads through camp, you'll see few hikers along this little-used route.

Past this point, the trail is sketchy and not recommended. In spots, poison oak, rocks, brush, and large debris encroach on or obscure the tread. Although crews recently cleared much of the brush and slide debris from the trail, slopes along the creek's upper headwaters are prone to future slides. In fact, just past camp the trail crosses gullies past two major slides in an area known as **Big Slide** (4.9 miles, 1800').

Hardy hikers will continue along arid south-facing slopes where chaparral species such as coyote brush and chamise thrive. The revitalizing sound of water heralds your arrival at the South Fork (6.8 miles, 1880'). The trail crosses the rocky canyon on a fallen redwood and climbs a **ridge** (7.8 miles, 1950') between two of the headwater drainages. You'll veer north for the next 0.1 mile, switchback east 100 yards, then drop south into **Kelly Camp**.

Beyond the South Fork headwaters, the trail descends the remaining 3.5 miles to its southern trailhead at the **Pacific Valley Station**. If you parked your vehicle at the northern trailhead, you'll need to hike 0.8 mile north along Highway 1 to the turnout.

Trip 68

ALDER CREEK CAMP TO VILLA CREEK CAMP

LENGTH AND TYPE: 4.2-mile out-and-back, 4.7-mile point-to-point (Highway 1), or 8.4-mile point-to-point (Salmon Creek Station)

RATING: Strenuous

TRAIL CONDITION: Passable, poison oak

HIGHLIGHTS: Pause for unobstructed coastal views as you follow glassy creeks through peaceful groves of alders and redwoods.

TO REACH THE TRAILHEAD: Willow Creek Road is on the east side of Highway 1, 8 miles south of Nacimiento-Fergusson Road, 62 miles south of Carmel, a mile north of Gorda, and 8.4 miles north of the southern Buckeye Trailhead at the abandoned Salmon Creek Station.

Climb this rugged dirt road about 7 miles to an unmarked four-way junction and stay straight on the right fork, which makes a steep 1.5 mile descent into the Alder Creek drainage. The road ends at Alder Creek Camp, though it may be impassable during heavy winter rains. In summer it's a dry, dusty road. The signed northern Buckeye Trailhead lies on the north bank, 100 feet downstream from the main campsite.

TRIP SUMMARY: This route offers several day-hike or overnight options, including: (1) 4.2 miles round-trip to Villa Creek Camp; (2) 4.7 miles point-to-point from Alder Creek Camp to Highway 1 via the Buckeye and Cruikshank Trails; and (3) 8.4 miles point-to-point to Salmon Creek Station via the Buckeye Trail. If you can arrange a shuttle vehicle, consider the point-to-point treks, which offer unobstructed coastal views.

This hike is best enjoyed in spring and fall, when fog banks roll well offshore. Colorful spring wildflowers paint hillside oak savannas, while in fall, creekside alders and maples flash vibrant yellows, oranges, and reds. Seriously consider wearing pants on this hike to protect against ubiquitous poison oak and ticks.

Trip Description

From its northern trailhead at **Alder Creek Camp** (2240'), the **Buckeye Trail** enters the creek's lush corridor, where poison oak is a common trailside companion. You'll quickly cross **Alder Creek** and begin climbing the canyon walls southwest through dense oak woodlands and encroaching ceanothus thickets.

Sections of this trail may be overgrown. (For the latest trail conditions, contact the Pacific Valley Station, (805) 927-4211, or the Ventana Wilderness Alliance, (831) 423-3191.)

After half a mile, the well-graded trail tops a grassy ridge between the **Villa Creek** and Alder Creek drainages. In spring, pause to picnic amid these wildflower-strewn slopes and watch as hawks kite over the tall grass in search of small prey. In 2003, flags marked the faint tread across the open slopes past stands of pines and oaks.

From the ridge, you'll veer right into the Villa Creek drainage, forging briefly through dense thickets of chaparral, primarily ceanothus. The trail abruptly switchbacks right and reenters the Alder Creek drainage, then heads toward a conspicuous serpentine outcrop at the divide.

From the divide, the trail skirts the western edge of open slopes 0.6 mile and drops past a seeping spring that supports thriving willows and exotic pampas grass. Onward, past a cluster of fragrant bays and a dry wash, the trail steepens on its final descent to the banks of Villa Creek. You'll emerge at **Villa Creek Camp** (2.1 miles, 1050), perched atop a small creekside bench.

There's room for up to three small tents in the shade of redwoods beside the year-round creek. You'll also find a table and a fire ring. In summer, the shade offers welcome respite from the sun-drenched upper canyon. During the wet season, colorful fungi sprout from the lush forest floor, though the camp may be damp and cold.

Trip 69

HIGHWAY 1 TO VILLA CREEK CAMP

LENGTH AND TYPE: 5.6-mile out-and-back

RATING: Moderate

TRAIL CONDITION: Clear, poison oak

HIGHLIGHTS: Gorgeous coastal views en route to a redwood-lined camp

TO REACH THE TRAILHEAD: The Cruikshank Trailhead is on the east side of Highway 1, 0.6 mile south of the Villa Creek bridge, 66 miles south of Carmel, and 4.5 miles north of the abandoned Salmon Creek Station. Park at the small turnout on Highway 1 adjacent to the trailhead. There are no facilities or water at the trailhead.

TRIP SUMMARY: From Highway 1, you'll climb the Cruikshank Trail east along Villa Creek's steep south canyon wall, then descend the Buckeye Trail north to cool, redwood-fringed Villa Creek Camp.

Trip Description

From the signed **Cruikshank Trailhead** on **Highway 1,** you'll quickly climb steep switchbacks through dense coastal scrub. Pause often to catch your breath and take in the dramatic coastal views. After a strenuous 600-foot ascent in less than a mile, the grade eases.

Continue along the south wall of deep, V-shaped **Villa Creek** canyon through shallow redwood-lined gullies. You'll cross a small creek fringed with redwood sorrel, starflowers, and ferns, then a minute later pass a few eucalyptus trees, probably planted here by early homesteaders. Two miles from the trailhead, you'll cross logs over a small creek and enter

Lower Cruikshank Camp (see TRIP 70 Cruikshank & Silver Camps, on the following page, for details). Just past camp lies the signed **Buckeye Trail junction** (2.2 miles, 1440').

At the junction, turn left onto the northbound **Buckeye Trail**. Past an open meadow that marks the **Cruikshank homestead,** you'll make a steep 450-foot descent in half a mile to **Villa Creek** (2.7 miles, 1070'), amid a narrow band of redwoods.

At the southern limit of their range, these redwoods are only able to find adequate moisture for survival along such small creeks. Drier conditions prevent the trees from obtaining the colossal size more commonly associated with old-growth stands farther north. Other than a few small patches of redwood sorrel, sword ferns, and seasonal wildflowers, the forest floor here is also comparatively bare.

Crossing to the north bank, you'll briefly follow the year-round creek downstream to a trail junction and seasonal side drainage. From this junction, the left fork descends to **Villa Creek Camp** (2.8 miles, 1050'), which offers a table, a fire ring, and room for up to three small tents.

The Buckeye Trail continues north along the right fork. If you're bound for **Alder Creek Camp**, refer to TRIP 68 Alder Creek Camp to Villa Creek Camp (page 281) and follow that trail description in reverse.

Fresh signs of mountain lion are commonly found along the Cruikshank Trail.

Trip 70

CRUIKSHANK & SILVER CAMPS

LENGTH AND TYPE: 6.2-mile out-and-back

RATING: Moderate to challenging

TRAIL CONDITION: Clear to difficult, poison oak

HIGHLIGHTS: This scenic trail climbs past fragrant coastal scrub and vibrant spring wildflowers to lush redwood forests.

TO REACH THE TRAILHEAD: The Cruikshank Trailhead is on the east side of Highway 1, 0.6 mile south of the Villa Creek bridge, 66 miles south of Carmel, and 4.5 miles north of the abandoned Salmon Creek Station. Park at the small turnout on Highway 1 adjacent to the trailhead. There are no facilities or water at the trailhead.

TRIP SUMMARY: The Cruikshank Trail climbs the Villa Creek drainage 6.5 miles to its headwaters below Coast Ridge Road. Due to poor trail conditions, including encroaching poison oak and fallen trees, it's best to avoid the trail beyond Silver Camp.

Depending on your stamina and susceptibility to poison oak, this route offers several day-hike or overnight options, including: (1) 4.4 miles round-trip to Cruikshank Camp (trails are clear and well maintained); (2) 6.2 miles round-trip to Silver Camp (trails passable with some poison oak); and (3) 9 miles round-trip to Buckeye Camp via the Cruikshank and Buckeye Trails (see TRIP 71 Highway 1 to Buckeye Camp, page 286). If you can arrange a shuttle vehicle, consider a point-to-point trip from the lower Cruikshank Trailhead to the abandoned Salmon Creek Station (refer to TRIP 72 Salmon Creek Station to Buckeye Camp, page 288), although sections of the lower Buckeye Trail may be overgrown.

Trip Description

From the signed **Cruikshank Trailhead** on **Highway 1,** you'll quickly climb steep switchbacks through dense coastal scrub. Pause often to catch your breath and appreciate the stunning coastal views. After a strenuous 600-foot ascent in less than a mile, the grade eases.

Continue along the south wall of deep, V-shaped **Villa Creek** canyon through shallow redwood-lined gullies. You'll cross a small creek fringed with redwood sorrel, starflowers, and ferns, then a minute later pass a few eucalyptus trees, likely planted here by early homesteaders. Two miles from the trailhead, you'll cross logs over a small creek and enter **Lower Cruikshank Camp** (1300').

In the shade of redwoods and bays, the first campsite is equipped with a fire ring. The trail continues 0.2 mile to a shady second campsite (2.2 miles, 1400'), equipped with a fire ring and a bench in the shade of sprawling oaks. Just past the second site, you'll reach the signed **Buckeye Trail junction** (2.2 miles, 1440').

From this junction, the northbound **Buckeye Trail** leads to **Villa Creek and Alder Creek Camps** (see TRIP 68 Alder Creek Camp to Villa Creek Camp, page 281), the eastbound **Cruikshank Trail** leads to **Silver** and **Lion Den Camps,** and the southbound Buckeye Trail leads first to **Buckeye Camp,** then 3.4 miles farther to the abandoned **Salmon Creek Station** (see TRIP 72 Salmon Creek Station to Buckeye Camp, page 288).

Continue east on the Cruikshank Trail to **Cruikshank Camp,** amid a small open meadow, site of the former **Cruikshank homestead** and an **American Indian midden** dating back to the Salinian Indians. Poison oak encroaches on the trail beyond this point.

Southeast of camp, the trail ascends 510 feet over the next 0.9 mile to **Silver Camp** (3.1 miles, 1950'), amid a picturesque grassland.

Past camp, poison oak and debris obstruct the narrow trail, which is hard to discern from the many deer paths that cross the route. If you're determined to hike farther, the trail leads 2.5 miles farther to **Silver Peak Road,** 2.9 miles to Lion Den Camp, and 3.4 miles to the junction of **Coast Ridge Road.**

Trip 71

HIGHWAY 1 TO BUCKEYE CAMP

LENGTH AND TYPE: 9-mile out-and-back or 7.9-mile point-to-point

RATING: Moderate to strenuous

TRAIL CONDITION: Clear to difficult, poison oak

HIGHLIGHTS: In spring, sprawling Buckeye Meadow boasts a carpet of colorful wildflowers.

TO REACH THE TRAILHEAD: The Cruikshank Trailhead is on the east side of Highway 1, 0.6 mile south of the Villa Creek bridge, 66 miles south of Carmel, and 4.5 miles north of the abandoned Salmon Creek Station. Park at the small turnout on Highway 1 adjacent to the trailhead. There are no facilities or water at the trailhead.

TRIP SUMMARY: This route to Buckeye Camp via the Cruikshank and Buckeye Trails is ideal in spring, when wildflowers and other budding plants blanket the open meadow. The trails are passable, though poison oak and washouts are common in places.

Other options include a 4.4-mile round-trip to Cruikshank Camp (trails are clear and well maintained) or, if you can arrange a shuttle vehicle, the 7.9-mile point-to-point trek from the abandoned Salmon Creek Station to the lower Cruikshank Trailhead (refer to TRIP 72 Salmon Creek Station to Buckeye Camp, page 288).

Trip Description

See TRIP 70 Cruikshank & Silver Camps (page 285) for the first 2.2 miles of this route to the signed **Buckeye Trail junction** (1440').

Turn right at the junction and head south on the **Buckeye Trail.** You'll climb the north slopes of **Villa Creek** canyon past oak and pine woodlands and across redwood-lined dry gullies. Unfortunately, trail conditions deteriorate, as encroaching plants obscure an already diminished tread.

In scattered shade, the trail climbs to an open saddle along **Redwood Gulch.** On my hike, red and pink flagging marked this indistinct stretch, which climbs south from the saddle toward a pine-rimmed minor ridge (3.1 miles, 2200'). Pause atop the ridge for far-reaching views.

From here the trail contours through dense coastal scrub past five gullies, dry in all but the heaviest rains. It's best to wear long pants along this stretch, as ticks are common during the wet season and poison oak is a year-round nuisance. Past the fifth gully, the route drops along poor tread to a small creek (4.1 miles, 1890') that's usually dry by summer. An easy hop across leads quickly to a second creek that also runs dry by summer. Onward, the trail leads north from the pleasant shade of maples and oaks to a large rocky outcrop, then southeast to the edge of **Buckeye Meadow.**

Entering the oak-rimmed meadow, you'll reach the smaller of **Buckeye Camp**'s two sites (4.5 miles, 2050'). Marked by a fire ring and a weathered table, this site offers room for up to

Sprawling oaks and buckeyes line the carpet of wildflowers each spring in Buckeye Meadow.

two tents. Onward, the trail threads between two large valley oaks and leads 100 yards farther to the large main site (2060'), which can accommodate several tents in the shade of a large fragrant bay. This is an ideal spot for a group outing, with plenty of room to play Frisbee or frolic in the broad meadow. A reliable spring-fed creek passes just south of camp, though in summer the shallow murky water may lose its appeal.

Scattered large ponderosa and Coulter pines and eucalyptus trees border the meadow, which in spring is painted with deep purple lupines. Enjoy the beautiful surroundings before returning to the trailhead. If you're after a grander tour of the wilderness, refer to the following trip and reverse the trail description.

A BLESSING & A CURSE

While the dedication of Highway 1 in 1938 opened the Big Sur wilderness for all to enjoy, the construction project was also the source of devastating environmental damage, as crews dynamited and bulldozed coastal slopes to forge road cuts and bridges. Some of these scars remain, requiring continual maintenance and retrofitting. In stretches, heavy winter storms spawn landslides that can close the highway for extended periods. Invasive plant species compound the problem, as they choke out native flora, which loosens soil and boosts the potential for further slides.

Residents have long lobbied on behalf of the region, motivated by environmental concerns and fears that tourism might lead to rampant development and commercialism. Soon after the highway opened, residents lobbied the local board of supervisors and county planning commission to ban billboards and similar visual noise. As a result, visitors today can still enjoy stunning, uninterrupted vistas from the many turnouts along Highway 1.

Trip 72

SALMON CREEK STATION TO BUCKEYE CAMP

LENGTH AND TYPE: 6.8-mile out-and-back, 7.9-mile point-to-point (Cruikshank Trailhead), or 8.4-mile point-to-point (Alder Creek Camp)

RATING: Strenuous

TRAIL CONDITION: Difficult, poison oak

HIGHLIGHTS: Another route to spectacular Buckeye Meadow, whose spacious grasslands burst forth with new life in spring

Salmon Creek Station to Buckeye Camp

TO REACH THE TRAILHEAD: The signed Buckeye Trailhead is at the abandoned Salmon Creek Station, 100 yards north of a tight bend in Highway 1, 8 miles south of Gorda, and 1.5 miles north of the posted San Luis Obispo County line. Park at the station. The trailhead is immediately west of the parking area. There are no facilities or water at the trailhead.

TRIP SUMMARY: The Buckeye Trail offers some of the best day-hike and overnight options in the Silver Peak Wilderness. If you can arrange a shuttle vehicle, point-to-point trips include: (1) 1.5 miles to Soda Springs Trailhead via the Buckeye and Soda Springs Trails; (2) 7.9 miles to the Cruikshank Trailhead via the Buckeye and Cruikshank Trails; and (3) 8.4 miles to Alder Creek Camp via the Buckeye Trail. Regardless of your itinerary, Buckeye Camp is a highlight. Perched amid an open meadow, the camp is roomy enough for a group outing.

Unfortunately, most of the trail beats through fast-growing coastal brush that each year aggressively overruns the trail. Those susceptible to poison oak should think twice, as this toxic plant is common along the coastal slopes.

The best time to hike the trail is between October and May, when fog banks roll well offshore, migrating gray whales spout within sight of land, and the meadows bloom anew. However, the wet months (November through April) also bring an onslaught of ticks, which wait alongside trails for unwary passersby. Wear light-colored pants and a long-sleeved shirt to help spot them. Though not breathable, rain pants or nylon pants may thwart these pesky hitchhikers altogether.

Summer is less desirable, as fog often obscures coastal views and warmer temperatures (usually above 70°F) bring an onslaught of nagging flies that persist through late fall.

Trip Description

The signed **Buckeye Trailhead** (230') lies just west of the abandoned ranger station's dilapidated garage. You'll cross a cattle guard and climb behind the station to a gated barbwire fence. Be sure to close the gate behind you.

After a steep, short climb past interwoven branches of poison oak and morning glory, the trail reaches a piped **spring** (0.2 mile, 410') that pours into large metal barrels. Continue climbing along a minor ridge to open slopes of fragrant coastal scrub, including sagebrush, yarrow, hedge nettle, and ceanothus. The ridge leads to a minor saddle (0.5 mile, 760') directly above Highway 1 for spectacular, unobstructed views of the coast.

Spring often brings windy, fogless days, exposing a dramatic convergence of land and sea.

From the saddle, the trail crosses arid slopes flanked with open grasslands and scattered yuccas, climbing northwest past a barbwire fence to the **Soda Springs Trail junction** (1 mile, 860'). While the **Soda Springs Trail** leads a half mile to Highway 1, offering a shorter route to Buckeye Camp, the trail is steeper and often overgrown.

Past the junction, the trail crosses a bay-lined minor gully, which in wet season supports a small waterfall 30 feet northeast of the trail. You'll quickly cross three more gullies fringed with oaks, maples, bays, toyons, and buckeyes, offering shady respite from the exposed coastal slopes.

Just past a cascading creek, you'll reach an oak-clad minor ridge with impressive views. Cross another shady gully to a stand of ponderosa pines for views south toward **Piedras Blancas,** near Hearst Castle. Views open up to the north as you climb open oak and pine woodlands past a dry gully (3.3 miles, 2060'). From here the trail crosses a typically dry creek past a fence to the signed **Buckeye Camp** entrance at spacious **Buckeye Meadow.**

Skirting the oak-rimmed meadow, the trail reaches the main site (3.4 miles, 2060') in the shade of a large bay. This is an ideal spot for a group outing, with plenty of room for several tents. A reliable spring-fed creek passes just south of camp, though in summer the shallow murky water may lose its appeal. To reach the smaller second site, continue northwest, threading a pair of valley oaks at meadow's edge. The site lies just downslope, offering a fire ring, a weathered table, and room for up to two tents.

You can either return the way you came or loop north on the **Buckeye Trail** to the **Cruikshank Trailhead** along Highway 1 (refer to TRIP 71 Highway 1 to Buckeye Camp, page, 286 and follow that trail description in reverse). Be aware that this route may be overgrown and the tread obscured in places.

Trip 73

SALMON CREEK TRAIL TO SPRUCE CREEK & ESTRELLA CAMPS

LENGTH AND TYPE: 6.5-mile out-and-back or 6-mile point-to-point (Coast Ridge Road)

RATING: Moderate to strenuous

TRAIL CONDITION: Clear to difficult, poison oak, overgrown trail conditions past Spruce Creek Camp

HIGHLIGHTS: Follow mossy, forested Salmon Creek to impressive waterfalls, majestic oak woodlands, and vibrant spring wildflowers on the upper slopes.

TO REACH THE TRAILHEAD: The signed Salmon Creek Trailhead is at the tight bend in Highway 1, 8 miles south of Gorda, 27 miles south of Big Sur Station, 1.5 miles north of the posted San Luis Obispo County line, and 3.7 miles north of Ragged Point. Park at wide turnouts on either side of Highway 1. There are no facilities or water at the trailhead.

TRIP SUMMARY: This route offers several day-hike and overnight options. Don't miss the 0.2-mile round-trip day hike along Salmon Creek to Salmon Creek Falls. Though the falls are visible from the highway, be sure to brave the crowds on this popular trail. Another spectacular day-hike destination is Upper Salmon Creek Falls, 2.6 miles up the Salmon Creek Trail, between Spruce Creek and Estrella Camps. A short, steep unmarked spur leads down to the thundering falls, which cascade over large moss-covered boulders into an iridescent pool. Pause for an invigorating swim in spring and summer. Expect a quick dip, as water temperatures reach the high 50s Fahrenheit at best.

Backpackers can hike 2 miles to Spruce Creek Camp or 3.25 miles to Estrella Camp for year-round camping in the heart of the Salmon Creek drainage. Base yourself at either camp for day hikes farther into the wilderness. One favorite destination is Dutra Flat along the San Carpoforo Trail (see TRIP 74 Dutra Flat & San Carpoforo Camps, page 297).

Heavily overgrown trails and prevalent poison oak near Coast Ridge Road may limit your loop trip options. Trails descending from Coast Ridge Road are also in poor condition, as is the road itself in places. While the roadbed from the unmarked Willow Creek Road/Los Burros Road junction is sound, encroaching brush will scratch even the narrowest vehicles. Fallen trees, washouts, and heavy rains may make the road impassable. Check with the US Forest Service before attempting to drive the road (see Phone, page 277, for contact information).

Trip Description

From its trailhead on **Highway 1,** the **Salmon Creek Trail** climbs a moderate grade along the south bank of **Salmon Creek** toward the clearly audible falls. In 0.1 mile you'll reach the unmarked **Salmon Creek Falls Trail junction** (0.1 mile, 230'). No matter where you're headed, don't miss the 200-foot spur to the base of the falls, which winds past fragrant bays and large mossy boulders amid the cool mist.

After exploring the falls, carefully retrace your steps to this junction if you're bound for Spruce Creek Camp, the Spruce Creek Trail, or Estrella Camp. Don't be taken in by the heavily used, steep spur that continues up Salmon Creek to rocky promontories above the falls. Many hikers (perhaps misreading the USFS map that shows the trail following the river's course) mistake this spur for the Salmon Creek Trail, following it until it disappears into oblivion a mile upstream.

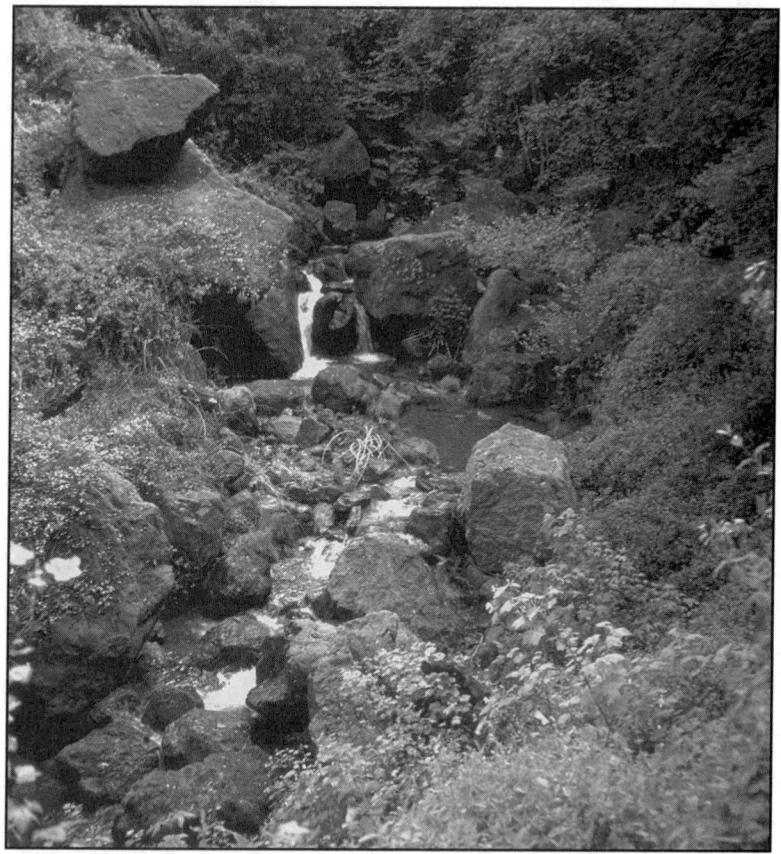

Spruce Creek flows past moss- and fern-covered boulders shaded by a lush riparian forest.

From the unmarked spur junction, you'll continue climbing a moderate grade up the south canyon wall. The trail soon switchbacks past a seasonal creek to a rocky viewpoint (0.3 mile, 760') that overlooks Salmon Creek's downstream passage to the **Pacific.** Fog may obscure the view in summer.

Notice the diverse plant life and dramatic vegetation shift in the canyon. A lush riparian forest of alders, maples, and bays along the canyon floor gives way to coastal scrub of fragrant sagebrush, sticky monkeyflowers, and coffeeberries, followed by a rocky, arid zone of succulents such as Our Lord's candle. The latter, a yucca, dies soon after sprouting a large stalk of cream-colored blossoms.

Onward, the trail switchbacks past a conspicuous mound of light-green, slippery **serpentine** (0.5 mile, 760'), California's state rock. Formed of basalt sediments from ancient seafloors, this stone slithered along fault lines to the surface. Many geologists believe this

explains serpentine's slick appearance. Few plants can survive in shallow, nutrient-poor serpentine soils. A few "serpentine endemics" have adapted, including California poppies, yucca, and other tenacious succulents. Pause to enjoy unobstructed ocean vistas across Highway 1 and west down Salmon Creek's sheer V-shaped canyon.

The trail continues to climb the north-facing slopes through dense coastal shrub into the shade of sprawling live oaks and bays. Past a gradual turn east, you'll reach an easily overlooked **spur junction** (0.8 mile, 940'). This spur leads northeast 40 feet to two small unofficial camps. Each can accommodate up to two tents, though neither is as pleasant as Spruce Creek or Estrella Camps. The nearest reliable water is back down at Salmon Creek.

The main trail continues its moderate climb past fragrant black sage and sagebrush thickets and mats of hedge nettles, which boast deep lavender blossoms in spring. Just past an unreliable creek (dry in all but heavy rain), you'll reach a **crest** (1.5 miles, 1050'), then gradually descend past groves of Douglas firs, tanoaks, and bays amid dense huckleberry bushes. The trail contours along the south canyon wall, passing two more **seasonal creeks** (1.8 miles, 1010'). Even in winter, these crossings will be an easy hop.

Fifty feet past the last creek, you'll reach the signed **Spruce Creek Trail junction** (1020'). From here the **Spruce Creek Trail** leads southeast 2.5 miles to **Dutra Flat Camp,** 4 miles to **Turkey Springs Camp,** and 6 miles to **San Carpoforo Camp** (see TRIP 74 Dutra Flat & San Carpoforo Camps, page 297). The **Salmon Creek Trail** continues northeast a quarter mile to Spruce Creek Camp, 1.5 miles to Estrella Camp, and 4 miles to Coast Ridge Road. The trail past Estrella Camp may be overgrown with brush and impassable to Coast Ridge Road.

From the Y-junction, bear left and head steadily downslope past large old-growth Douglas firs and vine-like poison oak a quarter mile to **Spruce Creek Camp** (2 miles, 750'). This idyllic backcountry camp offers three sites at the confluence of **Salmon and Spruce Creeks**.

The trail leads directly to the first site, atop a flat on Spruce Creek's south bank. There's room enough for up to two tents, as well as a fire ring and a few large logs for seating. Do not use the abandoned pit toilet 100 feet downstream along Salmon Creek, as the steep topography and winter runoff pose a problem. Until the toilet is replaced, bring a shovel and dig a waste pit at least 6 inches deep and 100 feet from water. Watch where you sit, as poison oak is prolific.

The second site lies across Salmon Creek, just below the confluence. Though usually just a boulder-hop, this crossing may be wet or even impassable during heavy winter rains. Use a walking stick or handy branch to keep your balance. Once across, take a short spur north 20 feet past a rope swing to the site, which offers a table, a fire ring, a grill, and room for up to three tents.

The third site sprawls across adjoining flats along the Salmon Creek Trail, 40 feet upstream from the first site. There's a fire ring and room for up to three tents.

Beyond the third site, the trail begins a moderate climb of the north-facing slopes in the shade of young Douglas firs, bays, oaks, and ceanothus, whose blue blossoms fill the air with a lilac aroma in spring. You'll skirt high above the creek past small rapids and swirling emerald pools. While this stretch of the trail is clear of overgrown brush, a few small washouts between Spruce Creek and Estrella Camps require careful footing.

As you cross steep minor gullies, the sound of cascading water will lead you on. Just before a bend in the trail (2.6 miles, 1140'), a steep spur drops 150 feet to the base of **Upper Salmon Creek Falls**. More reminiscent of a deer trail, the precarious spur slides down loose rock past poison oak. Despite the challenging trail conditions, the alluring waterfall and swimming hole tempt many hikers down to the banks of Salmon Creek.

A few yards past the spur, you'll veer south 200 feet up a minor gully, cross its small seasonal stream, then switchback north up the Salmon Creek drainage (2.7 miles, 1150'). Skirting a few fallen trees, the trail opens on fine views of the canyon's forested slopes and the often-fogbound coast. Onward, the trail veers southeast away from the creek to a spur junction (3.1 miles, 1340'). This short spur leads to a grassy flat where deer commonly graze, an excellent place to stargaze a few paces from **Estrella Camp**.

Just past the junction, you'll arrive at the first two sites (3.25 miles, 1360'), perched on the west bank of Estrella Creek just above its confluence with Salmon Creek. The open first site has room for up to three tents, while the second site can accommodate up to four tents in the shade of a sprawling live oak. Both sites are equipped with a fire ring, and drinking water lies just downslope at year-round **Estrella Creek**.

Few people hike farther due to encroaching brush and poison oak a mile past camp to trail's end at **Coast Ridge Road**. For current trail conditions, call the Pacific Valley Station

A mound of serpentine creates a barren landscape where only endemic species survive.

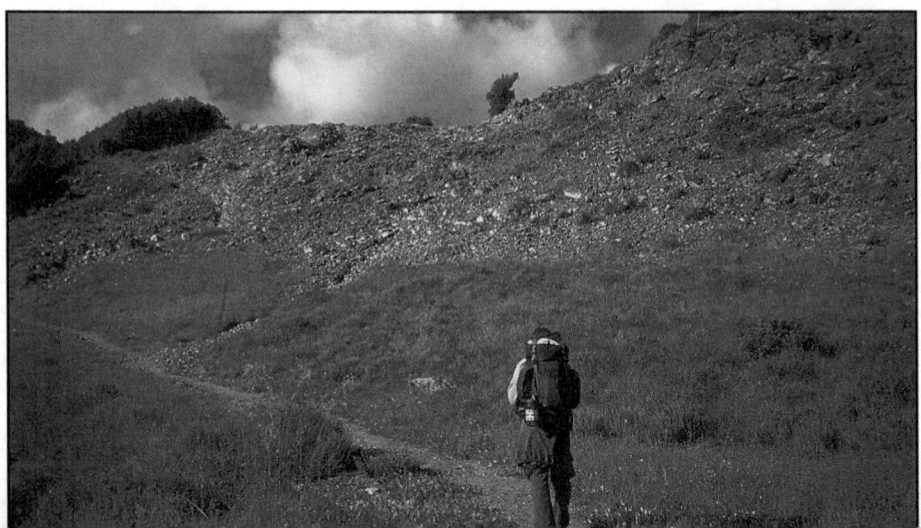

at (805) 927-4211. If you'd like join a volunteer maintenance crew, contact the Ventana Wilderness Alliance: (831) 423-3191, ventanawild.org. Though hard work, maintenance outings take in a spectacular loop trip up the Salmon Creek Trail to Coast Ridge Road and down the **Buckeye Trail**.

Trip 74

DUTRA FLAT & SAN CARPOFORO CAMPS

LENGTH AND TYPE: 15.6-mile out-and-back

RATING: Strenuous

TRAIL CONDITION: Passable to difficult, poison oak, cattle trails, faint tread

HIGHLIGHTS: Find solitude amid oak-studded golden hills, peaceful pine groves, and open meadows blanketed in fragrant spring wildflowers.

TO REACH THE TRAILHEAD: The signed Salmon Creek Trailhead is at the tight bend in Highway 1, 8 miles south of Gorda, 27 miles south of Big Sur Station, 1.5 miles north of the posted San Luis Obispo County line, and 3.7 miles north of Ragged Point. Park at wide turnouts on either side of Highway 1. There are no facilities or water at the trailhead.

TRIP SUMMARY: This route offers several out-and-back day hikes and overnight options, including: (1) 4 miles round-trip to Spruce Creek Camp, (2) 8.4 miles round-trip to Dutra Flat, (3) 12.2 miles round-trip to Turkey Springs Camp, and (4) 15.6 miles round-trip to San Carpoforo Camp. The Spruce Creek Trail becomes the San Carpoforo Trail at Dutra Flat.

The hike begins on a gentle ascent of the Salmon Creek drainage with views down-canyon to the often-fogbound coast. Onward, the trail climbs to the headwaters of the Spruce Creek drainage. Across the divide between the Spruce Creek and Dutra Creek watersheds, the San Carpoforo Trail winds past historic homestead sites and golden hills. You'll find a rich array of vegetation and terrain along the way, from riparian forests, to oak savannas, and wildflower-strewn open meadows.

Visit in spring to witness spectacular wildflower displays along the slopes of the San Carpoforo watershed. In winter, rain-saturated hillsides sprout vibrant green grasses and herbaceous plants. Year-round water sources are available at each camp in all but the driest years. Ticks are prolific during the wet season (November through April), flies and gnats are persistent in summer, and poison oak is unavoidable along the lower sections of the Spruce Creek Trail. On my hike, the last 100 yards to San Carpoforo Camp were overgrown with willow thickets and head-high stinging nettles.

Trip Description

See TRIP 73 Salmon Creek Trail to Spruce Creek & Estrella Camps (page 291) for the first 1.8 miles of this route to the **Spruce Creek Trail junction** (1.8 miles, 1020').

From the junction, turn right onto the less-traveled **Spruce Creek Trail,** which traces the slopes northeast of **Spruce Creek.** Unfortunately, poison oak is a common trailside companion along the overgrown trail.

Half a mile ahead, the trail breaks through the dense canopy of hardwoods and conifers to an open rocky barren (2.3 miles, 1200') and views north across the **Salmon Creek** drainage to 3590-foot **Silver Peak.** Past the barren, you'll turn south and follow year-round Spruce Creek past moss-covered boulders in the shade of bigleaf maples, sycamores, and oaks.

As you climb, notice how the vegetation changes from a riparian woodland to a mixed woodland of madrones, oaks, bays, and conifers. As you reach the divide between the Spruce Creek and **Dutra Creek** drainages (3.2 miles, 1950'), you enter a zone of brushy ceanothus, manzanita, and sage. The trail meets a gated barbwire fence at the saddle marking the divide. Be sure to close the gate behind you.

From here the vegetation and terrain shift dramatically from the steep, heavily forested canyons of Salmon and Spruce Creeks to rolling grasslands dotted with solitary oaks and stands of Coulter pines amid various seeps, springs, and meadows. The onward trail is virtually all downhill on a gentle to moderate grade.

Passing beneath a crimson canopy of tree-like manzanita, the trail descends to spacious meadows laced with small seasonal creeks and springs that are often dry by late spring. After 2.3 miles on the Spruce Creek Trail (called the **San Carpoforo Trail** from this point on), you'll arrive at **Dutra Flat Camp** (4.2 miles, 1930').

Once the site of an old homestead, this camp rests on a broad flat along a south-facing slope amid four large planted Monterey cypresses. With room enough for up to three tightly grouped tents, the site comes equipped with two fire rings and grills along with a table and bench. Rusty barbwire runs the perimeter, built to keep out cattle that feed on the grassy clearing above camp. In drier months, head uphill to find water at a spring-filled trough in the clearing.

A hundred feet south of camp is a marked junction with a spur that leads east 3 miles to **Coast Ridge Road.** Continue south on the San Carpoforo Trail. Ponderosa pines form small stands along these grassy slopes. In summer, go in search of several fruit trees on the south end of the flat. Reminders of the homestead that once occupied Dutra Flat, these trees still blossom and bear fruit.

Within sight of the dirt road from private **Baldwin Ranch,** which crosses the ridge to your west, you'll reach a minor gully. In wet months, water saturates the ground here, creating muddy seeps that preserve the tracks of visiting animals. Common visitors include bobcats, coyotes, gray foxes, and the occasional mountain lion.

Farther east the trail skirts a minor slide (4.7 miles, 1790'), so watch your footing. In spring this hillside supports decadent fields of purple lupine. Ahead, you'll veer southeast and descend a scenic ridge toward a notable lone oak on a small grassy knoll. Pause along the ridge for astounding views south across the **San Carpoforo drainage** and southern boundary of the **Silver Peak Wilderness.**

Before reaching the lone oak, you'll switchback south and descend to a minor gully (5.4 miles, 1560'), where several cattle paths cross the trail, headed north toward a creekside meadow. The trail contours to a minor ridge and the junction with another well-worn **cattle path** (5.8 miles, 1530') that hikers often mistake for the main trail. On my hike, pink flagging hung from a gray pine with a prominent forked top, marking this easily missed junction.

The cattle path leads straight past the gray pine, then plunges 0.7 mile down the southwest-facing walls of Dutra Creek canyon to **Baldwin Ranch Road.** From here, you could follow the less-scenic road 1.7 miles to the San Carpoforo Camp Trail.

If you prefer to continue on the main trail, turn left at the flagged junction just past the gray pine. In 0.3 mile, the trail crosses a small stream amid an open valley and arrives in **Turkey Springs Camp** (6.1 miles, 1410'). The peaceful site offers room for two tents in the shade of oaks and bays along a small spring-fed creek.

Beyond camp the trail meanders through the valley, crossing the creek four more times on its descent to Baldwin Ranch Road (7.3 miles, 740'). The trail merges with the well-graded road 0.3 mile farther to the signed **San Carpoforo Camp Trail junction.**

Turn right off the dirt road to cross a broad meadow to **San Carpoforo Creek.** This crossing is usually a knee-deep ford, though heavy winter rains may swell the creek, rendering it impassable. The trail continues downstream through dense willows and thickets of stinging nettles.

Brushing carefully past the nettles, you'll cross the creek once more to reach **San Carpoforo Camp** (7.8 miles, 650'), which offers room enough for up to five tents in the shade. In summer, swimming holes along the creek offer respite from the heat.

Note that the spelling of *San Carpoforo* on trail signs varies from "Carpoforo" to "Carpojo." USGS maps list it as Carpoforo, while locals pronounce it Carpojo.

APPENDIX

Trips by Theme

Epic Views

Day Hikes

- **#2** Carmelo Meadow, Granite Point, & Moss Cove Trails
- **#3** Cypress Grove Trail
- **#4** South Shore, Bird Island, South Plateau, & Pine Ridge Trails
- **#6** Rocky Ridge Trail
- **#8** Soberanes Point Trails
- **#9** Point Sur State Historic Park
- **#10** Trail Camp & Headlands Trails
- **#12** East Molera Trail
- **#15** Bluffs, Spring, Panorama, & Ridge Trails
- **#16** Valley View Trail
- **#20** Manuel Peak Trail
- **#24** Tan Bark Trail & Fire Road Loop
- **#25** Ewoldsen Trail
- **#26** McWay Falls
- **#32** Ragged Point Nature Trail
- **#33** Piedras Blancas
- **#42** Manuel Peak & Pfeiffer Big Sur State Park
- **#57** Junipero Serra Peak
- **#62** Cone Peak Trail

Backpacking Trips

- **#37** Devils Peak & Mt. Carmel
- **#38** Ventana Double Cone via Ventana Trail
- **#47** Ventana Double Cone via Big Pines Trail
- **#51** Ventana Double Cone via Pine Valley

- **#53** Black Cone Trail to Arroyo Seco
- **#65** Cone Peak Loop
- **#66** Highway 1 to Vicente Flat
- **#67** Prewitt Loop Trail
- **#70** Cruikshank & Silver Camps
- **#72** Salmon Creek Station to Buckeye Camp

Waterfalls

Day Hikes

- **#17** Pfeiffer Falls Trail
- **#26** McWay Falls
- **#28** Limekiln Falls Trail
- **#32** Ragged Point Nature Trail
- **#73** Salmon Creek Trail to Spruce Creek & Estrella Camps

Backpacking Trips

- **#40** Coast Road to Pico Blanco Camp
- **#41** Pico Blanco
- **#45** Hiding Canyon & Round Rock Camps
- **#49** Pine Valley
- **#50** Hiding Canyon & Round Rock Camps
- **#73** Salmon Creek Trail to Spruce Creek & Estrella Camps

Wildflowers

Day Hikes

- **#25** Ewoldsen Trail
- **#30** Pacific Valley Trail
- **#36** San Simeon Nature Trail

Backpacking Trips

#40 Coast Road to Pico Blanco Camp

#44 Bluff & Carmel River Camps

#45 Hiding Canyon & Round Rock Camps

#56 Willow Springs & Strawberry Camps

#58 Ventana Camp

#59 Sykes & Redwood Camps

#74 Dutra Flat & San Carpoforo Camps

Swimming
Day Hikes

#1 Carmel River State Beach

#4 South Shore, Bird Island, South Plateau, & Pine Ridge Trails

#13 River Trail Loop

#21 Gorge Trail

#22 Pfeiffer Beach

#34 Hearst Memorial State Beach

#35 San Simeon State Beach

Backpacking Trips

#39 Little Sur & Jackson Camps

#40 Coast Road to Pico Blanco Camp

#41 Pico Blanco

#44 Bluff & Carmel River Camps

#45 Hiding Canyon & Round Rock Camps

#49 Pine Valley

#50 Hiding Canyon & Round Rock Camps

#55 Tassajara Hot Springs

#56 Willow Springs & Strawberry Camps

#58 Ventana Camp

#59 Sykes & Redwood Camps

#73 Salmon Creek Trail to Spruce Creek & Estrella Camps

Redwood Forest
Day Hikes

#7 Soberanes Canyon Trail

#17 Pfeiffer Falls Trail

#18 Nature Trail

#24 Tan Bark Trail & Fire Road Loop

#25 Ewoldsen Trail

Trips #27–29   (all trails)

Backpacking Trips

#39 Little Sur & Jackson Camps

#40 Coast Road to Pico Blanco Camp

#59 Sykes & Redwood Camps

#60 Highway 1 to Terrace Creek Camp

#64 Vicente Flat Trail

#69 Highway 1 to Villa Creek Camp

Oak Woodland
Day Hikes

#24 Tan Bark Trail & Fire Road Loop

#25 Ewoldsen Trail

#36 San Simeon Nature Trail

#60 Highway 1 to Terrace Creek Camp

#61 Highway 1 to Coast Ridge Road

Backpacking Trips

#37 Devils Peak & Mt. Carmel

#38 Ventana Double Cone via Ventana Trail

#54 Church Creek to Pine Valley Camp

#56 Willow Springs & Strawberry Camps

#65 Cone Peak Loop

#67 Prewitt Loop Trail

#72 Salmon Creek Station to Buckeye Camp

By the Ocean
Day Hikes

Trips #1–4   (all trails)

#5 Coastal Access Trails

#8 Soberanes Point Trails

#9 Point Sur State Historic Park

#10 Trail Camp & Headlands Trails

#11 Beach & Creamery Meadow Trails Loop

#15 Bluffs, Spring, Panorama, & Ridge Trails

#22 Pfeiffer Beach

#23 Partington Cove Trail

#26 McWay Falls

#30 Pacific Valley Trail

#31 Sand Dollar Beach & Jade Cove

#32 Ragged Point Nature Trail

#33 Piedras Blancas

By the Ocean *(continued)*

Day Hikes (continued)

#34 Hearst Memorial State Beach

#35 San Simeon State Beach

Backpacking Trips

Backcountry camping west of Highway 1 is not permitted except at Andrew Molera State Park's walk-in campground, a half mile from Molera Beach and 0.3 mile from the parking lot.

Surfing

#1   Carmel River State Beach

#11 Beach & Creamery Meadow Trails Loop

#22 Pfeiffer Beach

#30 Pacific Valley Trail

#31 Sand Dollar Beach & Jade Cove

Less-Traveled Destinations

Day Hikes

#12 East Molera Trail

#19 Buzzards Roost Trail

#24 Tan Bark Trail & Fire Road Loop

#61 Highway 1 to Coast Ridge Road

Remote Wilderness

Backpacking Trips

#38 Ventana Double Cone via Ventana Trail

#45 Hiding Canyon & Round Rock Camps

#47 Ventana Double Cone via Big Pines Trail

#48 Miller Canyon & Pine Valley Loop

#51 Ventana Double Cone via Pine Valley

#54 Church Creek to Pine Valley Camp

#74 Dutra Flat & San Carpoforo Camps

Accessible by Public Transportation

Day Hikes

Trips #1–4   (all trails)

Trips #5–9   (all trails)

Trips #10–15 (all trails)

Trips #16–21 (seasonal)

Trips #34–36 (all trails)

Backpacking Trips

Trips #58 & 59 (seasonal)

Author's Favorites

Day Hikes

Trips #1–4   (all trails)

#6   Rocky Ridge Trail

#8   Soberanes Point Trails

#9   Point Sur State Historic Park

#10 Trail Camp & Headlands Trails

#15 Bluffs, Spring, Panorama, & Ridge Trails

#16 Valley View Trail

#21 Gorge Trail

#22 Pfeiffer Beach

#23 Partington Cove Trail

#25 Ewoldsen Trail

#26 McWay Falls

#31 Sand Dollar Beach & Jade Cove

#61 Highway 1 to Coast Ridge Road

Backpacking Trips

#38 Ventana Double Cone via Ventana Trail

#40 Coast Road to Pico Blanco Camp

#41 Pico Blanco

#49 Pine Valley

#51 Ventana Double Cone via Pine Valley

#53 Black Cone Trail to Arroyo Seco

#55 Tassajara Hot Springs

#62 Cone Peak Trail

#64 Vicente Flat Trail

#65 Cone Peak Loop

#72 Salmon Creek Station to Buckeye Camp

#74 Dutra Flat & San Carpoforo Camps

Recommended Reading

Plant & Animal Identification

Evarts, John and Marjorie Popper (editors), *Coast Redwood: A Natural & Cultural History.* Los Olivos, CA: Cachuma Press, 2001.

Hensen, Paul and Donald Usner, *The Natural History of Big Sur.* Berkeley, CA: University of California Press, 1993.

Johnson, Sharon G., Pamela C. Muick, Bruce M. Pavlik, and Marjorie Popper, *Oaks of California.* Los Olivos, CA: Cachuma Press, 1991.

Johnston, Verna R., *California Forests & Woodlands.* Berkeley, CA: University of California Press, 1994.

Keator, Glenn, Ruth M. Heady, and Valerie R. Winemiller, *Pacific Coast Fern Finder.* Rochester, N.Y.: Nature Study Guild, 1981.

Lanner, Ronald M., *Conifers of California.* Los Olivos, CA: Cachuma Press, 1999.

Lyons, Kathleen, and Mary Beth Cooney-Lazaneo, *Plants of the Coast Redwood Region.* Boulder Creek, CA: Looking Press, 1988.

McMinn, Howard, and Evelyn Maino, *An Illustrated Manual of Pacific Coast Trees.* 2nd ed. Berkeley, CA: University of California Press, 1981.

Peterson, Roger Tory, A *Field Guide to Western Birds.* Boston: Houghton Mifflin, 1972.

Spellenberg, Richard, *National Audubon Society Field Guide to North American Wildflowers,* Western Region. New York: Alfred A. Knopf, 1998.

Stuart, John, and John Sawyer, *Trees & Shrubs of California.* Berkeley, CA: University of California Press, 2001.

Watts, Phoebe, *Redwood Region Flower Finder.* Berkeley, CA: Nature Study Guild, 1979.

Geology

Alt, David D., and Donald W. Hyndmand, *Roadside Geology of Northern & Central California.* Missoula, Mont.: Mountain Press Publishing Company, 2000.

Earnst, W.G. (editor), *The Geotectonic Development of California.* Englewood Cliffs, N.J.: Prentice Hall, 1981.

Howard, A.D., *Geologic History of Middle California.* Natural History Guide 43. Berkeley, CA: University of California Press, 1979.

Oakeshott, G.B., *Guide to the Geology of Pfeiffer Big Sur State Park,* Monterey County, California. California Division of Mines & Geology Special Report 11, 1951.

Page, B. M., *Migration of Salinian Composite Block in California & Disappearance of Fragments.* American Journal of Science, 282: 1694-1734. 1982.

Trask, P., *Geology of the Point Sur Quadrangle,* California. University of California Publications, Bulletin of the Department of Geological Sciences, 16(6): 119-186. 1926.

Van Andel, T.H., *New Views on an Old Planet: Continental Drift & the History of the Earth.* Cambridge, Mass.: Cambridge University Press. 1985.

Cultural History

Breschini, Gary S., *The Indians of Monterey County*. Carmel, CA: Monterey County Archaeological Society, 1972.

Breschini, Gary S., and Trudy Haversat, *An Overview of the Esselen Indians of Central Monterey County*. Salinas, CA: Coyote Press, 1993.

Brown, William S., *History of the Los Padres National Forest,* 1989-1945. San Francisco: US Forest Service, 1945.

Fink, Augusta, *Monterey County: The Dramatic Story of Its Past*. Santa Cruz, CA: Western Tanager, 1978.

Goodman, Judith (editor), *Big Sur Women*. Big Sur, CA: Big Sur Women's Press, 1983.

Kroeber, A.L., *Handbook of the Indians of California*. Berkeley, CA: Reprint. California Book Company, 1953.

Margolin, Malcolm, *The Ohlone Way: Indian Life in the San Francisco–Monterey Bay Area*. Berkeley, CA: Heyday Books, 1978.

Wall, Rosalind Sharp, *A Wild Coast & Lonely*. San Carlos, CA: Wide World/Tetra, 1992.

Regional Guides

Heid, Matt, *101 Hikes in Northern California 2nd edition*. Berkeley, CA: Wilderness Press, 2008.

Hensen, Paul and Donald Usner, *The Natural History of Big Sur*. Berkeley, CA: University of California Press, 1993.

Lorentzen, Bob, and Richard Nichols, *Hiking the California Coastal Trail: Volume 2*. Mendocino, CA: Bored Feet Publications, 1998.

Puterbaugh, Park and Alan Bisbort, *California Beaches*. San Francisco: Foghorn Press, 1996.

Ventana Chapter, Sierra Club (editors), *Trail Guide to Los Padres National Forest Northern Section*. Carmel, CA: PIP Printing, 1996.

INDEX

■ ■ ■ ■ ■ ■ ■ ■ ■ ■ ■ ■ ■

MAP INDEX

ABOUT THE AUTHOR

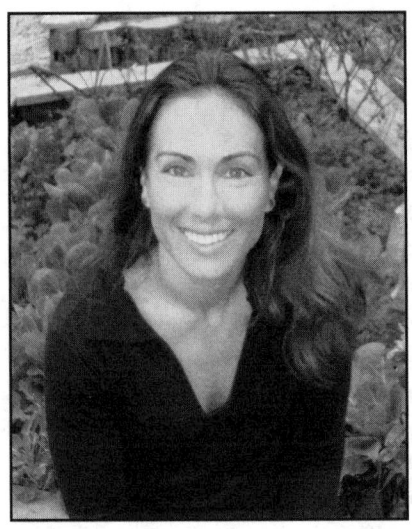

An avid hiker, backpacker, and naturalist, **Analise Elliot Heid** has pursued an outdoor lifestyle both professionally and recreationally. She currently works as an environmental educator, science teacher, and school garden program director along the California coast. Analise holds a B.S. in forestry from U.C. Berkeley, a M.A. in education from San Francisco State University, and works as a master teacher in the Cal State University Science Teacher and Researcher Program.

PART I

Striking

The majority of violent situations you will find yourself in will occur face-to-face (*Panim-a-Panim*), regardless of whether you are dealing with a sexual assailant, a mugger, or a drunk in a bar. This means that in most situations, your solutions will involve striking (preferably preemptively) to a greater or lesser degree, and so you should therefore learn to strike hard and accurately.

If you look at what you are attempting to do in a violent altercation, 80 to 90 percent of it will be to try to deliver pain and concussive force through striking, with the goal of emotionally and physically debilitating your assailant so that they are either unable or unwilling to continue the fight. To this end, your striking should be conducted as an all-out assault against them, to be carried out with full emotion and aggression. It should look very different from the way that you spar—sparring is something you do with a partner; real-life striking is something you do against an assailant.

Your striking will be given its power and potency through your aggression and your emotion; a poorly executed strike delivered with full emotion and aggression will be more effective than a technically perfect one that lacks any emotional commitment.

Upper-Body Combatives

Many people who practice punching on focus mitts are surprised when they're not able to generate the same type of power when striking the head with bare knuckles. The same will often be experienced by individuals who train/spar wearing gloves—the bigger the gloves they wear, the more difficult they will find the transition. When you strike a focus mitt, you are hitting a flat surface, so you are able to hit it square on and deliver driving force through the target. Gloves create the same effect by "flattening" the striking surface and spreading the force into the target. When you punch bare-knuckled to the head, you are rarely striking a flat surface—especially if you are striking someone who is directly in front of you. If, on the other hand, you move to the side of the person and strike, you can present the face as a flatter surface, and you can deliver greater concussive, damaging force. The effect of punching a face positioned directly in front of you is that your punches will often "roll" off the tar-

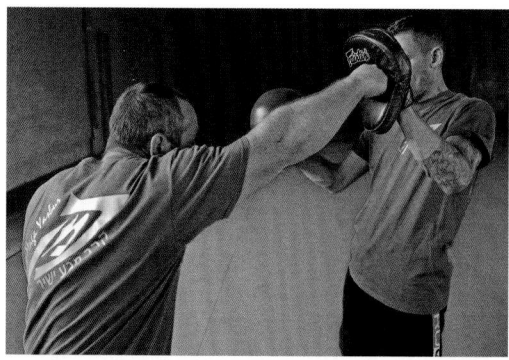

When you practice on striking surfaces that offer you a flat target, you can generate and focus power relatively easily. This is the purpose of such training aids. The problem is that in real-life altercations, where you are aiming strikes at the face/head, and other targets, you aren't striking a flat surface, so it isn't always possible to focus your power in the same way.

When you strike the face/head you are punching a spherical surface rather than a flat one. This may result in your fist rolling off the target rather than driving through it. It is also worth noting that a human head isn't fixed; it is able to rotate on the neck, which may also cause your punch to roll off the target.

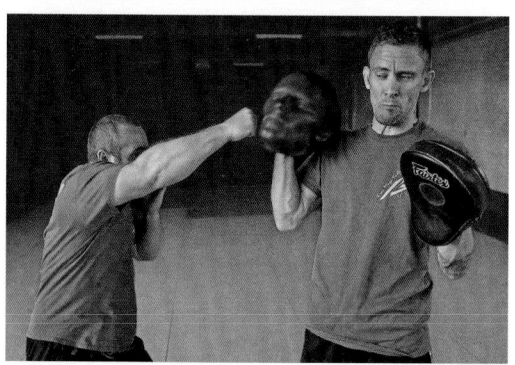

If you move to the side and strike the face/head at an angle, you will be striking a flatter surface than you would be if you were face on. This means you will be able to deliver driving force into the target. This is one reason you need to position yourself correctly before you deliver a punch.

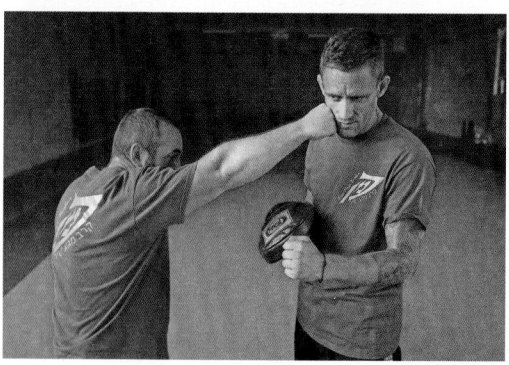

It is not always possible to get into such a position, so it is worth having other striking tools that can be delivered when directly facing your assailant.

get. The risk of this increases if the head moves with the initial impact of your strike. This is why, if you are going to deliver straight punches, positioning yourself before striking is so important.

Because of this, it is good to have other striking options/tools in your arsenal that can often be more effective at delivering force into an irregularly shaped target such as the face/head.

Thumb Strike to Eyes

A thumb strike to the eyes is a very effective initial strike for a variety of reasons. Firstly, it doesn't require a great deal of force to be effective, which means that you can throw it without having to first get your body aligned and into a position from which it can deliver real power. In the first moments of a fight, being able to do something that will disrupt your attacker is essential, as once an assailant gets some momentum and a rhythm to their assault, even relatively simple punches and strikes can be difficult to defend against. If you can interrupt your attacker's momentum and flow at the outset, they will find it difficult to put a series of strikes together. Getting a thumb into one of their eyes is a great way to do this, as it will prevent them from moving forward into you and will allow you to move into them, taking the role of attacker from them and assuming it for yourself.

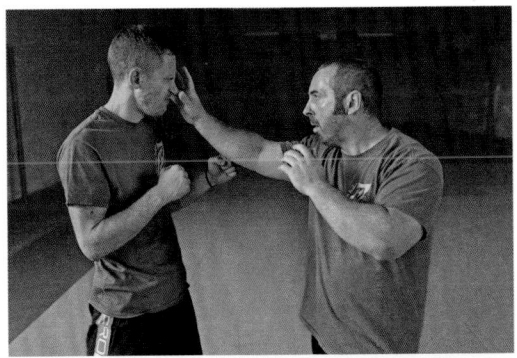

There are few strikes that are as simple and as effective as eye strikes—and one of the simplest ways to deliver an eye strike is to use the thumb. Simply moving your hand toward your attacker's face at speed will usually result in them closing their eyes, which means that even if your aim isn't good you will have caused them to pause/hesitate, allowing you the opportunity to follow up with other attacks/assaults.

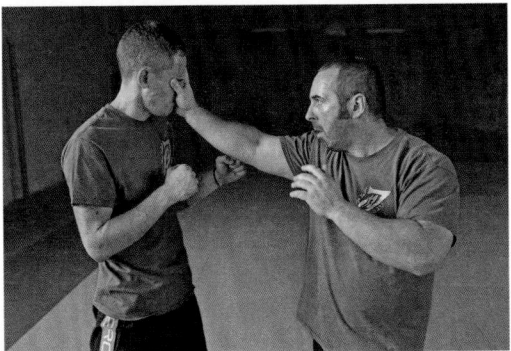

If you aim your palm at someone's face and stick the thumb out, it will find one of your attacker's eyes. Once you have made contact, simply drive your thumb into their eye socket with all of your strength. Don't try to measure the force you use; simply push into their eye as hard as you can. This is not a subtle technique. It is a great opening attack, as it doesn't require much accuracy or force to be effective.

Eye strikes are painful—you are aiming to drive your thumb as far into your assailant's eye socket as possible—there are no half-measures when it comes to dealing with violence. They are also disruptive: if you can affect your attacker's vision, you will be depriving them of one of the tools they would be using in order to attack you. Even after the initial pain subsides, the eye(s) will be watering, making it difficult for your assailant to see you.

Another reason eye strikes are effective is that the type of pain they elicit is hard to gear yourself up for. When we become adrenalized and ready to fight, we switch on various "pain management" systems, because we expect to get punched, kicked, hit, etc. If your attacker is fully adrenalized and highly aggressive, they may not initially feel or experience the actual pain that a blunt-trauma strike such as a punch should deliver. In my time working in the security industry I have been hit with beer bottles, pool balls, and similar objects, and have been able to continue fighting, only to experience the true pain of these strikes after the event. Sticking a thumb into an eye bypasses these pain-management systems and "wakes" your assailant up to the sensation of pain, within the fight.

Palm-Heels to Nose

Palm-heel strikes are extremely underestimated, and for some reason tend to only get taught as a second-class type of strike to the closed fist. Yet the palm-heel strike is highly effective, and should be part of everyone's toolkit. In my belief, it is wrong to rank the effectiveness of strikes against each other; it is more practical and useful to look on them as different tools, which are used to accomplish different goals and solve different problems. The open-palm strike should not be compared to a closed-fist punch and looked on as the "poor man's" alternative to it; rather, it should be looked on as a standalone strike with its own advantages and disadvantages.

I often see the palm-heel strike taught with the hand being a very rigid unit, with the fingers pulled back and the palm exposed as a relatively "flat" striking unit that should be targeted against the chin in order to both deliver concussive force and direct the head back, akin to a closed-fist punch. While this can be an effective way of striking, I prefer to deliver the palm-heel strike with the hand being looser, and in more of a "cupping" fashion that wraps around the face, both obscuring vision (masking the face) and pushing upward against the nose—directing the head back, in preparation for harder, more concussive strikes.

Delivered in this way, as a "softer" strike against the nose, the fingers and thumb can also be driven into the eyes, making for a more disruptive strike.

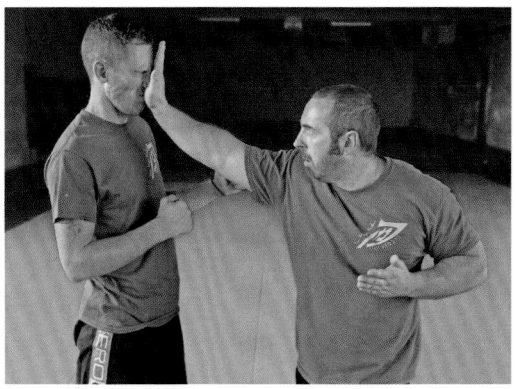

There are many different ways to deliver a palm-heel strike, and all are valid; they simply accomplish different things. A rigid palm-heel strike to the face will not deliver as much concussive force as a punch, but it is less likely to damage the knuckles and bones of the hand.

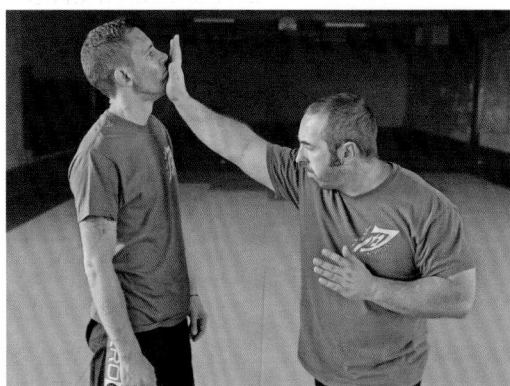

By throwing a palm-heel strike against the chin, you are able to move your attacker's head back, disrupting their balance and thus creating opportunities for further attacks.

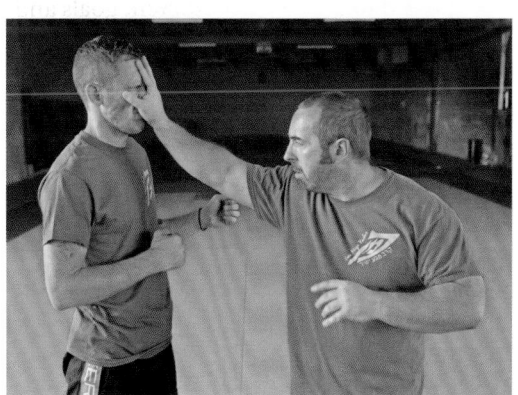

You can also use the palm-heel strike in a less rigid fashion, with the idea of quickly getting a hand/strike into your attacker's face so that their vision is obscured. Quickly getting a strike or hand into your attacker's face, whether your thumb hits their eye or not, is an easy way to disrupt an assailant's attack, and set up your own.

Cradle-Strike to Throat

The throat is a target that doesn't move. An assailant can turn their head away, moving the eyes as a target; however, the throat and neck stay in place, meaning that they are always available to be attacked. Striking the throat causes shock and pain (it's an unexpected pain), and can result in serious trauma; it can cause the internal cartilage of the trachea to collapse, resulting in difficulty breathing. A hard strike will also cause a degree of swelling around the throat, which will further affect breathing. This is one of the reasons why, in a fight, you should keep your chin tucked down so that the throat is protected (keeping your chin down will also direct your face downward, making you less vulnerable to a head-butt).

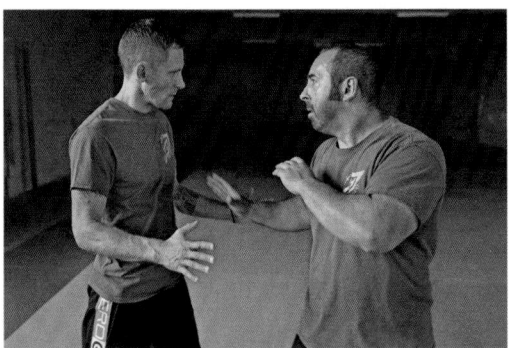

There are three soft and vulnerable targets that don't require any force for a strike to be effective: these are the eyes, throat, and groin. Sometimes the eyes are not an effective target because an attacker turns their face away to avoid being hit there. It doesn't matter how far a person turns their face/eyes away, however, the throat/neck will usually remain available. The best way to attack the throat is in an upward direction.

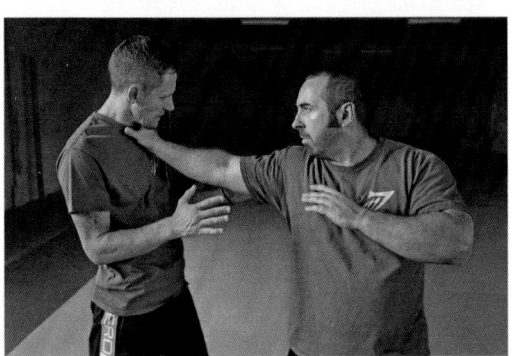

When you strike the throat, hit it hard. Your goal is to cause trauma and swelling to the throat so that your attacker's breathing is impaired. An attacker who can't breathe properly will not be able to fight effectively.

The throat can still be a target even if your attacker turns their face away, which would make an eye strike difficult/impossible. The throat can be a difficult target for an attacker to defend—unless they keep their chin tucked to their chest at all times.

The Initial Strike as a Range/Distance Finder

Your initial strike can be used as a tactile "marker" to set up further strikes. In a dynamic, fast-moving situation where there are many changes in movement, punches and strikes often won't land because the distance and position between the striking unit (e.g., the fist), and the target (e.g., the face), change as the punch/strike is being delivered. By not retracting the initial strike—such as the thumb to your assailant's eye(s)—you can not only control their head (the target), but also give yourself another tool for judging distance/range. You just have to deliver the second strike roughly where your first hand is, as it's already on the target. Using this method of zoning in on your targets makes it almost impossible to miss with your subsequent

When your attacker is backing away quickly, it can be difficult to judge range effectively. In such situations, you can use your eye strike as a range finder to make sure that your other strikes land with full force. As you move toward your attacker, make an eye strike with your left hand.

Rather than retract the strike, keep your hand pressed into your attacker's face as you set up a power strike. If your attacker tries to move toward you, your hand in their face will prevent them from doing so; if they continue to move back, or adjust their position, you will be able to feel their movement and follow them.

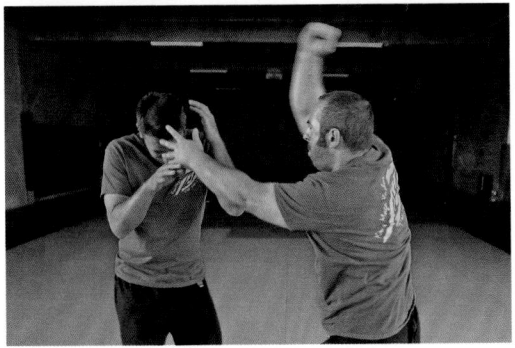

Keep your hand glued to your assailant as you strike them, so that you can keep delivering multiple power strikes against them. If your hand is on the target area, remove it as you strike with the other hand.

strikes. As long as you keep your hand on their eyes, you will always know where to hit, regardless of whether they move in to you, pull away, turn their head, etc.

The Krav Maga Yashir system works off the continuum: Disrupt, Damage, Destroy, and Disengage. This means that your first goal is to disrupt your attacker (something that can be accomplished by an easy-to-deliver "soft" strike to the eyes or throat) before going on to damage and destroy them with concussive/forceful blows ("hard" strikes).

Hammer-Fists

The hammer-fist is one of the most versatile striking tools that you have, as it can be delivered at multiple angles, and uses the bottom of the fist as the striking surface. In this fashion the relatively delicate bone structure of the hand is protected by the adipose tissue, meaning that it is unlikely that any damage to the hand will be sustained when using this type of strike—something you are always at risk of when punching with a closed fist.

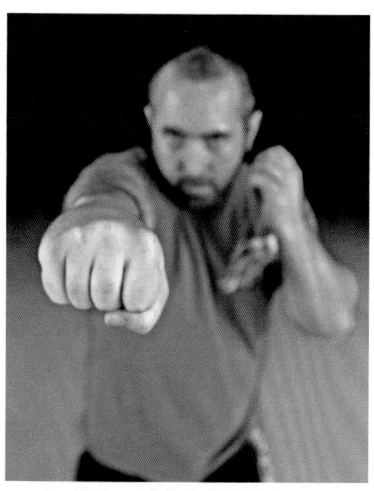

To strike with a closed fist without risking injury to the hand, it is wise to condition your hands. If you always wear wraps and/ or gloves when you train, you may develop bad habits with your striking, such as not closing your fist fully on impact, etc. These bad habits could see you injuring your hands in a real-life confrontation; for example, if your assailant should duck their head, you may end up striking the skull rather than the face, and if your hand/fist is not properly conditioned for this type of potential impact, it is likely that you'll damage it, as there would have been no consequence for this in a glove.

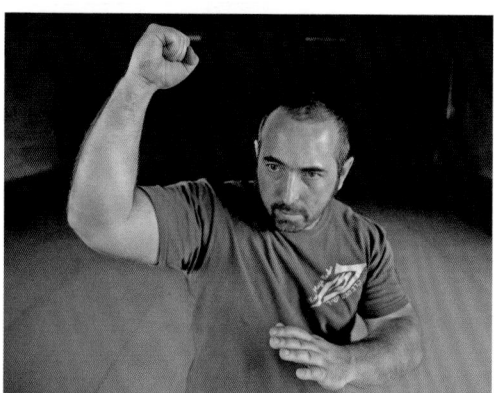

With the hammer-fist strike, you are making impact with the bottom of the fist. The fist is still tightened on impact, but instead of striking with the knuckles (which can also bruise quite easily), you are striking with the tightened soft tissue at the base of the fist, which doesn't damage easily; this protects the relatively fragile bones of the hand.

Downward/Forward Hammer-Fist

This strike derives its power from the dropping of the hand, assisted by the body, onto whatever target has been selected. It can be delivered straight down, against a target such as the back of your assailant's neck (if they are bent over), or it can be angled straight into an attacker's face if they are standing/facing you.

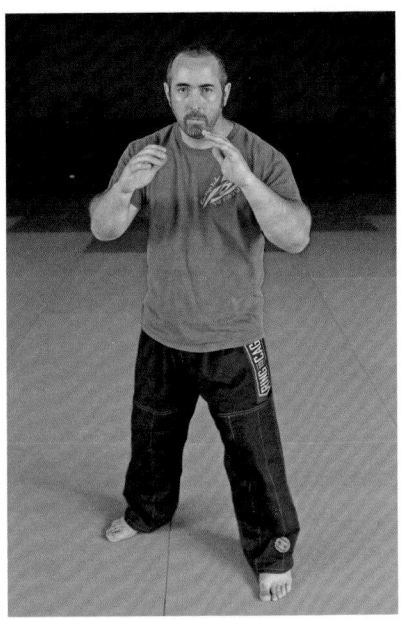

In real-life situations there is no time to get into a "fighting stance." If you try to do so, you will have both wasted time and informed your aggressor of your intentions. However, to practice hammer-fists, and understand how they work, a fighting stance is a good position to start from. In reality, your "fighting stance" is one that adheres to certain principles: weight distributed 50/50 between the feet, head over shoulders, shoulders over hips, feet on opposite corners of a rectangle, etc.

Turn the heel of your front foot outward (away from the centerline of your body), so that your body turns. At the same time, pull the elbow of your rear hand directly upward. The reason for the turning motion is that when you go to make your strike, you can "unwind" your body, to deliver more power into the strike.

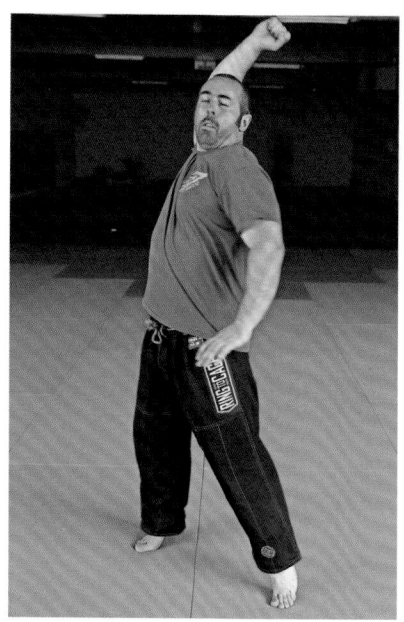

Once your elbow has reached its maximum height, start to extend your arm. As you reach upward with your hand, raise your weight off your front foot, transferring it to the rear—your front leg should hold about 30 percent of your weight; your rear, 70 percent. This will allow you to move weight forward as you deploy your hammer-fist, adding power to the strike.

Once your arm is fully extended, your weight transferred, and your body fully bladed, you will be ready to make the strike. Although it may seem that this process takes a long time, when all the movements are done simultaneously, it will be extremely fast.

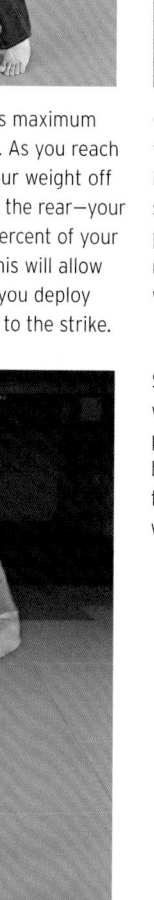

Start to unwind your body, and shift your weight forward (your right hip should be pushing forward into the strike), as you bring your fist down. You should have the feeling of the body pushing your hand forward and down.

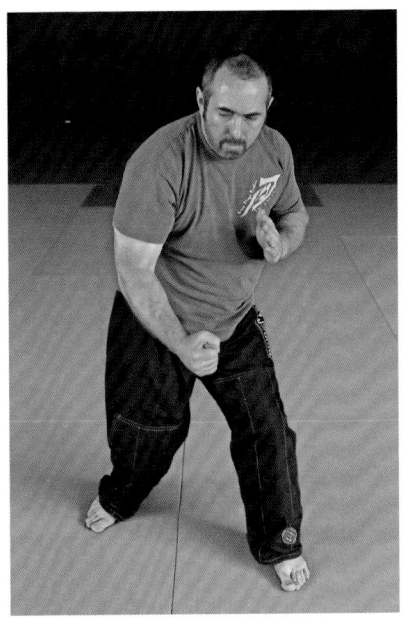

As you deliver the strike, start to bend the knees and sink your weight in order to add more power to your strike.

Rather than "bouncing" the strike off the target, drive through it, and prepare to raise the elbow again, in a cyclical fashion, to deliver another strike. Another advantage hammer-fist strikes have over straight punches is that it is much easier to move forward throwing multiple hammer-fist strikes than it is to move forward throwing full-force straight punches.

This is an extremely powerful strike, which sees your extended arm, held overhead, crash downward (and sometimes forward) into the intended target (nose, back of head/neck, clavicle, etc.). The same strike can be made while holding a pen, flashlight, etc., so that all the force of the strike is concentrated through a harder and much more focused striking surface.

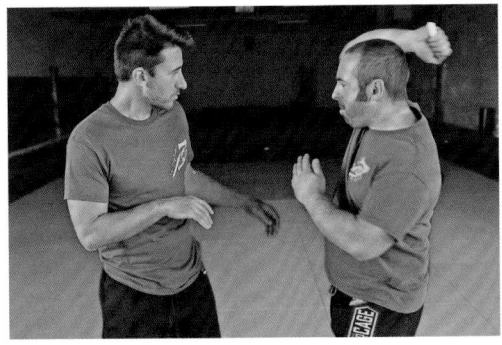

If you can find a solid object, such as a pen, a flashlight, a mobile phone, etc., you can use this to focus the power of your hammer-fist strike. Simply hold the object in your hand—with your thumb over the top to prevent it slipping when it makes impact—and deliver a hammer-fist strike against your assailant. If you aim for the chest, make sure you rip/scrape the object down the body after it has landed, in order to cause maximum trauma.

It may seem that the extension of the arm overhead is a little contrived, even theatrical, and more befitting of a martial-arts technique than one that should be used in a real-life situation. After all, do you really have time to extend the arm that high when dealing with an aggressor who is coming at you with full force and full speed? The real answer is no; however, in training we should enlarge and exaggerate our movements, making them as big as possible, for one simple reason: under stress and adrenaline, our movements shrink and become contracted. If we try to train our techniques as we think we would execute them in reality, it is likely that when we are called upon to use them in a real-life confrontation where we are adrenalized/stressed, they will be too small, and will not contain enough power to be effective.

When you train, you should look to make movements—however exaggerated—that will deliver the maximum amount of power and energy possible, with the awareness that adrenaline may well cause them to shrink and become less powerful.

Cycling Hammer-Fist Strikes

Striking combinations, from a self-defense perspective, do not have to be complex; in fact, there is no reason to throw a myriad of different strikes at your assailant if repeating the same strike over and over again is effective. Because the strike and recoil of the downward or vertical hammer-fist are circular in nature, the hand/fist can easily be pulled back up, ready to make another strike, without there having to be a break in the movement of the arm. This means you can land multiple hammer-fist strikes in quick succession, without giving your assailant an opportunity to attack/counterattack.

By moving forward, and, if necessary, using your left hand to push/strike your attacker's face (in order for it to be in place for your next strike) you should be able to land a large number of powerful strikes using just a hammer-fist.

Combining Eye/Throat Strikes and Range-Finders with Hammer-Fists

While a good eye or throat strike is effective at disrupting an attacker, at some point you will need to deliver forceful concussive strikes that will start to cause extreme pain and trauma to your assailant. A good follow-up strike to these strikes is to use the hammer-fist in a cyclical fashion to repeatedly beat down on your attacker. This may not seem like a particularly sophisticated solution; however, it is a simple and effective one that sees you laying down a lot of firepower in an aggressive and determined manner. If you can strike in such a way that there are few spaces and gaps between your strikes, it will be almost impossible for your assailant to launch any assault of their own. Your goal is not to fight your attacker, but to assault them with an all-out blitz that they are unable to cope with. Simplicity and aggression are often better friends than sophistication, where violence is concerned.

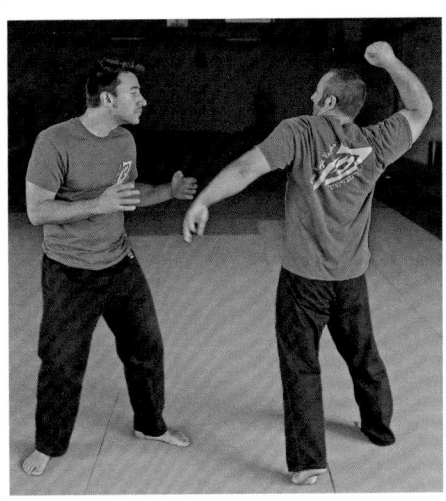

Eye strikes are good first strikes, as they don't need to be well placed or delivered with force to have an effect. Unfortunately, they don't deliver concussive force, which is necessary to cause your assailant the type of pain and trauma that will make them want to disengage from the fight. As you throw the eye strike, start to bring up the elbow of your rear hand in preparation for delivering a hammer-fist strike.

The eye strike will provide cover for the time it takes to raise the arm up to make a strong hammer-fist strike.

 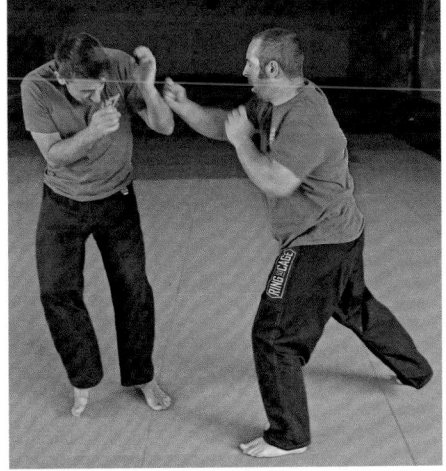

This time, instead of simply turning and dropping your weight, turn and step forward to bring your bodyweight into the strike.

Drive through with your hammer-fist. As you start cycling it through to throw another, start to move your left hand forward.

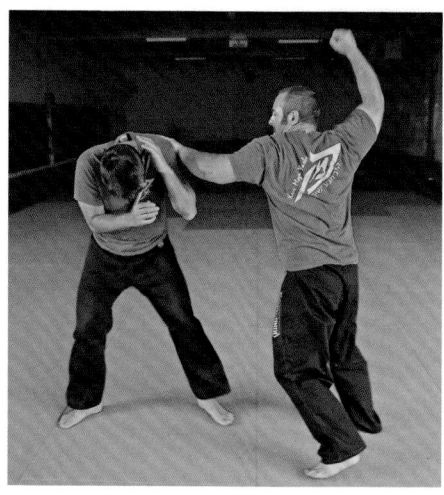

Your left hand can do one of several things: it can make an eye strike or a cradle-strike to the throat, or it can act as a range finder for your next strike. Bring your rear leg forward so that you are ready to step forward when you make your next hammer-fist strike.

Your goal is to keep your assailant moving backward as you overwhelm them with strikes. While they are moving backward and defending themselves, they will have few opportunities to make an attack of their own.

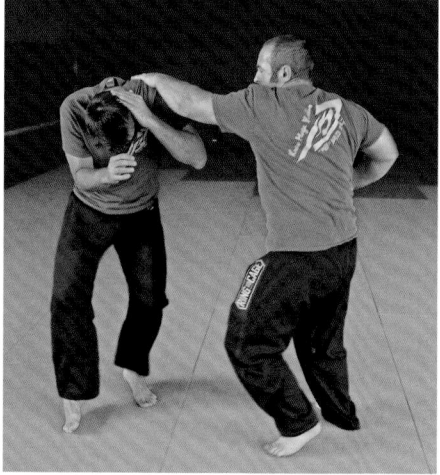

Drive through with your hammer-fist strike, stepping forward as you do. With your attacker bent over, the back of the neck is a good target to aim for. As you strike, pull your left hand back so that it can be used to make another strike.

Once again, bring the rear foot forward and make another eye strike or cradle-strike while setting up your hammer-fist strike.

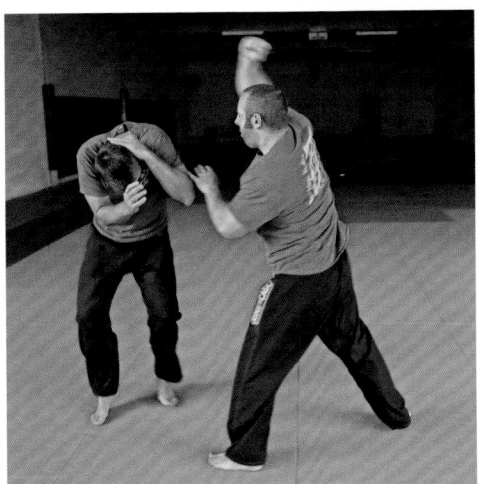

This process can be repeated over and over again. You don't have to alternate every hammer-fist with an eye/throat strike; it may be more effective to throw several hammer-fist strikes and only use the eye/throat strike as a way to move them back if they aren't moving fast enough in response to your hammer-fists, causing you to get jammed up. As soon as it is safe to do so, disengage. If you end up forcing your assailant into a wall or similar where they don't have an opportunity to disengage, they will be forced to come back at you fighting. It is rarely a good idea to stay too long attacking an assailant in such a position.

Horizontal/Outward Hammer-Fist Strikes

Hammer-fists can be thrown at virtually any angle, due to the ability of the forearm and shoulder to rotate and present the bottom of the fist in many directions. There are, of course, certain directions from which more power can be generated than others. One direction in which an immense amount of power can be generated is outward, away from the body. If this is coupled with the hips turning and/or a step out, so that the hips can be opened and the bodyweight transferred, then the entire movement of the body can be applied to the strike.

The outward hammer-fist strike comes into its own when your assailant tries to move out of the way of your linear striking. If an assailant is moving backward against someone cycling hammer-fists, they will soon realize that moving backward in a straight line only sees them remaining in the path of the onslaught, and that it would be better/safer if they moved to the side—offline and out of the line of fire. If you are attacking with momentum, it may be that as they move to your side, you initially continue moving forward. Your goal should now be to change direction while still striking, using something like a horizontal hammer-fist strike. You won't want to turn and then resume your striking, as this would create time and space for the assailant to recover and possibly initiate their own attack.

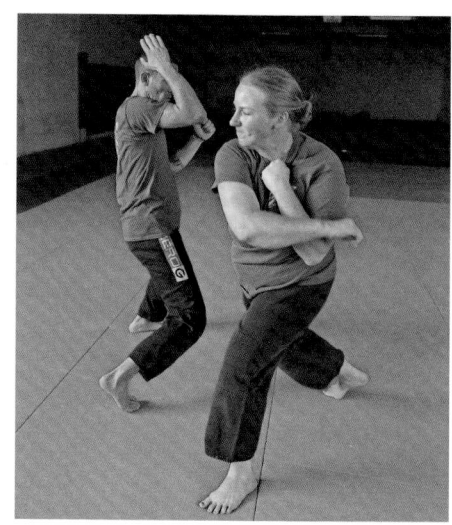

Just because you have a plan doesn't mean that your attacker will cooperate with it by reacting in the way you predict (or possibly the only manner in which you've trained). If you only train for one outcome, you will be surprised and caught flat-footed when your assailant doesn't respond as you expected. It may be that as you rain hammer-fist strikes down on your assailant, they will manage to step off to one side in order to avoid further strikes.

As soon as the target changes direction, so must your attacks—this is necessary in order to keep your assailant under pressure, not giving them any time or space to launch a counterattack against you. Immediately pull your arm across your body, and prepare to extend it horizontally toward your assailant.

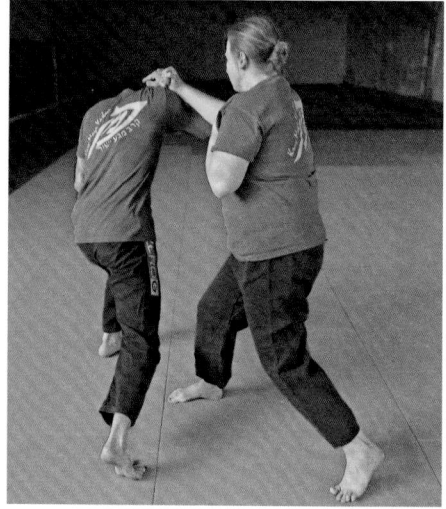

Turn with your body and hips to unwind your strike into your attacker—you can use your back muscles to assist with this turning action. Shift your weight from your left foot to your right in order to help get your bodyweight into the strike.

Strike your attacker's face or neck, connecting with the bottom of your fist, and drive through the strike.

The horizontal hammer-fist can be used effectively when you recognize that an assailant is coming toward you from the side or rear. One of the assumptions you should always work from is that your primary assailant is not alone; that they have friends and third parties who can come and assist them. This means that while you are dealing with an attacker who is in front of you, another can approach from the side, or from behind you. (This is one of the reasons you should move and scan, so that you have a 360-degree field of vision and know what is happening in your environment.) If you detect movement coming toward you, you should assume that it is hostile, as people generally move away from fights unless they have an interest in them. If it is a friend of yours coming to assist you, it's hard luck for them; in a fast-paced, dynamic conflict, you may not have time to make a full assessment of whether the movement belongs to someone coming to help you—and the only safe assumption is that it doesn't. If you are in a group where people might want to assist you in the case of a physical confrontation, plan with them beforehand the best way to do this.

Not all situations will involve single attackers, and it may not be evident who in the environment is an attacker, and who is not. In this situation, you are dealing with an aggressive individual who you are pretty sure is intending to attack you. Put your hands up in a placating manner as you try and de-escalate the situation, but also be ready to defend yourself. You may be aware of another person in the environment, but may not have enough time and space to move away from them.

The aggressor in front of you suddenly starts to move toward you. Your de-escalation stance, with hands raised, has prepared you to move to make an eye strike in order to set up your hammer-fist strikes. At this point, the second person has not indicated whether or not they are going to get involved.

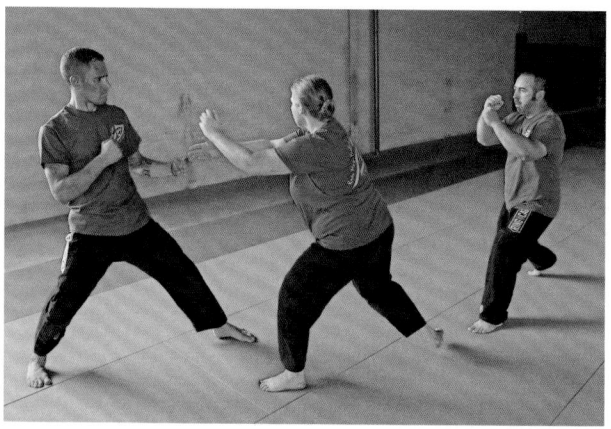

Your eye strike and first hammer-fist strike have caused your initial assailant to back away; however, as you were launching your assault on them, you realize that the second person has begun to move toward you.

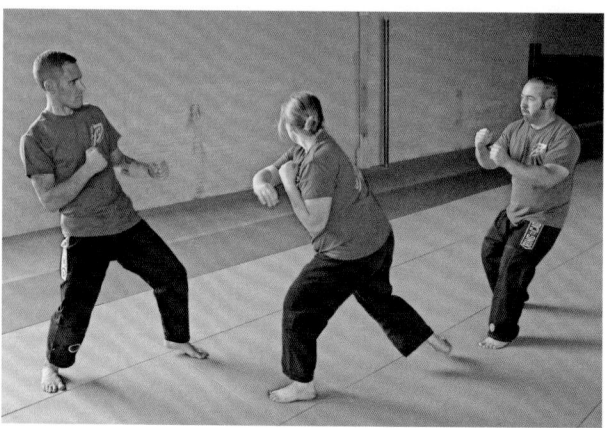

You don't have the time to work out whether they are coming to assist you or attack you, and your only safe option is to assume the latter. Because they are moving toward you, and your other attacker is moving away, the second person should now become your primary target. Bring your right hand across your body in preparation for delivering a horizontal hammer-fist.

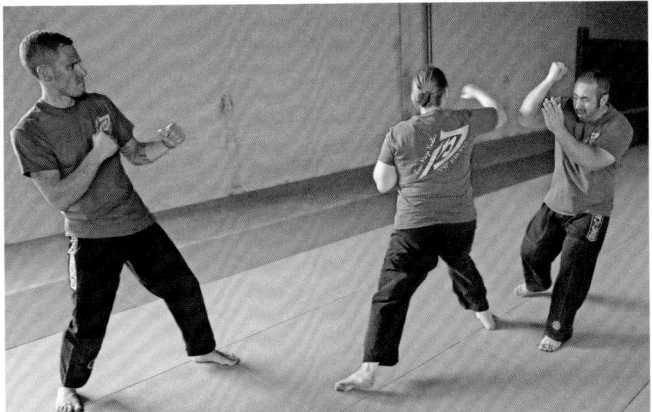

Step toward them and deliver a hammer-fist into their neck or the side of their face.

Once you have struck them, immediately turn back toward your original assailant. If they haven't already started to move toward you, they are likely to now. Use the follow-through motion of your strike to set yourself up to make a downward hammer-fist strike.

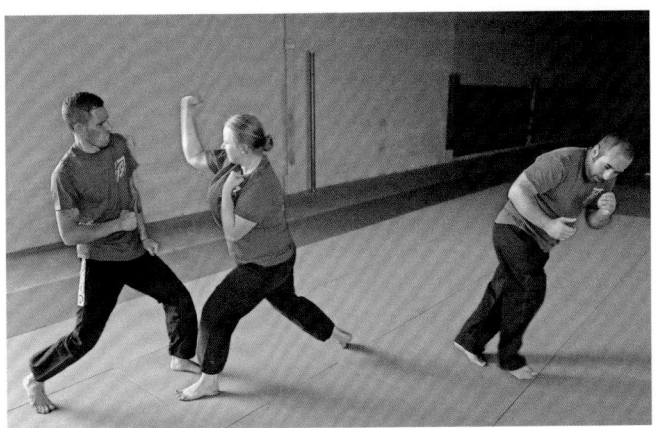

Step toward your first attacker and start to deliver downward hammer-fist strikes against them. Keep driving forward and delivering strikes so that you have dealt with them before the second attacker recovers. In multiple-assailant situations, you should try to take one attacker out at a time, rather than dividing your efforts and attention among them.

Forearm Strikes

The forearm can also be used as an effective striking tool, in a similar fashion to the horizontal hammer-fist. Although it is a slower-moving strike, it requires less accuracy, as is has a much larger striking surface—and it has the advantage of bringing the whole weight of the arm to bear. It can also be used at a closer range, making it an effective tool for creating space. A forearm strike works extremely well when it is brought down at a 45-degree angle against the neck and throat. You may also end up connecting with the forearm by chance if an attacker moves toward you as you are throwing a hammer-fist strike against them.

 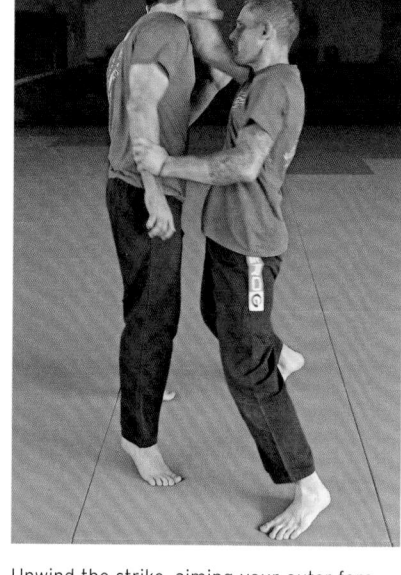

Forearm strikes against the neck are extremely powerful; they can be delivered with such force that it feels like the head is being torn off the body. Wind the arm around/across your body as if you were going to make a hammer-fist strike; of course, you will be much closer to your assailant when you are striking with the forearm.

Unwind the strike, aiming your outer forearm at your assailant's neck. Power should come from the turning action of your hips, coupled with the pulling action of your back muscles. It should be the body moving the arm, not the other way around.

Strike at a 45-degree angle, hitting downward into the base of the neck.

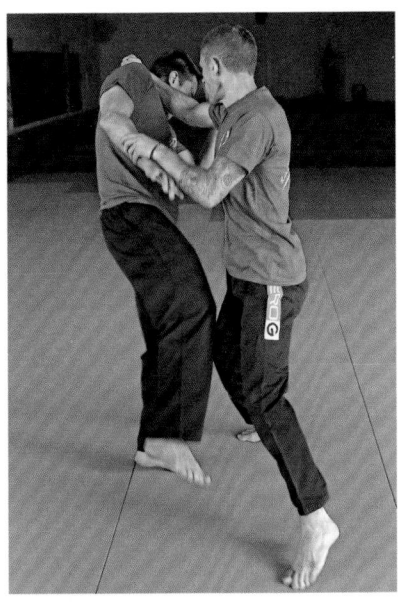

Keep transferring your weight into the strike and driving through your target. With a solid, driving strike you should be able to knock your attacker to the ground.

Hook Punches and Slicing/Circular Elbow Strikes

The toughest striking tools you have on your body are your elbows, knees, and head; and at some point you will be looking to move into an effective range to use these. (In reality, most fights either start at this range or soon close distance to it.)

Most people fail to make contact with circular elbow strikes because they underestimate how close they need to be to the target (their aggressor's head), and either miss completely or lean forward to make sure that they connect. When throwing any strike, the head should remain over the shoulders, and the shoulders should stay over the hips. If your body leans forward, not only will your balance be compromised, but you won't be able to fully utilize the power of the back muscles, which should help turn the torso and power the strike.

It is harder to get the timing and distance right with a circular strike than it is with strikes and punches that are directed forward. It is easier to judge distance and timing when your strike is traveling in a straight line, as opposed to a strike that travels in an arc, because the point at which that arc intersects the target has to be calculated. It is worth noting this, because in any physical confrontation you will want to keep things as simple as possible, and circular strikes—especially those delivered with the forward arm/hand—can be difficult to pull off successfully in a dynamic situation.

The power of the circular elbow strike comes from the hips and torso, rather than from the arm and shoulder; however, not a great deal of power needs to be generated for the strike to be successful. If the elbow can make impact and then drag across the face, digging into flesh and cutting skin, it will be an extremely effective strike, generating a lot of pain. One of the big myths about cutting the flesh/skin of the face is that you can cause a great deal of blood to run into the eyes, and so affect your aggressor's vision. This really only happens in a prolonged fight, after the effects of the adrenal fight/flight response have worn off. This is because when a person becomes adrenalized, the blood moves from the surface skin and peripheries to the larger muscles. This means that in the first 15 seconds or so of the fight (and most fights are shorter than this), there isn't a great quantity of blood in the forehead.

Rear Slicing Elbow

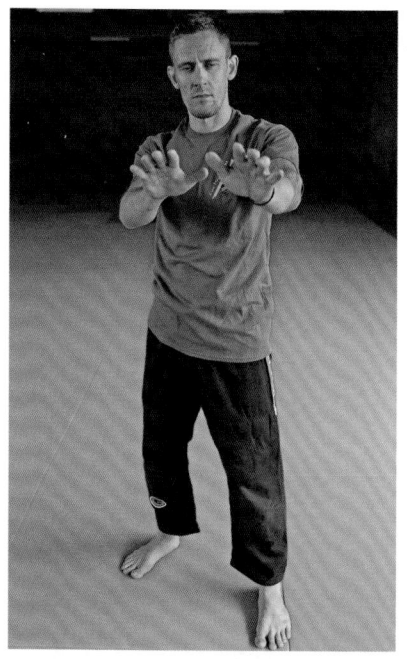

If you are facing an aggressive individual who has yet to launch an attack, you should adopt a de-escalation/interview stance. Your head should be over your shoulders, with your shoulders over your hips (i.e., you are upright, rather than bent forward or backward). Your hands should be out in front of you, controlling range and distance in a placating, non-aggressive manner. This is a good stance from which to launch many different attacks without giving your intentions away to an aggressor.

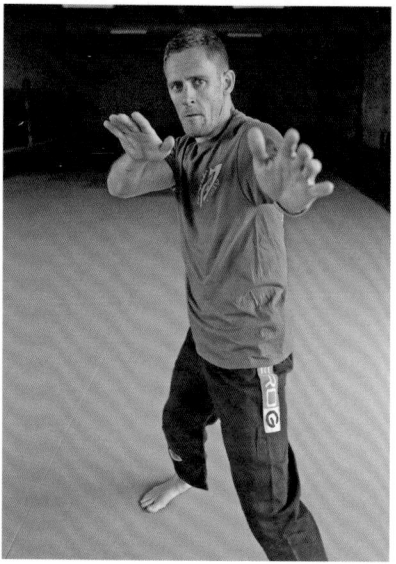

To throw a rear slicing elbow strike, first turn your left hip inward as you pull your arm back to make the strike. You should also shift some of your weight onto your back foot so that you can transfer it forward when you make the strike.

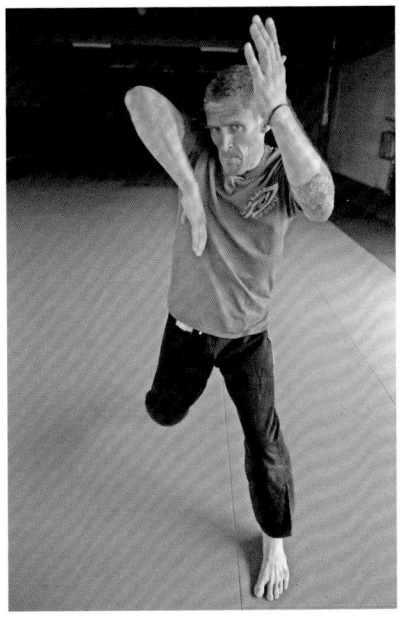

Start to pull your left hip back and drive your right hip forward as you turn at the waist to start bringing the elbow forward.

Start to roll the elbow over so that it can cut down at a 45-degree angle, as you drive your right hip forward and shift your weight toward the target.

You should be looking to cut across your assailant's face at a 45-degree angle, driving your strike into them and downward.

When you make the strike, continue to drive through the target, rather than recoiling it—from here, you will also be in a good position to deliver a horizontal hammer-fist strike with your right arm.

Forward Slicing Elbow

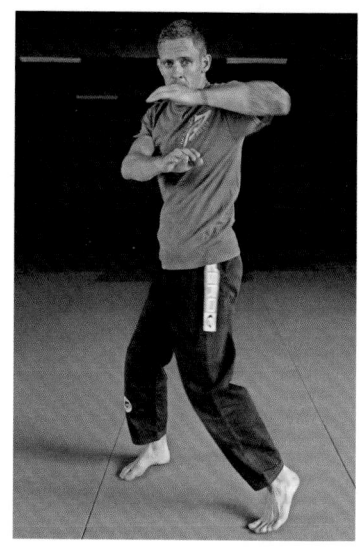

Assume a neutral but prepared stance, with your hands out in front of you. Position your feet on opposite corners of a rectangle, with your weight distributed evenly. This is a non-threatening, non-challenging stance that also displays confidence and self-assurance due to your upright posture.

Turn your forward hip in and pivot on the toes of your front foot. At the same time, pull your forward hand toward your chest and swing your elbow out.

Keep turning to bring your elbow into the target. As you do this, raise your other hand up to protect your head. You should still be looking ahead at your assailant.

Don't immediately recoil the strike on impact, but continue to drive through with your elbow. From here, you could swing your left arm back toward your assailant, using a hammer-fist or forearm strike.

When you are striking someone with a series of blows, you need to be able to work their response(s) into your strikes. It is unlikely, for example, that their head—the target—will remain in the same place, especially if you are effective in your striking: some people will duck; some will try to close distance with you to clinch and cover; others will move back, etc. This is the dynamic nature of a fight, and you must be able to adapt and alter your strikes based on your assailant's movements and responses. It may be that as you go to launch a forward slicing elbow, your aggressor has already moved back as a result of to your previous strike. This means you must be able to make this strike on the move, rather than from a static position. Being able to strike powerfully and with effect while moving is something that many people in the self-defense community neglect in their training, thinking it is something that is only applicable in combat sports such as Boxing, Muay Thai, and MMA. Being able to strike with power while moving, however, is an essential fighting skill that you will need to train in order to be effective in real-life confrontations.

 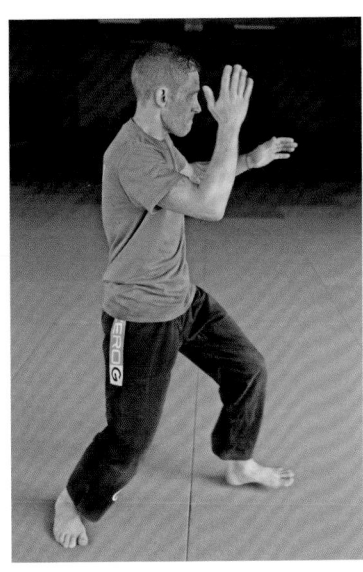

Assume your interview/de-escalation stance: hands out in front, feet on opposite corners of a rectangle, weight distributed 50/50, head over shoulders, shoulders over hips. Obviously, in addition to being used as an initial attack as shown here, this and all the other strikes described can be used as part of an attacking combination.

Move forward toward the target by pushing off explosively from your back foot, and stepping with your forward foot. Start to bring your forward hand to your chest and raise the elbow. Your rear hand should come up to guard your head as you do this.

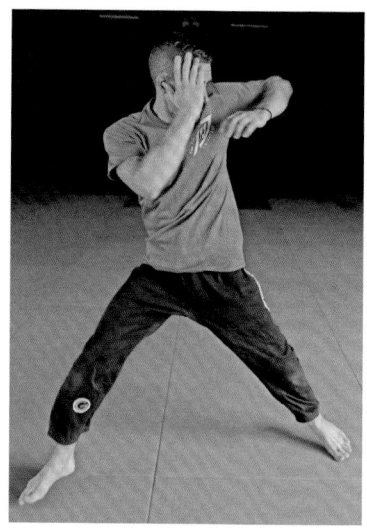

As you step and bring the elbow out, start to turn your body by turning your foot inward and rotating your torso. This will ensure that your weight is behind the strike.

Keep turning your body so that it is bladed/turned sideways to your attacker. Your weight should still be shifting forward at this point.

As your elbow connects, you should be positioned sideways to your attacker, and your weight should have been transferred into the strike.

Continue swinging/cutting through the target with your elbow and bring your rear foot forward—your weight transfer should naturally pull it with you. From here you can turn back out, either throwing a rear elbow strike with your back hand or a forearm/hammer-fist strike with your left arm. Even if you connect solidly with the target, don't assume the fight is now finished—your attacker may be drugged, adrenalized, etc., making them somewhat impervious to pain.

Hook Punches

Given the choice, you should look to throw elbow strikes to the head, rather than hook punches. Both are thrown from the same range, and the elbow is a much more devastating striking implement than the fist. However, there may be times when it is impossible to make a good connection with an elbow, making the hook punch a better tool to go with. One example would be when an assailant starts to cover their head with a high guard. In such a situation, your circular elbow strikes will not be able to make contact with your assailant's head, as they will be stopped by your assailant's arms. This means you will need a strike that is able to get behind their guard and reach the target. This is something that the hook punch is designed to do.

If a person has their hands up and is guarding their head, throwing circular elbow strikes is likely to be ineffective. It may be better to use a hook punch to get around your attacker's guard.

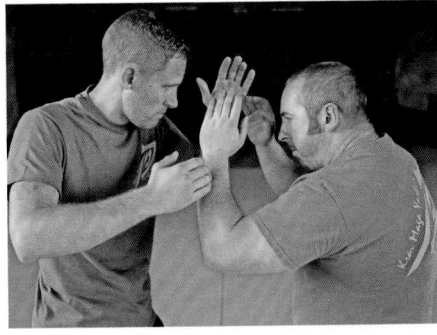

Rather than striking with the elbow, bring an arm up and prepare to make a hook punch around your attacker's guard.

Start to turn your torso just as you would when making a slicing elbow strike; the body movement for both these circular attacks is the same. Bring your arm up—it should have a 90-degree bend at the elbow to get around the arm of your attacker. Your hand should now be positioned to move behind your attacker's guard.

Keeping the arm in this position, continue to turn your torso to bring your fist toward your attacker's chin.

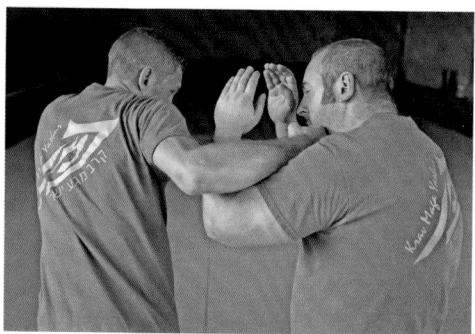

As you connect, start to extend the arm, driving your fist through the target. Don't keep turning the body beyond this point, as you risk turning away from your attacker and giving them your back.

The hook punch is delivered in much the same fashion as the slicing elbow. The body movement is exactly the same: the heel raises, the elbow comes up, the hips turn, and the torso twists. Instead of the elbow slicing, however, the fist is used to punch across the body into the attacker's head. The only real circular motion of the hook punch is made by the body turning; the arm itself extends in almost a straight line across the body, like a jab that is delivered sideways. It is the turning of the body that makes the arm motion appear circular.

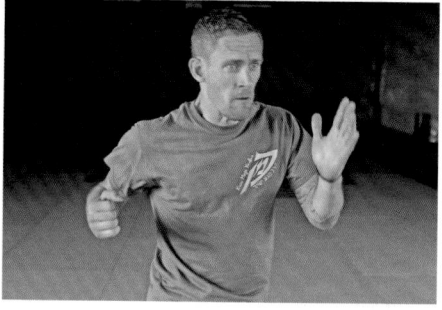

Pull your arm back and make a loose fist. Don't clench your fist tightly at this time, as this would tense the muscles of your arm and slow down its movement.

Hook punches work best as one of a combination of strikes; however, for the purpose of clearly illustrating the technique, it will be demonstrated from the interview/de-escalation stance.

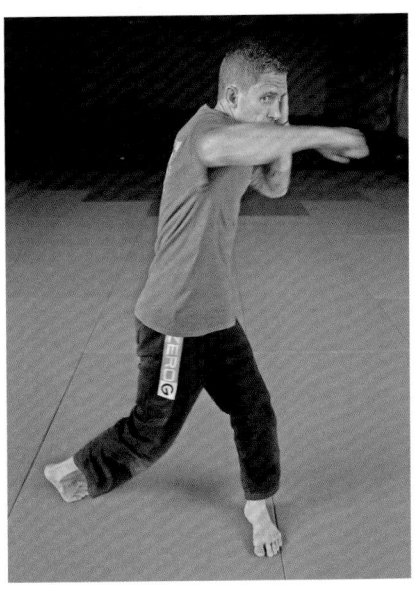

Imagine that you have a piece of string that runs from your elbow and attaches to your heel. As you raise your elbow it pulls your heel up, so that you can pivot on the ball of the foot. This will allow you to drive your hip into the strike.

Keep turning your body, with the arm bent at the elbow. At this point, all of the power should be generated by the turn of the body.

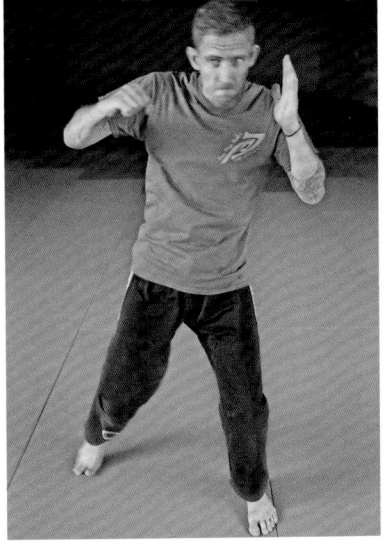

As your fist connects with the target, stop your body turn and start to extend your arm; think of it as making a jab punch across your body. This will allow you to drive your fist through the target without having to keep turning, which would expose your back to your assailant.

Once you have extended the arm, recoil it and start to pull your body back by sharply pulling your right hip backward.

By continuing to pull the hip back, you should end up back in the position you started from.

If the arm itself were to make a circular motion, rather than be moved by the body, two things would happen. For one, the punch would hit the target at an angle and force would be transmitted in several directions; for a strike to have maximum power, all the force should be directed into and through the target in a straight line. The other problem with the arm moving in a circular fashion is that if you miss, it will pull your body around, exposing your back to your attacker. If the body turns enough to put power into a "sideways" jab, but isn't pulled around by the arm in a circular fashion, the hips will stay square and facing your assailant.

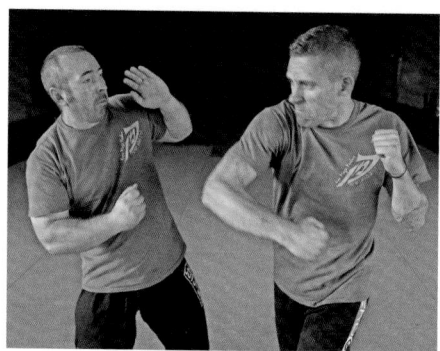

When you throw a hook punch, don't swing your punch and/or turn your body too far. If you fail to connect with the punch, you will end up in a vulnerable position. If your attacker pulls their head back from your strike, the momentum of your swing will see your fist travel past them—something that would not have happened had you extended the arm, jabbing it out across your body.

As you continue to turn, your back will now be exposed toward your attacker and your hands will not be in a position where they could be used to cover/block/protect you.

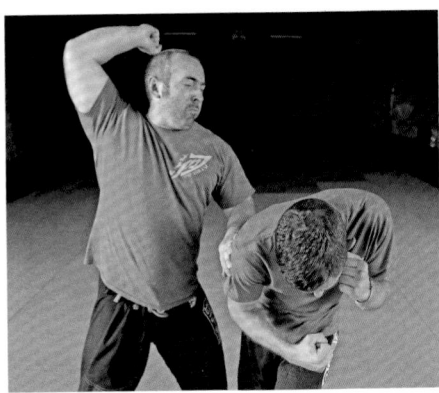

Your assailant will now be able to launch their own attack, striking vulnerable targets such as the back of your neck.

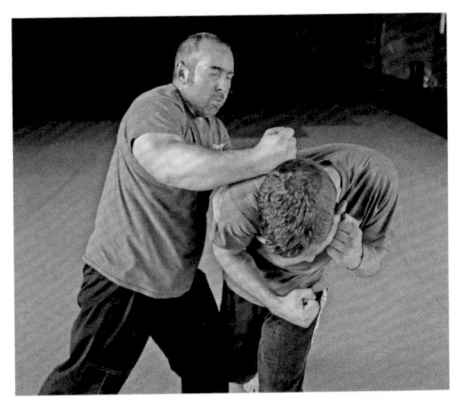

If your back is turned to your assailant, they will be able to drive into you, delivering strike after strike, before you can reorient yourself to respond.

I have been involved in many, many discussions concerning the orientation of the fist when throwing a hook punch; e.g., should the thumb be up (vertical fist), or should it be facing toward you (horizontal fist), etc.

If the fist is turned over so that the thumb is pointing toward you, you will generate more power. The rotation caused by such a movement engages the muscles of the shoulder to a greater degree than if no rotation had occurred. The issue, however, is that the larger knuckles, which you want to strike with, are now closer to you than to your assailant. If you are accurate with your hook punches, and your timing is good enough that your attacker isn't able to pull their head away from the punch to any degree, this won't be a problem.

If you strike with the thumb up, you will lose some power, but it is unlikely you will end up connecting with anything but the larger knuckles.

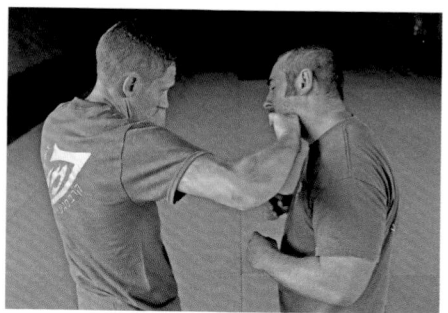

However, if your attacker flinches, or your range control isn't perfect, you will probably connect with your weaker knuckles, and if you hit the skull, they may break. The irony of punching is that the harder you punch, the more likely you are to injure your hand.

The only issue to be aware of when punching this way is that, although you are connecting with the largest knuckles, you may run the risk of damaging your wrist if your fist isn't clenched tightly and your wrist fixed and locked.

Although it's an interesting theoretical debate, when it actually comes down to it, the way you orient your fist doesn't really matter; each position has its pros and cons, and at the end of the day, the hand position probably only accounts for 5 percent of the final strike. The most important part of any punch is the way the body works as a unit to create power. If you are looking to maximize the efficiency and effectiveness of your punching, it would be better to concentrate on this, rather than getting caught up in the nuances around the orientation of the fist.

At the end of the day, the orientation of the fist should, in most cases, be affected by your level of proficiency in throwing the strike. If you believe you have the control and range to ensure that you can connect with the larger knuckles, rotating the fist and engaging the shoulder muscles will give your strike more power. Another consideration is whether or not you are carrying a weapon. If your primary tool of self-defense is a firearm, baton, pepper spray, etc., the risk of breaking a knuckle probably isn't worth it. If you break a bone in your hand during this process so that you are unable to draw/use these tools, then the strike will have failed to achieve its purpose in creating the time, space and distance to allow you to get to them.

If your assailant is effectively using a high guard to protect their head (possibly even against your hook punches), you may want to get them to drop their hands so that this target is exposed. Do not be fooled into thinking that because someone is acting in a defensive manner they are beaten/finished, or that you have the advantage. It may be that they are simply waiting for an opportunity to pull out a weapon and change the odds of the fight.

One way to get your assailant to lower their guard and drop their hands is to start attacking the body. Be aware that it is possible to condition the body to take a high degree of pain, so you may need to strike the same target several times in order to have an effect. If you can land your strikes to the kidneys, you will elicit a flinch response that makes your aggressor crunch up in such a way that the arms will drop down to protect the body. It can be difficult to strike so accurately in a dynamic context, though, and heavy clothing, such as a coat, can mitigate some of the effects of your strikes. However, if you repeatedly strike in roughly the same place, putting the full weight of your body into the strike, your assailant will be forced to start defending this area. As soon as the assailant's hands drop and you recoil your strike, you should turn your attention to the head.

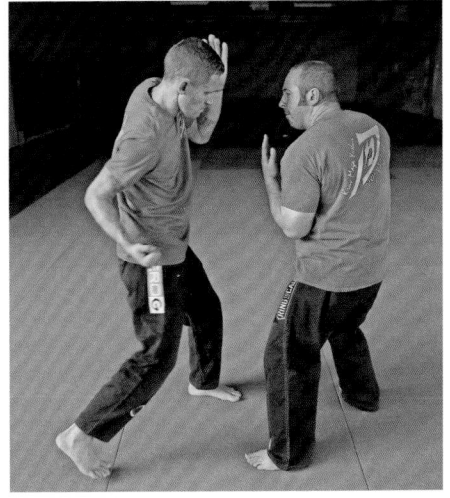

If your attacker is protecting their head well, and has a high and tight guard, it may be difficult to get an elbow—or even a hook punch—in.

One way that you may be able to get your assailant to drop their guard and open themselves up is to throw low punches/hooks at their body. To try to protect from these, they will need to lower their hands, which will make their head available as a target.

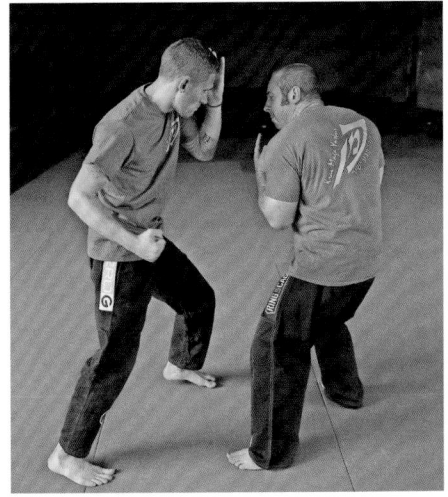

Although they have blocked your low hook, their head is now exposed.

Pull your punch back by recoiling your hip, so that you are now in a position to deliver a hook (or slicing elbow strike) to your assailant's head.

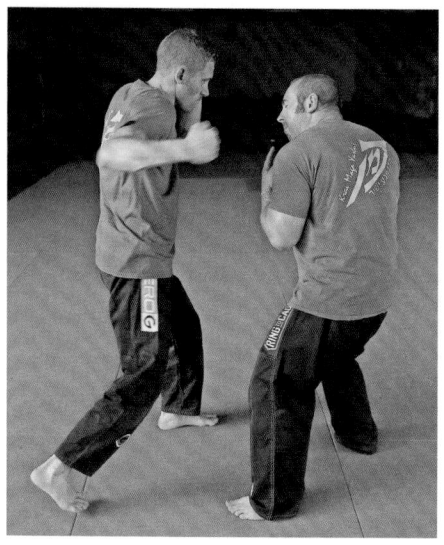

Push your hip forward, raise the elbow and the heel, and make a hook strike to the head.

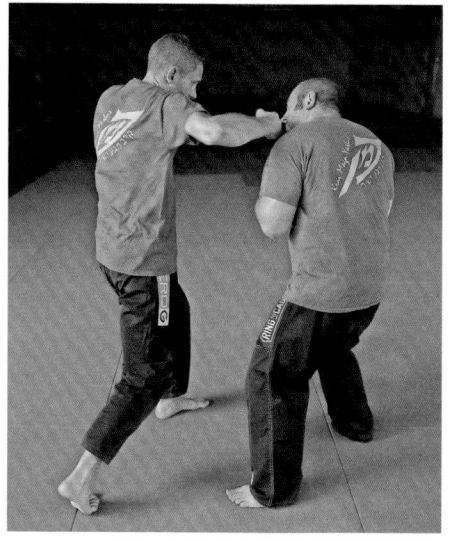

With your attacker's guard opened up and their head vulnerable, you can start to deliver further strikes to this target.

Although body shots are generally not the most effective type of strike (unless you are extremely accurate and able to target specific areas such as the liver) in a short conflict (lasting less than 10 seconds), they are useful for setting up other strikes and diverting an assailant's attention away from other areas. In longer-lasting incidents, body shots will end up tiring and exhausting an unconditioned assailant, and can be extremely effective at slowing them down. This is especially true if the person you are assaulting does not know how to control their breathing when they are punched.

Even if a person is guarding their face or head, making it difficult to throw elbow strikes at it, you don't necessarily have to use hook punches to get around their guard. A very simple solution is to use one hand to hook around and clear their blocking arms so that you are able to strike them.

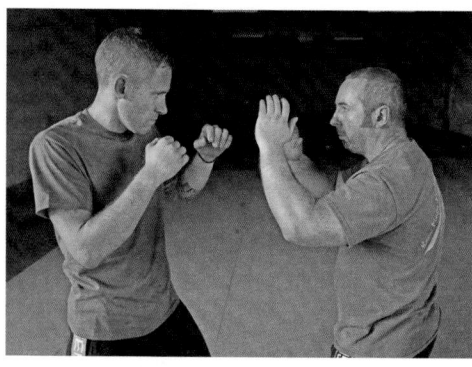

Another simple way to open a person's guard up...

...is to grab the wrist of one of the arms (it is often easier to grab their left arm with your left hand, and vice versa) and pull the arm down to expose the head.

This will allow you to throw elbow strikes and/or similar attacks toward your assailant's face.

If there is space between your assailant's arms, you could also come through the middle of their guard with a slicing uppercut elbow.

Assume your de-escalation/interview stance.

Step/slide forward with your left foot, turning your hand in, and start to raise your elbow. Your rear hand should start to pull back in order to come back and guard your head.

Keep raising the elbow in a circular fashion toward the target.

Once it hits, continue to drive it upward, while at the same time pulling your hand back behind your head.

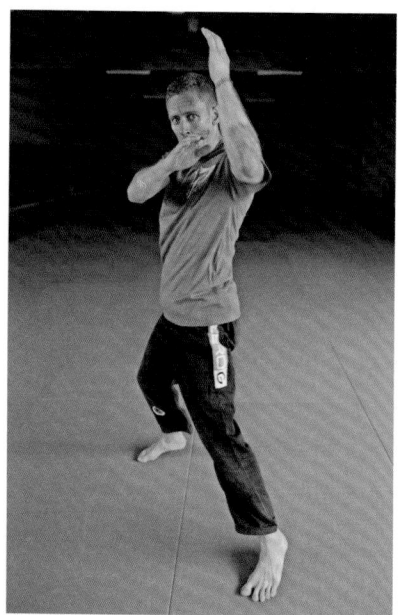

In this and the next photograph, you can see how the body turns inward to add power to the strike.

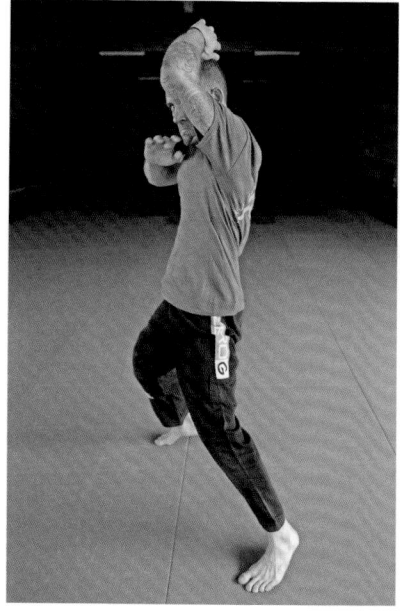

If you were square-on to your aggressor, your elbow will have now come directly to your assailant's center line; i.e., directly between their guard.

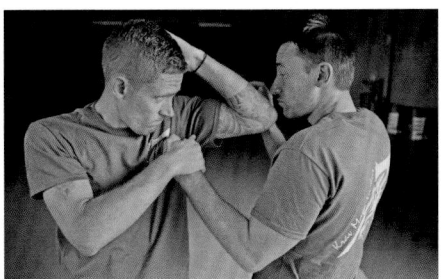

By continuing the upward arc of the elbow after it has connected, you will cause the head to be driven backward, and the elbow will be scraped upward into your assailant's face.

Combining Hook Punches with Hammer-Fist Strikes

The outward hammer-fist can also be thrown as a second strike after a hook punch or slicing elbow—it works especially well if either of these short-range strikes have missed—either because your attacker pulled their head back, or because you misjudged the range and distance (something which can easily happen in a dynamic situation).

If your assailant moves their head back to avoid one of these strikes, immediately turn your body back and extend the arm, throwing a horizontal outward hammer-fist at your attacker's head or neck. It is probably best to err on the side of caution and strike a little deeper than might be necessary to reach the target. This way, you will at least make contact with your forearm if your attacker pulls their head away again.

As you throw your hook punch, your attacker may pull their head back to avoid it.

If you have already committed to the strike, your hook punch will miss. So long as you don't swing the punch wildly, your attacker won't have the opportunity to attack your back.

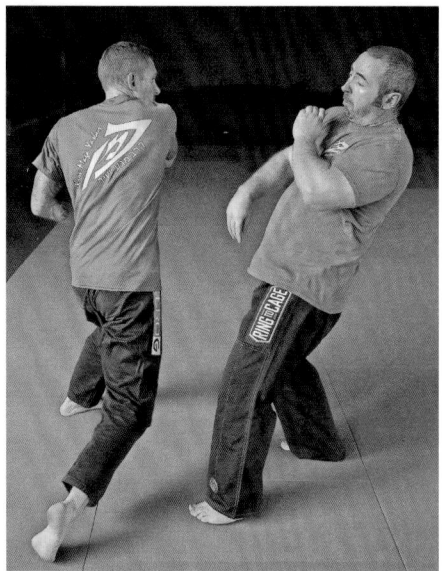

Bring your arm back across your body in order to deliver a hammer-fist or forearm strike.

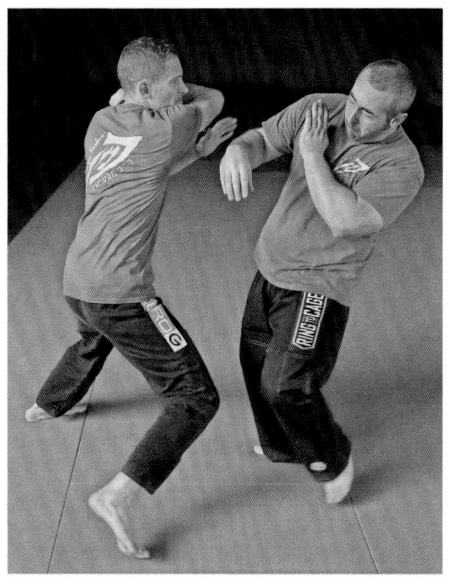

Transferring your weight forward and taking a step forward will move you toward your attacker. As you do this, unwind your arm from around you to deliver either a forearm strike or a hammer-fist strike, depending on the range.

Even if your attacker has their hands held up to guard their head, the power generated by your body unwinding and moving forward is likely to crash straight through them, hitting the target regardless.

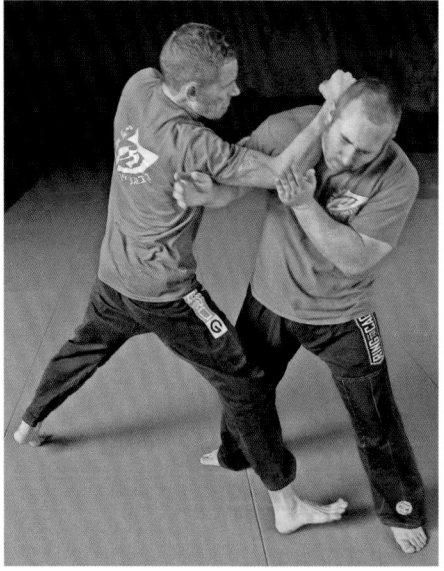

Continue to drive your strike into your attacker as if you are trying to use it to cut off their head.

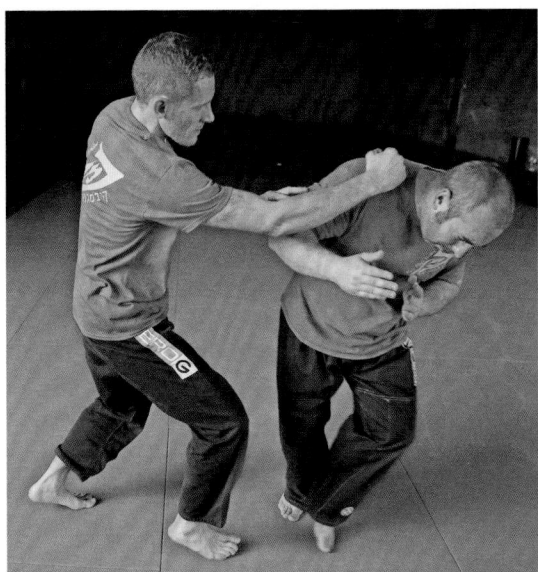

This should see them concussed, with their balance severely compromised. From here, you can either disengage or continue to deliver strikes until your attacker is no longer able to continue fighting, emotionally and/or physically.

It may be that you connect with the hook, and this moves the person's head back, which sets up the hammer-fist strike. If you strike in this rhythm, with both strikes occurring in quick succession, you may knock your assailant out, as the brain will receive a "double shake," being quickly moved one way and then the other. It is worth pointing out that knocking your assailant out is something that may happen in the course of striking, rather than something that you should aim to do. If you spend your time chasing/looking for an opening that will allow you the chance to knock your aggressor out, you will be wasting time that could have been spent delivering multiple strikes, which might have totally overwhelmed them and caused them to emotionally crumble, removing them from the fight much earlier. During your blitzing assault on your assailant, you may "get lucky" and physically knock them out, but don't waste your time looking for that one opportunity. You should lay down your strikes like a machine gunner, not a sniper.

Defending Against Punches with a Punch

One of the foundational principles of Krav Maga is that attack should follow defense at the earliest opportunity. One way to do this is to combine an attack with a defensive movement, such as using the same punch to both attack your assailant and at the same time defend against their punch. This particular technique works well against a circular punch when you are already in the fight. If you are "sucker punched" and taken by surprise, your natural reflexes will take over and you will perform a 360 defense; i.e., you will end up flinching, and bring your arm up to block.

You should only ever attempt to defend a punch with a punch when you are sure that your attacker doesn't have a knife, broken bottle, or other such implement in their hand. The trick to being successful with this is to ignore the punch that is being thrown by your aggressor, as the movement will draw both your attention and your strike away from its intended target and toward your assailant's attack. Instead, all of your focus should be on executing your own punch, and letting the movement of your arm perform a blocking action.

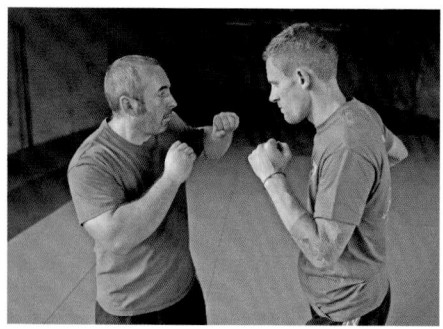

As your assailant begins to throw a circular punch toward you, start to raise your elbow upward while at the same time driving your fist forward toward your attacker's face.

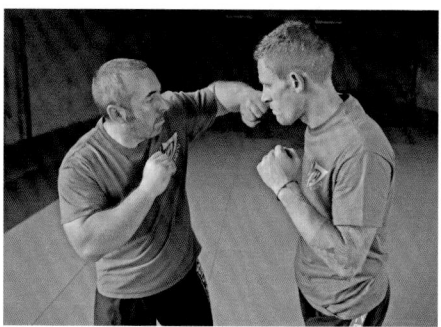

Keep raising the elbow up as you deliver the punch forward. Your fist will be corkscrewing round so that thumb is pointing toward the ground, rather than up.

Continue this rotation of the fist so that the elbow is lifted high. This means that your attacker's strike will be blocked by your punching arm.

Continue to extend your arm and drive your fist into and through your attacker's face. You can then follow up on this, using your left arm to deliver further strikes.

Be aware that this is not a "power" punch as such, because you will be connecting with the smaller, weaker knuckles of the hand—you should instead think of it as a "jabbing" punch that interrupts your attacker's assault and rhythm, and allows you the opportunity to set up further strikes of your own.

Other Attacking Tools

Biting

A real-life fight is a dirty thing, and as such, nothing can ever be ruled out. If you are fighting for survival—and this is the only reason you should be fighting—everything and anything should be used. This includes biting. Although we don't possess the jaw and bite strength of a Rottweiler or a pit bull, biting can be an effective tool for us to use. It is worth pointing out that clothing can often render biting ineffectual, so it should never be seen as a silver bullet, though it definitely does have its time and place.

Biting works very well for small children who are being abducted or pulled away by an adult assailant. A child should try to grab their attacker's arm with both hands to steady themselves, and then bite into it. As soon as they feel the grip loosen, they should move to get away/disengage. Understand that although this type of assault—a stranger trying to kidnap a child, for whatever purposes—is what we fear most, it is not the most likely way for an adult to get a child to go with them. Children need to be educated in identifying the grooming process that adult predators use, as well as learning physical self-defense techniques.

Biting is an effective tool for two basic reasons: firstly, a person who is bitten instinctively pulls away from the bite, making it a great way to create space to move/escape when held in a lock or control. Secondly, it sends a clear message to your attacker as to where your head space is, and what you are prepared to do in order to survive the fight—being bitten is something an attacker probably didn't expect when they decided to assault you.

If you are dealing with a multiple-assailant situation in which you want to send a clear message to the group—one that says they are not going to have an easy time dealing with you—biting the primary aggressor, and moving them so that they are between you and the others, can be an effective strategy. If those less-committed members of the group witness the most aggressive and determined member bleeding and in extreme pain, they will be less likely to want to involve themselves in the fight.

If you find yourself in a situation where you have no disengagement options and are dealing with multiple assailants, you should first see if de-escalation or acquiescing to your aggressors' demands (handing your wallet over if it's a mugging, etc.) will work as a solution. If your attackers seem committed to violence—i.e., they stay after you give them what they want, they continue to be verbally aggressive, etc., you will need to take decisive action.

Grab the attacker who is nearest to you—one hand grabbing the back of their head, the other their chin—and move rapidly and aggressively toward them. It is likely that the assailant nearest to you is the primary aggressor, and the other person(s) with them secondary aggressors who may or may not be motivated to get involved. They may simply be members of the group who will join in if necessary, but will not want to initiate an assault.

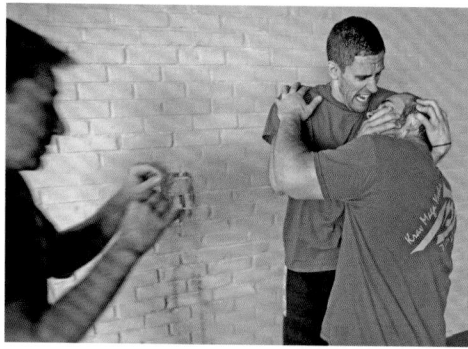

Turn your attacker's head so that their nose is in line with your mouth. Once those who are less motivated understand what is happening and what you are about to do, they may well back away, as they now know what the cost of involvement may be.

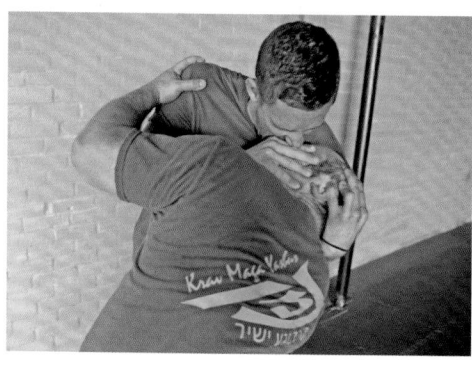

When you bite the nose, get a good grip on it (don't seal your mouth around it, though, for health and safety reasons), and while still holding the head, rip it from side to side. This may seem barbaric, but you will want to cause your assailant as much pain as possible. Ideally, you want everyone else in the group to hear your attacker's screams and shouts so that they hesitate to get involved. Still holding/biting your attacker, maneuver yourself to a position from which you can disengage.

When you bite, you should aim to "nip" at your assailant's exposed or unprotected flesh (i.e., that covered by a T-shirt or another type of clothing with sufficiently thin material), rather than making deep bites. Nipping and then pulling/ripping the flesh with the teeth causes much more acute pain than simply making a deep bite. Another advantage of nipping is that the mouth rarely forms an airtight seal around the flesh; this means that most blood-borne diseases such as HIV and hepatitis will present less of a risk.

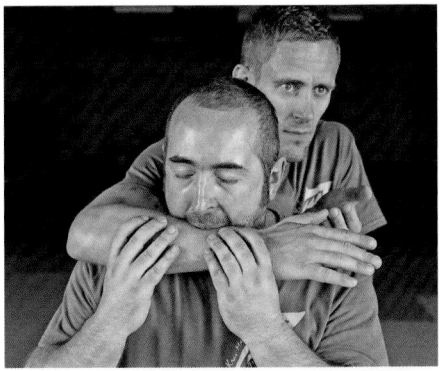

Another reason "full" bites are inadvisable is that they can end up allowing your aggressor to take advantage of the relative weakness of your jaw. A good example of this would be a rear strangle situation, where it might at first glance seem a good idea to bite the attacking arm.

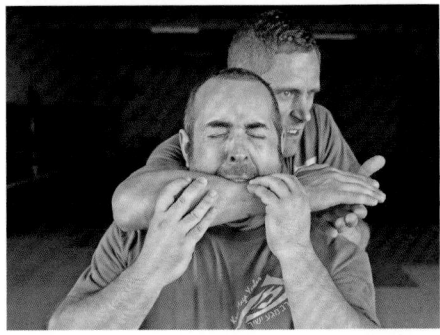

The problem arises when the attacker, rather than pulling away from the bite, pulls into it, extending and painfully opening the jaw, to the point where the bite no longer troubles them and they have control of your head—and therefore your body and movement.

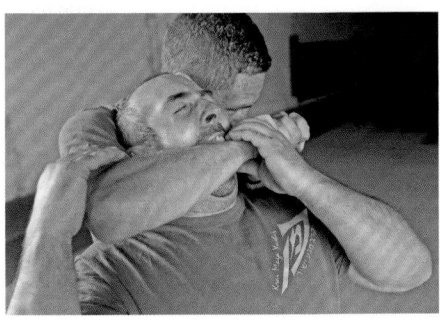

When an attacker pulls back violently, they move their arm backward toward your back teeth, where you have no leverage, and your bite will be ineffective. Having your jaw forced open in this way is extremely painful.

Head-Butts

The skull is extremely thick in certain places, and with the head comprising of about 8 percent of total bodyweight, using this area of the body to strike can be extremely effective. The toughest part of the skull is at the top of the forehead, at the hairline, and this is the area you want to direct toward your assailant's face/bridge of the nose (soft target areas).

There are two basic ways to deliver the head-butt. The simplest way is to "lock" the neck and simply drive your forehead into your attacker's face. The other involves swinging your head forward, toward your assailant's face. When swinging the forehead down, try not to just swing from the neck, but swing from the middle of your back as you push your head forward.

Driving Head-Butt

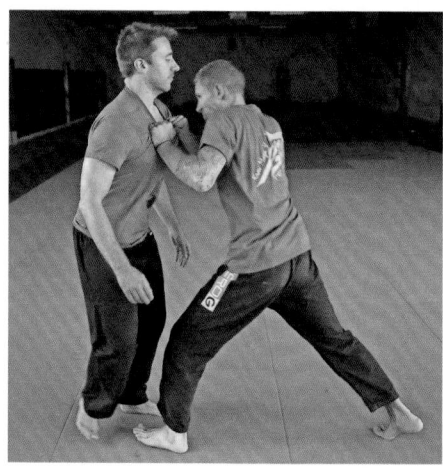

I have been head-butted twice in my life; on both occasions I was knocked unconscious, and I can still recall the exact pain I felt. In most cases, we are quick to forget extreme pain, but for some reason, I can still remember exactly what it feels like to be struck this way. One of the easiest ways to deliver a head-butt is to grab your attacker's clothing and aim the top of your forehead toward your attacker's face.

Take a step forward, pushing your attacker back while lowering yourself. When they are unbalanced, they are not in a good position to defend themselves.

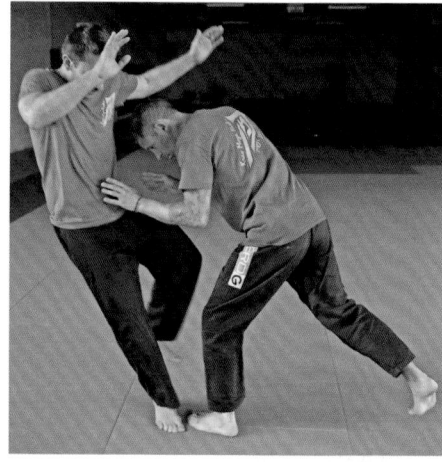

Strike with the top of your skull (normally around the front hairline) toward your attacker's nose, crushing it against your skull. Take this opportunity to drag your rear foot forward, so that you are in a good position to deal with their attacks and/or make your own further attacks.

The same head-butt can be delivered to an attacker's chest or upper-body in order to open them up and disrupt their balance.

Swinging Head-Butt

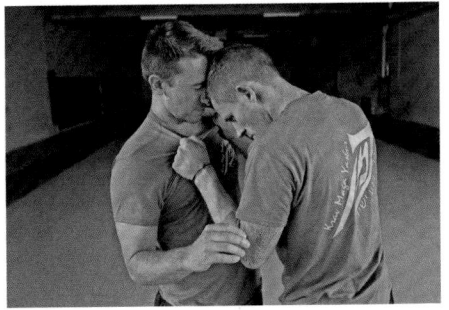

Take hold of your assailant's clothing and pull your head back. Rather than driving your head forward with the neck locked, swing your head toward your attacker.

You should aim to connect the solid, bony part of your skull—around the top of the forehead/hairline—with the bridge of your attacker's nose.

Lower-Body Combatives

Front Kick with Glisha

When you strike someone, whether it's a punch or a kick, you will ideally want them to either be rooted in place or moving onto your strike. This is why it isn't enough to just be able to punch and kick with power; you must also be able to control your assailant's movement so that your strikes produce an effect. If you kick someone as they are moving back, a lot of your power will go into pushing your attacker backward, adding to their movement rather than being absorbed by them. This may be your intention; however, if you want to inflict pain and damage on them, it will not be effective to kick them as they are moving backward.

Kicks can be delivered at close range, but they will generally be more effective at long range. Many systems will break down their techniques by range, saying that there is a kicking range, a punching range, a grappling range, etc. In reality, this is not the case, as a grappler can shoot in and tackle you from what would normally be considered outside of kicking range, and if you are dealing with a skilled Karateka from a style such as Kyokushin, they will be able to round-kick your head when you are in "grappling" range. The notion that different types of techniques are restricted by range is an erroneous one. That said, certain types of techniques are easier to deploy at particular ranges, and the front thrust kick is one that works best from distance, when an attacker is moving toward you, onto your kick.

The issue affecting the use of this kick is that most fights in reality start extremely close, denying you an easy opportunity to deploy such a kick. However, there are situations (albeit rare), where assailants do come at you from distance, as well as times when you can create the distance (more common) that will allow you to make such a kick.

If you have the space and time to back away from an assailant, you should. Getting to safety should be your number one priority in any situation. There are, of course, times when there is space between you and an attacker, but not enough space to be able to move away safely. In such situations, your better option may be to engage and take away the timing of your assailant's attack. In such cases, take a step forward toward them to start your movement into the kick.

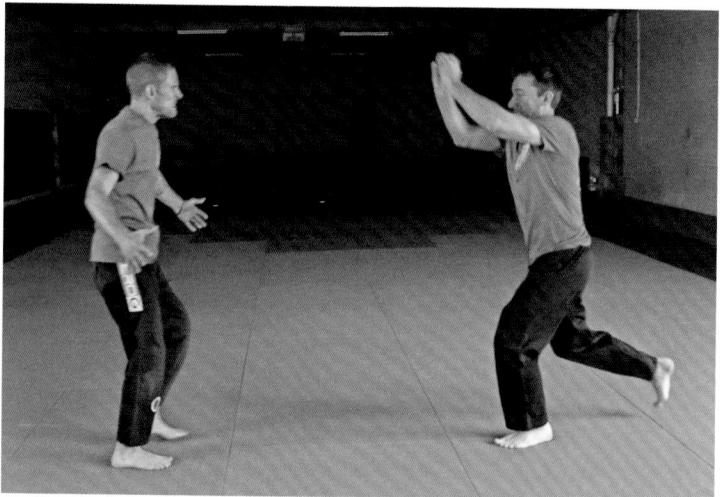

As you do this, transfer your weight onto your left leg and start to bring your right leg through in preparation for launching a thrusting kick.

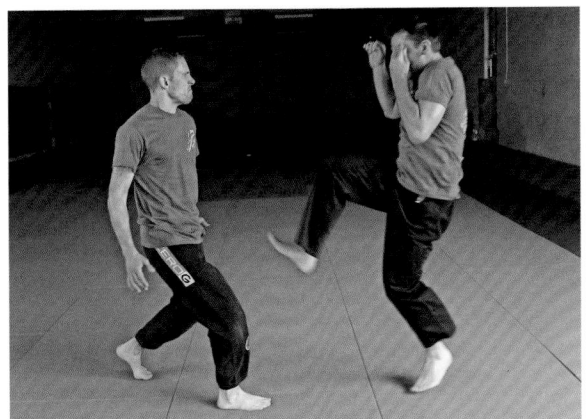

As you raise your knee up, slide on the foot of your supporting leg. This will transfer your weight forward, adding momentum to the kick. You shouldn't hop or jump, but instead slide the foot forward as part of your forward movement, making sure it stays in contact with the ground.

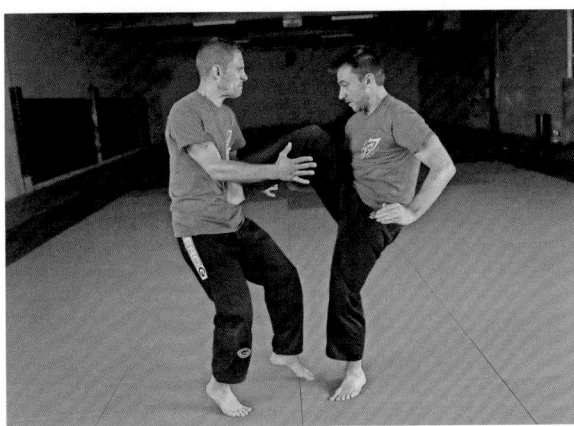

What gives the kick its potency is the timing. You want to still be moving forward as your foot impacts into your assailant; however, at the moment you extend your leg and drive/push into your attacker, you will need to root the supporting leg so as to have a solid platform to drive off from. The closer you are to your assailant when you connect with them, the deeper you can drive your kick.

Once you make contact, root your supporting leg and extend your kick, driving your assailant back. By turning the foot so that your toes are pointing to the side, rather than at your assailant, you will drive your hip a few more inches toward your attacker, adding to the thrust of the kick.

PART II

Armed and Unarmed Self-Defense Scenarios

De-escalation

When you find yourself dealing with an aggressive and emotional individual, you should start by asking yourself a simple question: is this a premeditated situation or a spontaneous one? In a premeditated act of aggression/violence, your aggressor has planned and/or orchestrated the situation and has an outcome in mind. They may, for example, be a mugger who has acquired a weapon, chosen a location, selected a victim, and is looking to take their wallet or purse, etc. In a spontaneous act of violence, the aggressor did not enter the situation with any plans to become aggressive. Rather, your actions or behavior—whether real or perceived—caused them to become angry and violent; perhaps you spilled a drink on them, or cut them off in traffic, or cut in front of them in line. The wrongdoing may be imagined or perceived on their part, but their belief in the injustice means that they have become aggressive and therefore dangerous. One of the big differences between spontaneous and premeditated acts of violence is that in spontaneous acts of violence, your aggressor has no predefined outcomes; they don't know what they want from the situation—unlike a mugger or sexual assailant, who has very clear objectives that they are looking to achieve.

In premeditated acts of aggression, you have two choices: you can either acquiesce to your aggressor's demands or you can resist them—that is, fight. If a mugger wants your wallet, you can give it to them, or you can attempt to deal with them physically; trying to talk them out of mugging you is not an option. Because an aggressor in a spontaneous act of violence doesn't come to a situation with a particular outcome in mind, you will in all likelihood have the opportunity to present other non-violent solutions and alternatives. If you have inadvertently spilled a drink on someone, they won't know what will make the situation right for them; they may feel in the moment that they have no alternatives but to act violently against you. If the option is presented in the right way, however, they may come to accept that other non-violent routes are open to them, such as accepting a replacement drink from you, having you pay for their dry cleaning, etc.

The only way an aggressive individual will be able to consider these alternatives to violence is if their high and volatile emotional state can be reduced, so that they are able to consider non-violent solutions to the situation. This is the goal and purpose of the de-escalation process.

A large part of our communication with others comes down to our body language—some studies suggest body language may account for up to 67 percent of our overall communication. If you are trying to de-escalate a situation and get an aggressor to consider non-violent alternatives, you will want to adopt a stance which is both non-threatening and placating, without at the same time looking overly submissive. You will also want to be well positioned and prepared to deal with your aggressor, should they indicate that they are going to launch an attack. If you look too aggressive (clenching your fists, etc.), you may well give your aggressor a reason to fear for their safety and pull a weapon or strike you.

You can alter your hand position depending on the exact message you want to convey to your aggressor. With the palms positioned downward, your "message" is more calming and placating.

If you put your palms directly out, you are sending a clear message to your aggressor that they should stop where they are and not come any closer. If you believe that your aggressor is about to get physical, you should move your hands to this position.

How People Interpret the World When Angry

If you spill a drink on someone, they are likely to become angry. They may feel uncomfortable and humiliated, and think that what happened to them wasn't fair and needs to be addressed and righted. This is a complex mix of thoughts and feelings that lack tangible direction; the individual knows what has happened to them is "wrong," but they don't know exactly what it is that will make things right, and therefore may consider violence as the only path open to them.

Having become emotional/angry, they will be using different parts of their brain to interpret what is going on around them, and determine how they should act, than those that they use when calm. In short, they lose the ability to rationalize and reason, and start using more animalistic, primitive ways of understanding their situation. "Triune Brain Theory" suggests that, depending on our emotional state, we work with one of three different brains: a reasoning one; a limbic/mammalian one; and a reptilian one. (It is important to note that when we are discussing Triune Brain Theory in this context, we are using it as a behavioral model, not as an evolutionary one, which is how it was first presented.) I like to think of the three brains as being a human brain (reasoning), a dog/wolf brain (limbic/mammalian), and a snake brain (reptilian). This allows me a good point of reference when dealing with aggressive/emotional individuals: how would a dog interpret my actions/behaviors, and how would a snake interpret them?

There are five ways that human beings can understand aggressive behavior and respond to highly emotional states. These are:

1. Reasoning
2. Posturing
3. Submission
4. Fight
5. Flight

When a person is angry and emotional, their ability to reason—that is, the reasoning part of the brain—switches off. When this happens, their mammalian or limbic system takes over; this part of the brain understands social interaction through displays of dominance/posturing and submission, just like a dog or wolf. If a person becomes highly emotional, their reptilian brain takes over, and everything is seen as being fight or flight. A snake, being a non-social creature, is unable to posture or act submissively; it can either attack or slither away when threatened. (Some snakes can give a warning signal that they're about to attack; they are not posturing, however, as there is no submissive response that would see them back down.) If you have ever asked someone to "calm down" during an argument or conflict, you have probably been met with the response, "I AM CALM!" This is because either their limbic or their reptilian brain is dominant at that point, and your request has been interpreted as an act of posturing or possibly even "fighting talk." You can ask/tell people to calm down, be quiet, stop shouting, etc., but each of these requests will be interpreted as commands, with you instructing your aggressor how to act (which is posturing or fighting talk). If you want to resolve the situation non-physically, you will need to get your aggressor to use their reasoning brain, which will allow them to consider alternatives to violence.

TRIUNE BRAIN THEORY & AGGRESSION

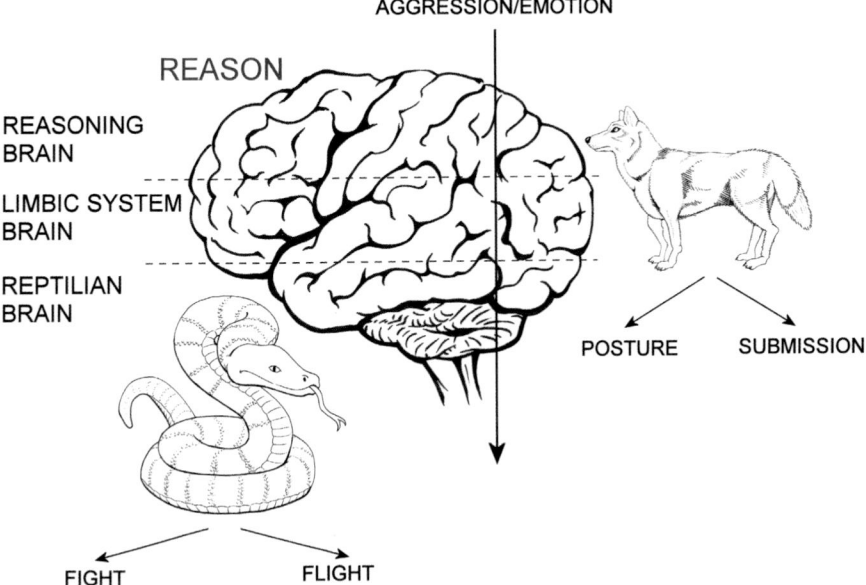

As a person becomes emotional or aggressive, their reasoning brain starts to switch off and they begin using their Limbic/Mammalian Brain (this "brain" understands conflicts and disputes in terms of posturing and submission, just as a dog or wolf does). If they become highly aggressive, they will interpret your actions and behaviors using their Reptilian Brain. This means they will understand everything in terms of fight and flight (the way a snake would interpret and respond to danger) and have their own responses limited to these two options. The purpose of de-escalation is to reduce a person's emotional state so that they can start engaging their Reasoning Brain and consider alternatives to violence.

Engaging the "Reasoning Brain"

We employ the Reasoning Brain most of the time. It is responsible for making informed, rational decisions and choices. The easiest way to get an aggressive individual to start using their reasoning brain again is to use open-ended questions. This compels the individual to think about what they are being asked and begin to consider alternatives. If, after you've spilled a drink on them, you ask them, "What can

I do to sort this out?" they will have to start considering what it is that will make the situation right for them. Such open-ended questions force people to think of non-violent alternatives for resolving the encounter. This thought process reduces the emotion in a situation, which is the goal of de-escalation. If this tactic is effective, they will begin acting with reason, rather than emotion. If an individual can be made to consider alternatives to violence, it will be hard for them to think of violence as either being justifiable, or as their only alternative.

There is a huge difference between you presenting a solution to a situation—such as offering to buy a person another drink—and them telling you that you need to buy them another drink. In the first instance, your offer will be seen as an act of posturing; that is, you are telling them what will resolve the situation. In the second, you are letting them posture to you—they are telling you what will end the conflict. By "accepting" their resolution of getting them another drink, you are responding submissively to *their* act of posturing—something that animals do in order to resolve conflict; and aggressive people interpret and view the world much as animals do.

Warning Signs

One of the reasons it is important to ask your aggressor—in spontaneous acts of violence—what will resolve the situation is that it will give you an idea as to whether de-escalation will be appropriate and/or successful. When people become overly aggressive, they switch off their ability to reason verbally; if someone is about to attack/assault you, they don't have a need to interpret verbal information. If, when you ask the question, "what can I do to sort this out?" you are met with one of the following responses, you should either preemptively attack or accept that you are about to be assaulted (and prepare for it):

1. Silence
2. Garbled words
3. Repetitive Looping

If an aggressive individual responds to your question, "What can I do to sort this out?" with silence, their reasoning, or mammalian brain isn't operating anymore, so they can't make sense of what you are saying. This means that they are about to assault you, and you should make a preemptive assault of your own. If they garble/mix up their words, saying something like, "You drink my spilled," they are only a few moments from responding physically. Repetitive Looping may happen when an aggressor isn't yet ready to assault you, but is gearing up to get themselves emotionally ready. To do this, they will keep repeating, over and over again, the accusation that justifies their acting violently toward you: "You spilled my drink! *You spilled my drink!* YOU SPILLED MY DRINK!"

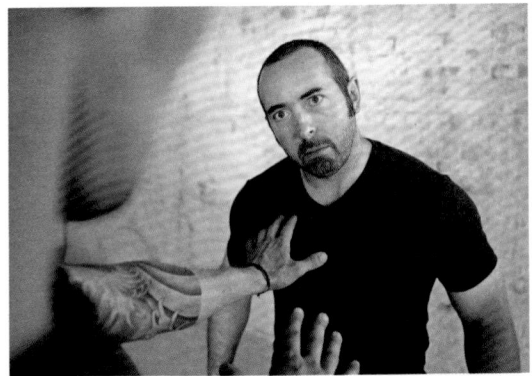

If you are met with silence when you try to talk to your aggressor and ask them what you can do to resolve the situation, then you can be almost certain that they are operating with their "Reptilian Brain," and are in fight-or-flight mode. It would be dangerous to assume that they are just going to walk away at this point. Your better option is to assume they are in fight mode, preparing to assault you. This is where it may be worth making a preemptive attack of your own.

A highly emotional and aggressive individual who is unable to interpret and respond to what you are saying—e.g., "What can I do to sort this out?"—and simply keeps shouting at you is not in a state of mind where de-escalate will be effective. They are simply too emotional for you to be able to communicate with them verbally.

When you engage the "Reasoning Brain" and are met with any of the aforementioned responses, you need to forget de-escalation. If an aggressive individual can still respond to reason (understand what you are saying), then de-escalation is a possible alternative to violence. If not, you should look to either attack preemptively or quickly disengage, as violence is inevitable.

Front Kick with Glisha from De-escalation Stance

When someone is clearly oblivious to every attempt you make to resolve a conflict in a non-physical manner (this only applies to spontaneous acts of violence), you may need to change your approach and make a strong, posturing display to them. From your Interview/De-escalation stance, move your hands rapidly toward their face while shouting in a firm voice, "Stay back!" As you do this, you should move backward and away from them. This will give you the distance and range from which to deploy a front kick, if necessary. This action is intended to prevent your aggressor from making an assault, while putting yourself in a stronger position.

We are born with two innate fears: loud noise and fast movement. Both of these trigger our startle/flinch reflex. By moving your hands rapidly toward your aggressor and shouting your command, you are hitting their startle reflex on two fronts. With many highly emotional people, these two actions will act as a "wake-up" moment, forcing them out of their aggressive state. By moving backward, you are creating distance that they will now need to cover in order to assault you—they can't just grab or punch you; they will need to take several steps toward you first. If you have "shaken" them up with your actions (loud noise and fast movement), they will need to somehow now get themselves back to their former emotional state and make the conscious decision to move toward you and attack you. In the majority of cases, unless the person believes the injustice committed against them is really significant, it won't happen. If they do attack, they will be moving forward and into space, which will give you the time to make an effective front kick. By creating this space, you are inviting them to move into it, and if they do, you will be well prepared to deal with them.

Glisha means "to slide" in Hebrew. When you add a sliding motion to your kick, you are effectively moving all of your bodyweight toward your attacker. As Krav Maga was originally designed as a system for the common soldier or infantry member, it was designed to be used by someone who had a pack on their back. This added weight would add power to the kick. The trick to making the front kick with glisha work is to slide forward, driving your weight into the attacker, and then root with the supporting leg as you extend the kicking leg. This means that there is an initial impact, followed by a solid extension of the leg.

It may be that you inadvertently knock into someone in a bar and spill their drink. You should immediately assume your de-escalation stance and ask them what you can do to resolve the situation. They may be fueled by alcohol, and may start shouting and swearing at you about how you should look where you're going, that you're disrespecting them, etc. Understand that this isn't a situation where de-escalation isn't effective; you will need another solution.

From your de-escalation stance, move your hands quickly toward your aggressor's eyes and tell them "Back off!" in a loud, strong voice. The fast movement and the loud noise should elicit a certain level of shock and surprise, causing them to flinch. This will give you time to move back and put distance between yourself and them.

As you move back, continue to face your aggressor. Stay in your de-escalation stance; you want to continue to demonstrate that you are not a threat to them. It is also useful to demonstrate this to anyone else in the environment who may be a potential witness if the incident results in legal ramifications. At this point you may have the time and space to fully disengage. If you have this opportunity, you should take it.

Your aggressor will now have to make a conscious choice to move forward and attack you. Hopefully, shouting something like "Back off!" will have shocked them out of their emotional state and taken away their inclination to act violently. If you continue to back away, they may be able to tell themselves and others that they were the dominant party in the confrontation and caused you to back away, and so not feel the need to continue the confrontation. If they do advance, however, you should move in to meet them.

As you step forward, start to raise your knee up in preparation for making the kick. Keep your hands up in front of your face/head.

Lift your weight off your supporting leg and slide it forward so that all of your bodyweight is moving toward your attacker.

As your foot crashes into them, root your supporting leg so that you have a solid base. If you haven't got a solid base when you extend the kicking leg, you are just as likely to push yourself off your attacker as you are to drive them back—and they won't have absorbed the full impact of the kick. The chest is a good target to choose when using this type of kick, as it forces a person's head and body back. If you strike the stomach or groin they may fold over your kick instead, and so remain close to you.

Extend your leg, and at the same time push the hip of the kicking leg forward to add power to the strike. This is accomplished by turning the heel of the supporting leg toward your attacker, pivoting on the ball of your foot.

After kicking, retract the leg rather than falling forward toward your assailant.

If your attacker is stunned and unable to respond right away, exit the situation as quickly as possible. There is no reason to stay and engage with them further, or deal with others who may want to join them in assaulting you.

PART III

Armed Assaults

Spoiling Weapon Draws

It would be wrong to train weapon defenses only for situations where the weapon has already been drawn. There may be times when your aggressor draws their weapon—be it a knife or gun—in your presence. If this happens, they are giving you an opportunity to spoil their draw and control them, and the weapon, before it is drawn and made operable. Even if drawn, a folding knife may still need to be opened, a firearm may have to have its safety released, or be racked to bring a bullet into the chamber, etc. If any of these actions can be prevented, then these weapons will not be able to be used as intended (a firearm that can't fire—if drawn—can still be used as an impact weapon against you, and this is something you should be aware of).

Nullifying a threat at the earliest opportunity is an important and obvious survival strategy, and although spoiling weapon draws can be difficult to perform when stressed and surprised, especially against a skilled and trained aggressor, it is a skill that you should look to develop. Fortunately, because most people don't train to draw their weapon at speed with the pressure of someone looking to prevent them from doing so, your success rate may actually be a lot higher than you experience in training. The important thing to remember is that if you fail to spoil the draw, you must continue to try and gain control of the weapon and/or overwhelm your attacker by striking them repeatedly.

You stand a better chance of spoiling a weapon draw if you are aware that the person is carrying a weapon in the first place. You should always assume that any individual you interact with is carrying. However, if you are certain that they are, your focus should be on preventing them from drawing that weapon and making it operational. When someone pulls a weapon, you will have no idea whether their intention is simply to threaten/intimidate you, or to actually use it against you. Preventing them from being able to do either will be your best course of action.

Signs That Someone Is Carrying a Weapon

The larger and heavier a weapon is, the more likely it is that you will be able to identify a person who is carrying. Firearms, especially if unholstered, can leave what is referred to as a "print" in the carrier's clothing (that is, the silhouette/shape of the weapon can be made out).

When carried unholstered in the rear of the pants, the weapon a person is carrying will be very obvious. The weapon may not be "on display" all the time, but as the person moves, and their clothing readjusts to their movement, it will pull against the weapon, revealing it. It could also be that the wind may blow the clothing against the gun. If someone is carrying to the rear and sits down in a chair, you may well hear the sound of the gun hitting the back of the chair, etc.

When a person carries a weapon to the front of their body, the "print" is usually smaller and less obvious; however, the person's movement may also reveal the weapon's presence. Most people will choose to carry their weapon in the front, whether it is a knife or a gun, because it is more accessible and easier to draw from this position. Because of this, you may need to be able to identify signs other than a "print" that reveal whether a person is armed.

If a weapon is large, bulky, and/or heavy, a person may change the manner in which they move to accommodate it. If someone's walking pattern is uneven and unnatural—favoring one leg over the other, for example—they may be having to adjust their movement and stride lengths to accommodate the weapon.

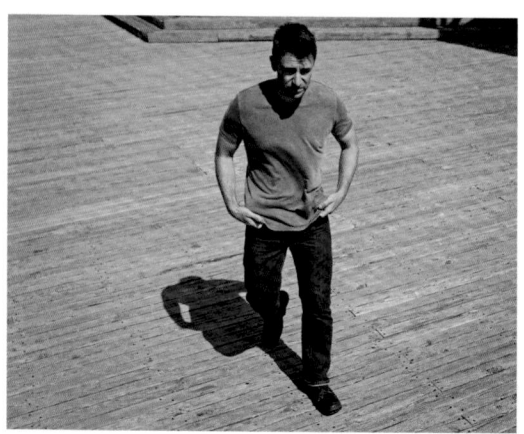

People who are unused to carrying a weapon will often find themselves continually checking it, possibly patting the weapon every so often as they move. They may also walk with their arms closer to their body than they would when walking normally. This is especially true if they are getting ready to draw the weapon.

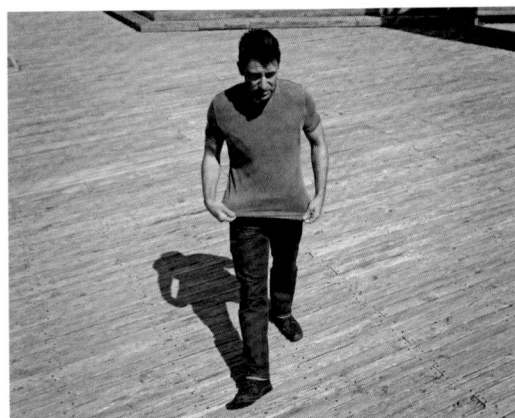

A person carrying a weapon may also adjust their clothing, "stretching it" so it is loose and will not get caught up with the weapon when they go to draw it. If their clothing is tight against them, it may be difficult for them to pull it up and gain access to their weapon.

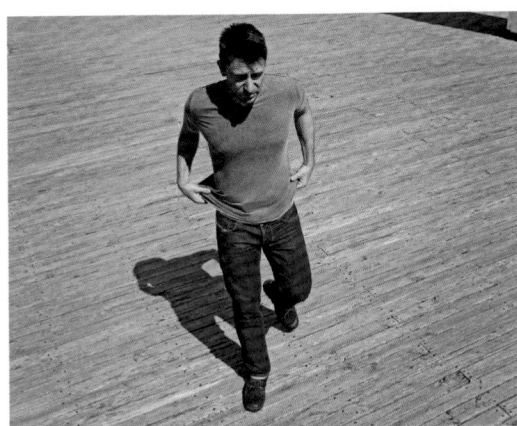

They may also "smooth" out their clothing so that the weapon doesn't leave a print, making sure that their clothing is not bunching up around the weapon.

In general, if a person is continually adjusting their clothing around the waistband area, or keeps their hands very close to their waistband as they move, it is wise to assume that they are carrying a weapon.

Spoiling the Draw at a Distance

Most incidents of violence, whether premeditated or spontaneous, happen at very close range—sometimes so close that you are unable to see a weapon being drawn in the first place. If you are nose to nose with an aggressive individual and they choose to draw a weapon from their waistband, it is unlikely that you will be able to see them do so. This is why it is important to control range and distance during any altercation, stepping back to a distance where you can see both the hands and feet of your aggressor. There are times, however, when you may spot an aggressive individual coming toward you, and recognize by their posture and determined movement that they have harmful intent toward you. As they walk, you may see them adjusting their clothing and reaching toward their waistband, which should alert you that they may be about to draw a weapon.

The individual may even be someone you know who has expressed an interest in causing you harm, or who has a strong dislike toward you. It would be a mistake to assume that you will only ever be attacked or assaulted by strangers.

The distance between you and your aggressor may not be sufficient for you to try to disengage to safety, or to have time to look for an improvised weapon or get a barrier, such as a parked car, between you and them. It may be that they are coming from the only entry/exit point available, cutting you off completely. If this is the case, acting preemptively may well be your best survival strategy.

As your aggressor approaches you from a distance, you may see them lift their clothing and reach for their waistband. Rather than wait for them to reach you, you should immediately start to engage.

If there is some distance between you and them, you can use a glisha (sliding step) to help you cover the ground quickly and add weight/momentum to your kick.

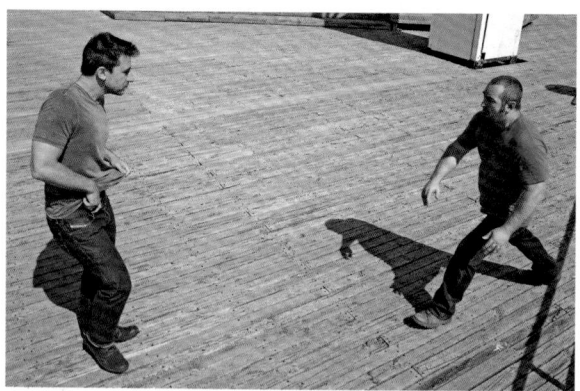

Favoring your dominant leg (in this case, the right), take a large step forward. This in itself will cover some of the distance between you and your aggressor.

This is also an unexpected response to your attacker's movement, and will start to put them under pressure to make a successful weapon draw. The more stress and duress you put your aggressor under, the more likely they are to fail in their attempt.

Instead of taking a step with your right leg, start to bring your right knee past your left leg. Ideally you want to bring your knee as high as you can. Raising the knee high gives you the option of kicking at any height, whereas keeping it low means you are restricted to only kicking low.

You should use this movement of raising the knee to lift weight off your left leg, so you can slide on it.

Start to throw your bodyweight forward, toward your attacker. Think of it not as a "hopping" movement, but one where your foot doesn't actually lose contact with the ground. You want all of your weight to be moving forward, rather than any being wasted on upward motion.

Your attacker will now be in the position where they will have to defend themselves from your obvious attack.

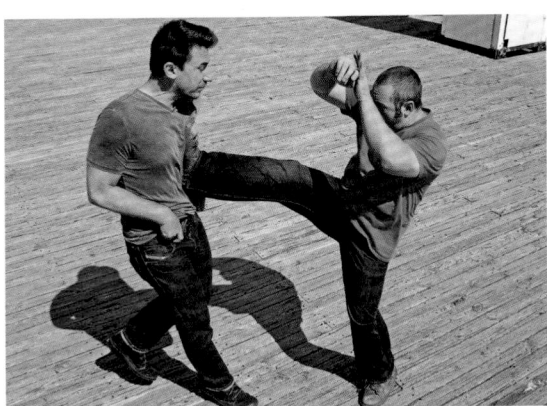

When you initially connect, you will want your weight to be moving forward so that the kick has your entire bodyweight behind it. Once you start to extend your kicking leg, however, you will need to be grounded in order to kick through the person; otherwise you may well push yourself backward.

You can add extra drive to your kick by turning the toes of your supporting leg outward, so that your heel and your hip are brought forward and into your strike.

Continue to extend the kicking leg, driving your attacker backward. You should have connected with their chest so that they are pushed backward.

Retract the kicking leg, rather than falling forward with it. You will want to keep distance between yourself and your assailant, which will allow you to disengage.

Most people have not practiced their weapon draws, and will be put under a lot of pressure when they see you coming toward them with a kick. Even if they are carrying a firearm and manage to draw it, they will still have to take aim. It is unlikely that they will have the time to do so successfully, especially if they hesitate in order to assess how they will deal with your preemptive kick.

Dealing with Weapon Draws Within Arm's Reach (Front Carry)

When a person first reaches to draw a weapon, you won't know whether it's a knife or gun; you just know they're pulling something. In a verbally aggressive altercation, someone reaching to their waist is unlikely to be going for a handkerchief or comb—it is fairly safe to assume that they are going for a weapon. It is important to have this clear in your head. If you hesitate, overthinking the situation, you will probably miss the opportunity to spoil the draw. Being decisive is largely what separates those who survive from those who don't, and trying to get too much information about your situation, such as what is it that a person is reaching for, will slow you down.

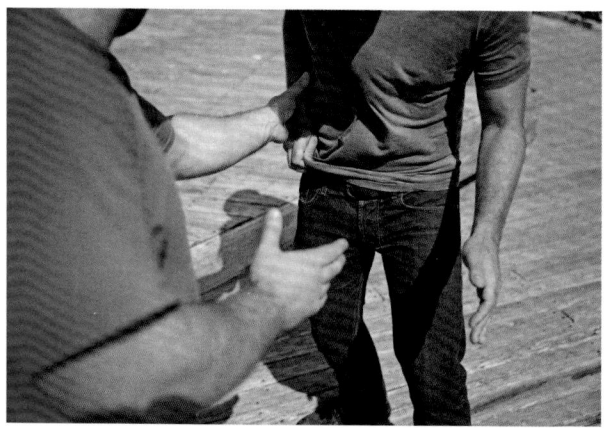

When someone goes to draw a weapon, they will need to in most cases, clear their clothing, in order to gain access to it.

When you go to spoil a person's draw, it may be that you react to the movement of the arm clearing the clothing, and end up controlling this, rather than the arm/hand that would be reaching for the weapon. This isn't an issue, as preventing the clothing from being cleared will also delay the weapon from being drawn.

It is far better to simply go for an arm, and be decisive, rather than to try and recognize in the high emotion of the situation, which arm is performing which function.

When controlling a person's arm/wrist around waist/hip level, it is often easier to use an underhand grip (with the thumb up, as seen in the above photo), for several reasons. The main one is that when a person's wrist is against their body, getting all of your fingers around their wrist/arm—which is what would happen with an overhand grip (thumb down)—can be difficult, as there simply isn't the room to do this.

In this situation, you may have observed the assailant readjusting their clothing and/or tapping themselves around the waistband—all signs that they have a concealed weapon.

Because of this, you should drop your hands to shadow those of your aggressor, so that you won't have to move them too far if your aggressor attempts to draw a weapon. If they were to move their hands up, away from their waist, yours would follow.

As you see both of their hands pull back—one to clear the clothing, the other to reach for the weapon—"blade" your body to get extra range/reach, and shoot your left hand out in an underhand grip to take hold of their wrist/arm.

At this point you will not have had time to register whether you are controlling the hand clearing the clothing, or the one drawing the weapon. This is not necessarily relevant at this point.

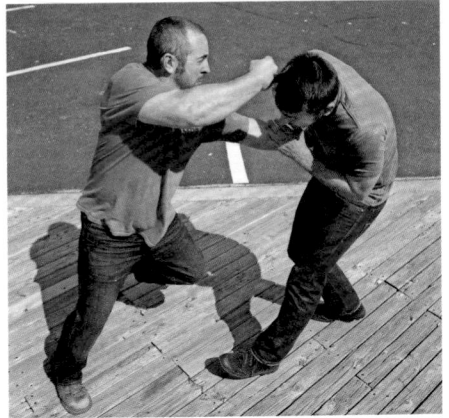

At the same time as you reach forward, you should pull your right hand back and prepare to strike them.

You should be leaning somewhat into them, so it is your weight, rather than your arm strength, that is preventing them from drawing the weapon. Don't lean so much that if they were to suddenly step back, you would lose your balance.

Start driving forward, and at the same time use this momentum to deliver power to your strikes. You want to stay bladed/side-on to your attacker, so that you can maintain downward pressure on their arm, preventing the weapon from being drawn.

This means you will be unable to turn your right hip into the strike, or turn the shoulder into it, so you will need to move your arm like a piston, back and forth, with a vertical fist.

Your striking arm should travel close to your body, both when it is pulled back and when it is driven forward. Power will come from your forward momentum, rather than from the hips, as would normally be the case when striking.

You will need to keep moving forward as you strike so that your attacker is unable to pull away from you and create the space necessary to draw their weapon.

Keep striking your assailant until you have a safe opportunity to disengage and/or they are no longer able to offer up any resistance.

Your goal is to exit the situation as soon as possible, before your assailant manages to find a way to neutralize what you are doing, or friends and third parties who may be with them come to their assistance.

Spoiling the Draw of Knives and Blades

Combative approaches, in which you strike and punch your aggressor, are generally effective. There are times, however, when striking an aggressor will not be effective, regardless of how well your strikes land. If you are punching a highly adrenalized assailant who is pain tolerant, your strikes may not result in the response you were expecting. This may also be the case when you are dealing with attackers who are drunk or on drugs; they simply won't feel the effect of your strikes. The definition of madness is doing the same thing over and over again, expecting a different result; if your strikes and punches aren't having much effect, it would be madness to continue with this approach.

In this scenario, we will look at a situation in which you are dealing with a pain-resistant assailant who is attempting to draw a knife or blade.

The majority of knives you are likely to face will have a folding blade rather than a fixed one. Folding knives are much more easily concealed than fixed blades, as the blade folds into the handle, making it a much smaller weapon to carry. The disadvantage is that, unlike a fixed blade, a folding knife needs to be opened and the blade locked into place, all of which makes it a slower weapon to deploy. Again, if someone has not practiced this under the stress of facing someone who is committed to stopping them, they may not have the time and space to perform these actions. This means you may end up working with a knife that has been pulled, but not opened. In this scenario, however, we will assume that the knife is already operational.

In striking an assailant to prevent them from drawing a weapon, you may start to recognize that your strikes are having little to no effect, and understand that continuing with this approach isn't going to be successful.

Instead of making the next strike, you should shoot your striking hand down toward your attacker's hand/wrist, using an underhand grip to gain control of it.

You now have two hands controlling their weapon arm. At the same time, you should close distance with your assailant, moving somewhat to the side. This will make it very difficult for them to use their other hand against you.

It may be that the weapon has not yet been fully drawn. If this is the case, you may not be aware whether you are dealing with a gun or a knife. This is one reason you want to be at your assailant's side, rather than in front of them and potentially in the line of fire.

You are now going to "assist" your attacker with their draw, pulling the hand that is holding the weapon upward.

Once the weapon is out, you will have the opportunity to assess whether it is a knife or a gun. In this scenario, it is a knife. You could choose to disarm; at this range, however, it is quicker and more effective to slash your assailant across their side while they still are still holding the knife, rather than trying to fight them for it. Trying to disarm a highly adrenalized and committed attacker is not as easy as it may seem; they will try to hold onto their weapon for all they are worth.

After cutting them, pull the knife arm down toward your hips. This motion should take your assailant's balance and cause them to stop thinking about using/controlling the knife, as their attention will now be on regaining their balance.

Once done, release your left hand and bring it around your attacker's weapon arm.

Pull their arm to you, clasping it against your body. You should now have full control of their weapon arm, and be behind the knife, with it pointing toward your assailant.

The knife should be pulled to your hips, with your feet square, and your hips back. You should be at your attacker's side, facing them. Your feet should be at a 90-degree angle to theirs.

Start to drive your hips forward while at the same time pulling your chest back. It should feel as though you are leaning back.

This motion will drive the knife toward your attacker and pull them toward the knife.

Keep driving with your hips and pulling your assailant onto the knife.

You can then pull your hips back, keeping their arm pinned to you, and repeat this stabbing motion until they are no longer a threat to you.

Spoiling the Draw of Firearms

It may be that when you go to control your assailant's weapon hand (after trying to deal with them combatively), you realize that you are dealing with a firearm, not a knife.

As you get your second hand around your assailant's hand/wrist, you may realize that you are dealing with a firearm rather than a knife.

You should deal with it in much the same fashion as you would the knife. In fast-moving and dynamic situations, it is important to reuse similar techniques and movements so that you can act without having to have all the information available to you from the start. Recognizing the exact nature of the threat can happen later on.

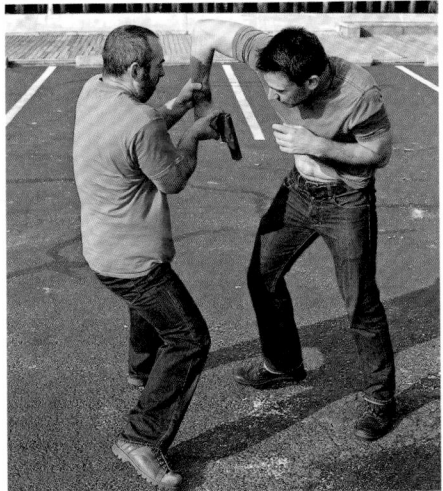

Once again, you would help your assailant complete their draw. The higher you can lift the elbow, the better, as this makes it harder for your attacker to train the gun back on you.

Stepping to the side will also mean that you are behind the weapon, rather than in front of it. In this position you are away from their free hand, making it difficult for them to punch or grab you with it.

You should now slip your right hand down toward the gun so that you are able to better control it, and in a good position to perform a disarm as well.

Grabbing the gun in an underhand fashion, means that your hand won't be muzzled—it will be as far from the end of the barrel as possible.

If it were a snub-nosed revolver or similar short-barreled weapon, using an overhand grip on the gun could mean that your hand would cover and be in front of the barrel. If that were the case, your hand could be shot if your assailant pulled the trigger.

Taking a solid grip on the wrist, the hand that is on the gun should now "punch" through, under your attacker's arm, so that you can cause them to release the gun from their grip.

If you compare the position of the rear leg/foot here with that in the next photo, you can see that the right hip drives forward, adding power to the extension of the arm.

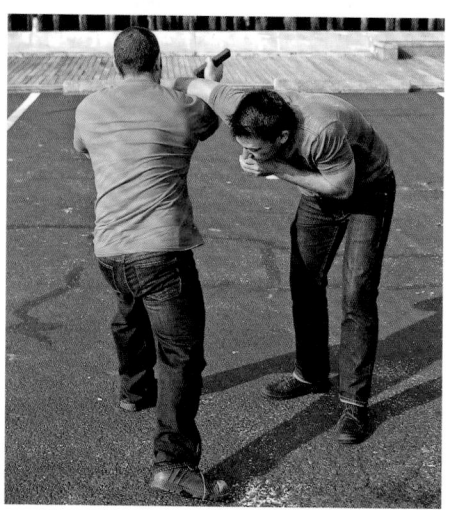

In the final position, your right arm should be fully extended, with the gun released from your assailant's grasp.

The body position is almost the same as if you had thrown a rear cross, and this should be the feeling that you go for—that you have thrown a rear punch, while holding the gun.

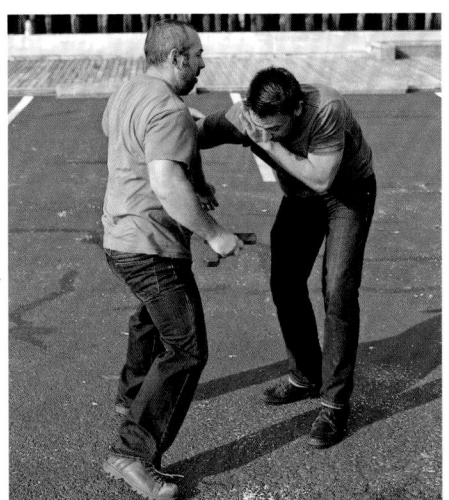

Once the gun is released, retract it/pull it back.

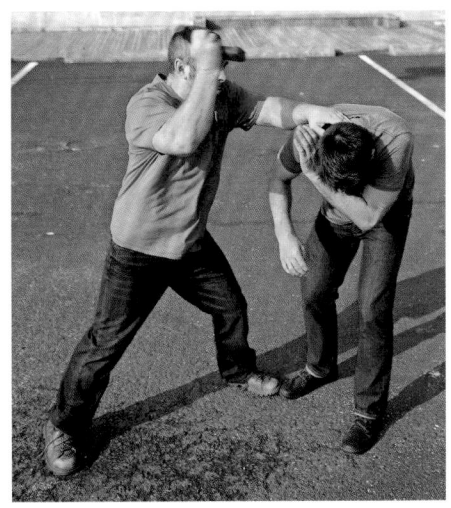

Now you should deliver a series of concussive strikes with the gun in order to disable your assailant.

In situations where you disarm at close quarters, it is essential not to assume that the gun you have in your hand is operational and can be used as a firearm. The person may have been carrying it with one in the chamber and with the safety on; or perhaps with the safety off, intending to rack the slide to bring a bullet into the chamber, etc. When you disarm, you may not be aware of what state the gun is in, and will probably not have the time to assess whether it is operable. It may be that the gun isn't even loaded or has been so poorly maintained that it isn't operable. At the end of the day, you have no real knowledge or experience of the weapon, and it would be unwise to rely on its capabilities as a firearm. This is why it is safer to use it as an impact weapon.

Even if it is operable, loaded, and fully functional, it may still not be the best idea to rely on the gun as a ballistic weapon. Depending on the caliber of the gun, its bullets may not have any real stopping power against an adrenalized attacker (unless you are extremely accurate in your placement of shots). Furthermore, at close range, you may not have the time to unload enough rounds to stop someone who is committed to causing you harm—it could be that they come at you with a knife after you have disarmed them of the gun. If you use the gun as an impact weapon, you will have a good chance of knocking your assailant unconscious with your first or second strike; at close range this may be a quicker way of disabling an attacker than attempting to shoot them.

Disengagement as Part of Spoiling the Draw

Things don't always go as planned in fast-paced, dynamic situations, and it is always good to have a bailout plan—something you can do when what you've tried hasn't worked out. Unfortunately, many self-defense techniques are promoted with the idea that there is only a successful outcome. Anyone who has any real-world experience will tell you that things often go wrong, and it is important to be able to adapt and implement another solution rather than persist with the one that isn't working.

The solution below is a good "last-ditch" attempt for when things start going wrong and you're unable to successfully spoil the draw. The technique works better against a knife than a gun, because you aren't performing a disarm, but rather disrupting your assailant and disengaging, leaving them with their weapon.

If your attacker has a firearm, you should really only attempt this if you have time and space to disengage safely and possibly put objects and barriers between yourself and your assailant (either as cover or concealment) to obstruct their firing line as you exit the situation quickly. Even when you aren't able to do this, however, if performed with speed and commitment, you should be able to put 10 to 15 yards between yourself and your attacker before they are able to respond. This is usually enough distance that they will not be able to get an accurate shot off (unless they have trained for such scenarios). Someone might be a great marksman against targets on the range, but that environment is one in which they aren't being disrupted, or asked to perform under stress and duress against a rapidly moving target. Handguns are really only accurate in the most trained of hands, and with every yard of distance they become less so. In most situations, you will be dealing with criminals carrying illegally owned firearms that they will not have had the opportunity to properly practice with.

This technique comes with no guarantees; however, it is always good to have something to do when everything else hits the fan.

In this situation, we'll assume the assailant has managed to draw their weapon and is in a good position to pull it back and/or step back, pulling it away from you. If they do this, it may not be possible to land a successful and effective strike. Instead, you should look to get both hands on the weapon arm in order to control it.

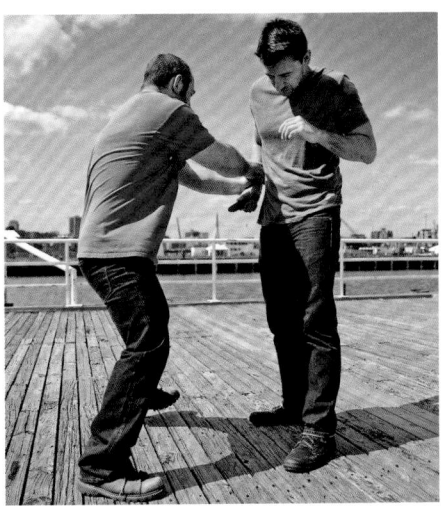

Instead of punching, quickly go to grab your attacker's wrist with your right hand so that you have two arms controlling their one.

Many people will get caught up in what the assailant might do with their free hand. In reality, most times this will be nothing, as they will be so focused on their weapon and retaining it that they will lack the awareness to use their free hand.

As you grab the wrist, step forward and slightly to the side. It is never a good idea to be directly in front of a weapon, whether it is a knife or gun, as this allows your attacker easy access to you as a target. If you are to the side, they will have to either turn themselves and/or the weapon in order to attack you.

Strongly pull down at a 45-degree angle, moving your attacker down and disrupting their balance. The success of this technique rests on your ability to unbalance your assailant to such a degree that they are unable to recover in time to use the weapon against you.

Keep pulling on the arm so that the weapon moves behind you.

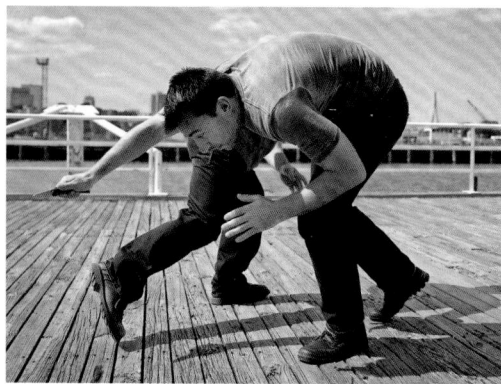

As soon as you start to feel that your attacker is also moving behind you and toward the ground, release your grip and start moving away from them as fast as you can.

When you run, don't look behind you; this will slow you down. The more distance you can put between yourself and your attacker, the greater your chances of survival. If you can put barriers and obstacles between yourself and them, you should do so. That said, distance is your best form of "cover."

If you pull your attacker hard enough and they find themselves falling, they may even release their weapon so that they can use their hands to break their fall.

It may also be that their weapon hits the ground as they fall, therefore becoming dislodged or forcing them to readjust their grip in order to keep hold of it. This can slow your attacker down and hinder their ability to make a second attack, especially if their weapon is a firearm.

This tactic can be used any time you get two hands onto your aggressor's weapon arm/hand and believe that you have a "safe" disengagement opportunity. Although disarming the aggressor may be part of an overall survival strategy, it should not become a goal in and of itself. The situation that you are in will determine the solution: if you can disengage safely without disarming, you should do so.

Gun and Knife Threats

When someone puts a knife to your throat, or points a gun at your head (or any other body part), it is not always clear whether they intend to use the weapon. There has to be a reason why they would show you the weapon rather than simply using it against you. They may want to intimidate you into complying with their demands—handing over a wallet, forcing you into their car, etc. With some demands, such as handing over your possessions, it is easier and safer to comply, while others, such as being told to move to another location, are usually best dealt with using a physical solution. There are five basic approaches you can take when dealing with weapons. They apply to firearms as well as knives. In no particular order, these approaches are:

1. Disengaging from your attacker
2. Controlling your attacker and their ability to use the weapon (rather than controlling the weapon itself)
3. Combatively assaulting your attacker
4. Disarming your attacker
5. Using the weapon against your attacker while they still hold it

Where weapons are concerned, people often get caught up in the belief that the only way to handle a weapon threat is to disarm their attacker. This is a very narrow and potentially dangerous way of looking at scenarios involving armed assailants. There are often simpler, faster, and more direct ways of dealing with such situations. You should let the situation determine the solution, rather than working to an inflexible plan such as performing a disarm, regardless of the situational components. It is always worth remembering that in threat situations, the attacker shows you the weapon for a reason, i.e., to force compliance with a demand. This means it is worth taking a moment to educate yourself about the situation rather than charging ahead with a predetermined plan that may actually prove disastrous. For example, you may have failed to identify the assailant's armed accomplice as you forged ahead with the disarm.

Always remember that reality is very different from a training environment. Techniques are not in and of themselves a solution to a situation or incident; they may be part of it, but surviving violence requires a lot more than simply the ability to perform a technique. It requires some degree of threat and risk assessment, along with decision-making skills, etc.

Many training scenarios are set up to end when a disarm is performed; for example, a student will perform the disarm, make the motion of tapping and racking the weapon as they back away, and tell their training partner, "Back off," "Get down," or something like that. This is not a realistic way to train. It is based on one or more of the following assumptions, none of which you should ever take for granted:

1. That the firearm is real, rather than an imitation or replica weapon
2. That it is loaded and operable (many firearms owned by criminals are not in the best condition)
3. That the person performing the disarm is conversant with the use of that particular model/weapon
4. That the round will be a "stopping" round (for example, a 9 mm round is unlikely to stop an adrenalized and committed attacker unless it is placed very well—something which is hard to do under stress and duress—and the person disarming the weapon is prepared to use such lethal force)
5. That the assailant will back away, rather than keep coming once they have been disarmed of their weapon.

The only person who really knows anything about the weapon is its owner: they know whether it is loaded, and have an idea of its condition, and whether it's a replica. You don't want to be pointing an imitation or unloaded/inoperable pistol at someone as they run at you with a knife. You should always assume the person you are dealing with has another weapon, even if you've disarmed them of the one they were primarily using.

Likewise, don't assume the situation has ended even if you have disarmed someone of a working firearm; they may still come at you, if they believe that their best survival option is to keep engaging with you. At close range an assailant whom you have shot may still be able to get to you (unless you have managed to hit a joint or an area of the body which controls nerve signals, such as the spine). In a training scenario, you may feel a sense of empowerment after disarming, but in reality, you will still be in a potentially deadly situation.

It is also worth understanding that weapon disarming in real life isn't as easy as it looks in a training environment. However hard you tell a training partner to hold on to a weapon, in a real-life situation an assailant will hold onto it ten times harder—they know/believe, that if you should disarm them, you are likely to use the weapon against them. For them, retaining it is a matter of life and death, and they will do everything possible to hold on to it. This means it is sometimes more efficient and effective to put your focus elsewhere, such as on disengaging, controlling them, or using the weapon against them while they hold it.

This is not to say that weapon disarming doesn't have its place, because it certainly does; however, it would be simplistic to say it is the first and only solution to dealing with weapon threats. You should also look at the other available options.

Disengagement as a Strategy Against Weapon Threats

Effective Decision-Making

When you are operating under high stress and duress, such as when you have a weapon pointed at you, you will need to be able to think and make decisions quickly. To do this, you need to use simple heuristics, or "rules of thumb." Working this way prevents you suffering from information overload; that is, taking in so much information about what's going on that you have too many things to consider and think about. Having a rule of thumb or heuristic will prevent this from happening.

Also remember that you are looking for effective solutions, rather than best solutions. If you find a solution that works, that's the one you should adopt, rather than wasting time looking for a better one.

The first solution I consider in any situation is whether I can disengage: Can I do something that allows me to quickly exit the situation?

Knife to Opposite Side of Throat

Imagine a situation in which you walk into an empty bar and sit down at an empty table. After a while, another person enters the bar and comes up to you, informing you that you are sitting in their seat. Your first assumption may be that you are dealing with someone who is just looking for a fight. This could be the case; however, this individual may also be operating in what we refer to as an *alternate reality*. Normal social convention would suggest that seats are allocated on a first-come, first-served basis; if a table is empty, it's your right to take it. However, another person's reality could be that for the past fifteen years, they and their friends/family have always sat at that table, which makes it their territory, and not a place where anyone else is allowed to sit. That is their reality, and it is unlikely that any argument you make will convince them that they are wrong. When people become territorial, they are not acting or thinking rationally; they are working from animal instinct.

You have a choice: you can find another table, or you can stay where you are. Understand that if you stay, you are not adopting a survival strategy; you are working from ego. Furthermore, studies have shown that people will work twice as hard to get back what they've lost (or perceive they've lost) than they will to try to gain/achieve something new. This means that the individual who believes you've taken their territory (i.e., the table) will be twice as committed as you are to continue holding on to it. Also, in their reality they are justified to use violence against you, because you are the one who is in the wrong and you aren't presenting them with any alternative courses of action.

Having worked in bar security for a number of years, these were the type of disputes that I used to see on a regular basis: one person acting according to their understanding of a situation, another to theirs, both feeling justified that they were right, and neither's ego letting them give up their claim to whatever the dispute was over. One person walking away would have solved everything, apart from the damage to their fragile ego. Recognizing when to fight (and not to fight)—i.e., for survival—is a critical threat-analysis and decision-making ability.

Imagine that you enter a bar you haven't been to before, and take a seat at an empty table. About twenty minutes later, someone taps you on the shoulder and informs you that you are sitting at their table.

If their posture and language are aggressive, you should recognize that the situation could turn violent.

Rather than having to deal with an aggressive and potentially violent individual while seated, you should immediately stand up.

From here you should assume your de-escalation stance and start the de-escalation process. If you fail to do this, you may find yourself adopting a more confrontational and argumentative stance. As you assert your claim that it is your right to sit at that table, your aggressor may feel threatened by your actions/behavior and reach into their back pocket.

When you miss your chance to spoil the draw, your aggressor places a knife to your neck.

You should immediately start to bring your hands up in a submissive manner, telling them that you don't want any trouble. This also gets your hands closer to the weapon, in case you need to enact a physical solution.

As you do this, you will need to assess your situation; you may be in an unfamiliar bar where your aggressor has friends they can rely on to assist them.

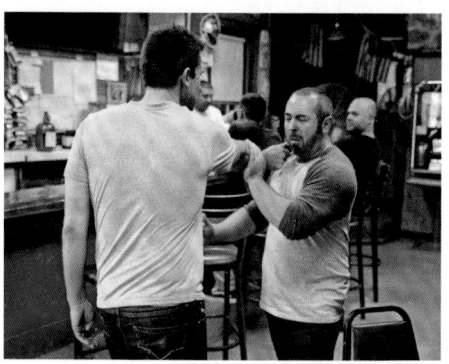

In such situations, it is unlikely that your aggressor will simply put their knife away without using it; the potential social embarrassment of having over-reacted is something that compels many people to continue acting aggressively and violently when it is obvious that the person they are dealing with is no longer a threat.

Because you are in an unfamiliar environment, disengaging may be the most effective solution. It keeps you from getting tied up with your assailant in a place where third parties might come to their assistance.

Turning/blading your body, you forcefully slap the weapon arm away.

Drop your other arm down and make a groin strike. This is a forceful slap upward toward the groin. Understand that this strike may not be effective if, for example, your assailant is wearing their jeans with the crotch hanging low, which will prevent your hand from reaching the groin.

Keep the hand that slapped the knife arm away up by your neck, in case your assailant makes a reverse slash. Also, stay tight to them so you are inside the arc of the slash if they do so.

As you take a big step past them, raise your rear leg. You should still have your hand guarding your neck, and be inside the arc the knife would make if it were to be slashed out at you.

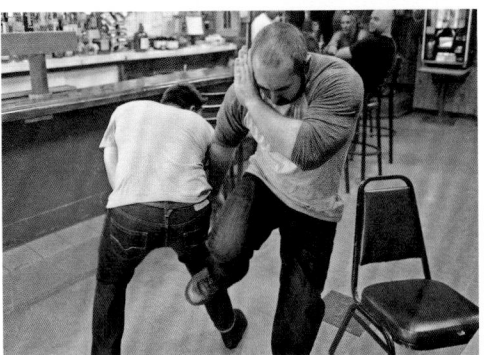

Perform a stomp kick to the back of your attacker's leg, driving it down so that their knee is driven into the floor. You are not looking to cause a devastating injury here; you simply want to prevent them from being able to immediately follow you to make a further attack.

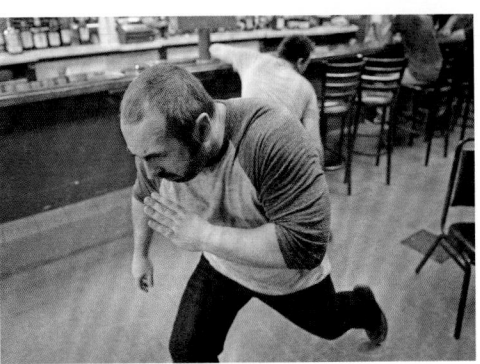

The stomp kick should be part of your running motion—it should occur as part of your natural movement to disengage.

Keep moving/running toward the entrance/exit of the bar. Your situational awareness should include not only understanding who in your environment is a potential threat/danger, but where entry, exit, and concealment points are, etc.

Short-Barreled Weapons—Pointed at Front of Head

The same technique will also work against a firearm that is pointed at your head. This is obviously a much riskier technique to perform against a gun than a knife, because making distance from someone armed with a gun doesn't mean that you are safe; they can still potentially shoot you. However, there are situations when disengaging, rather than controlling the weapon, may be an effective option.

When you grab the barrel of a semi-automatic, you should by default prevent the slide from moving (depending on the weapon, this requires about ten pounds of pressure), so that after it has been fired, the spent casing cannot be ejected, and the weapon effectively jams. More importantly, the hot gases that the bullet expels, which normally cause the slide to move, are contained within the gun, meaning that you can safely hold on to the weapon.

If you are dealing with a revolver, and the trigger is pulled while you are holding it, all of the hot gases (which in a semi-automatic are used to work the slide) will exit through the frame and burn your hand. It is possible to hold on, but it will be extremely painful, and you may end up releasing your grip on the gun because of the pain. It may be safer to not take the risk of this happening, and instead of grabbing the barrel of the revolver, pat it away and attempt to disengage. This should only be attempted if you believe the environment will allow you to do so safely.

You may also want to try a disengagement option if you are dealing with more than one assailant. Controlling and disarming a weapon takes time, and if your attacker has a friend with them, don't expect them to stand idly by while you take the time to perform a control and/or disarm.

It is always worth considering whether you are overestimating your own abilities and level of training. It takes a lot less skill to aggressively knock the gun away and disengage than it does to control and/or disarm the person wielding it—especially if they are much bigger and stronger than you. Be realistic in what you are able to perform and do, putting your ego aside.

This should certainly not be your default solution for dealing with firearms; however, in certain situations—such as those in which you can quickly get cover and/or concealment and can easily put distance between yourself and your assailant—it is perhaps the safest and most effective option.

Parking lots are an attractive proposition for many criminals, as cars can offer good concealment points, and a large number of potential victims are coming and going.

It may be that as you step out of your car, you are accosted by an assailant with a gun. Immediately raise your hands up—this is what your assailant will expect you to do when they point a gun at you.

At this point you could be suffering negatively from ASR (Adrenal Stress Response), which could affect your ability to get a good grip on the gun. Under high stress and duress, blood flows away from your body's peripheries, including the hands, and moves to the larger muscles.

To perform your body defense, you should sway/turn to the side while slapping the gun forcefully out of the way. At the same time, move your other hand down toward your assailant's groin.

Stepping forward with a large step so that you can reach, make a groin strike.

Part of the effect of the groin strike, whether it lands with any force or not, is that your aggressor will pull the hips back and bend forward. This will mean you end up moving further behind the gun (as the gun travels past you).

With your step, your foot should go past your attacker's foot, setting up your stomp to the back of their knee.

Stomp down with full force on the back of your assailant's knee, driving it into the concrete.

As well as striking your assailant, you should be looking to use the kick to propel you forward so that it both disrupts your attacker and aids your movement.

Immediately seek either cover or concealment. Concealment is that which will obscure your attacker's sightlines, but doesn't actually offer you any physical protection (you could hide behind the car door, for example but it wouldn't stop a bullet). Cover will offer you actual protection (the engine block of the car can stop a bullet).

It is all too easy to overestimate the accuracy of handguns and the proficiency of those who use them. Most trained firearms owners are not accurate with short-barreled weapons beyond 7 to 10 yards, especially against moving targets; and most have not trained to recover quickly after having their firearm knocked away and/or being driven to the ground. Even if an assailant is able to get a shot off after you have slapped the gun away, it is unlikely that it will be a good one, which means that even if they do hit you, it is more likely to be your peripheries—e.g., shoulders, arms, etc.—rather than your center of mass, where your vital organs are. When you consider that you are most likely to encounter an individual who is carrying an illegally owned firearm and who has had little or no training, disengaging in this manner can be an extremely effective solution.

Use of Your Environment

It is, where possible/feasible, always worth backing your car into parking spaces rather than simply driving in, front first.

By backing in next to another vehicle, when you open your door you create a protective space, which makes it difficult for a potential attacker to gain access to you—your door protects your front, the wall your back, and your car and the one next to you, your sides.

If you drive in front first, rather than reversing, you lose this protective space, and when you go to get in your car, your back will be vulnerable to attack.

It will also take you longer to leave the parking lot than if you had reversed in, because you will now need to back out. Though we will not go into the specifics of tactical driving, know that it is much more difficult to ram a car that is blocking you when driving in reverse.

Control of the Assailant as a Strategy Against Weapon Threats

There are times when it is not possible to disengage. It is sometimes easier and more effective to control the assailant, rather than their weapon. This doesn't mean that you should completely disregard the weapon; rather that you should put yourself in a position where you are safe from its use, and from which you can focus on disabling your attacker. You should consider taking this approach over, say, a combative one (that involves the use of striking to disable an assailant) when you believe you are dealing with an adrenalized and/or pain-resistant attacker—e.g., someone who may be drunk or high on drugs—who will not be affected by your punches and strikes.

Before we look at a technique that could be used to accomplish this, it is worth understanding how different environments, such as parking lots, affect violent crime. If we can understand why and how different predatory individuals use particular locations, we can start to develop strategies and tactics—e.g., the way we park a car—to make it difficult for them to target us as victims.

Every location where violent crimes take place has three components:
1. Crime Attractors
2. Crime Promoters
3. Crime Preventers

A location that attracts crime is one where there is a plentiful supply of victims. This is why dark, deserted alleys are not places where muggers will choose to commit their crimes. By and large, these individuals will pick locations that have the largest number of potential victims. A mugger is going to choose a place that is relatively highly trafficked; parking lots meet this particular requirement. There are also characteristics of a location that will help promote crime. One of these is a high number of potential escape routes (something alleyways don't have). A parking lot is basically a grid of cars; this structure offers numerous escape routes for a criminal.

In a parking lot it is relatively easy for a criminal to position themselves between two cars and remain unseen, especially if they can find an SUV or van to stand behind. The layout of the cars in a grid format allows a criminal to easily disengage between different cars in order to escape unseen after they have committed their crime. In such an open layout, it would be very difficult to restrict and confine a criminal's movement.

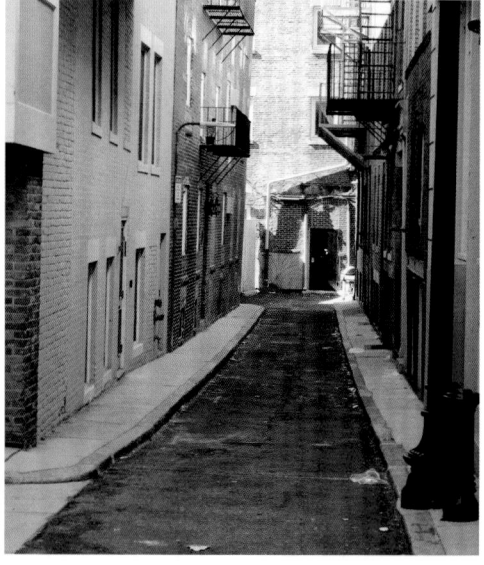

An alleyway offers neither a large number of potential victims nor a multitude of escape routes. In fact, a criminal who would commit a crime in such a location would have to exit the alleyway in order to escape, as there is only one way in and out. It would be extremely easy to "trap" a criminal working in such a location, as you would only need to block one entranceway. Only the most novice criminal would choose a rarely trafficked location with a single escape route.

Crime preventers are those things that deter criminals, such as the presence of law-enforcement personnel, security cameras, lighting, etc. One of the biggest crime preventers is natural surveillance—people being able to easily observe a crime taking place. Natural surveillance is more important than good lighting; it matters little that a place is well lit if it is obscured from view. It is also worth noting that crowded places don't necessarily offer good natural surveillance. If people are closely packed in a crowd, it is difficult for them to see what is going on next to them, even if it is only a few feet away. If you are looking to park your car in a place that enjoys natural surveillance, one of the best places to park is near parking lot entrances or exits. These spots have continuous traffic of people entering and exiting, and there are therefore a large number of eyes on both you and your vehicle.

Gun to Front of Head

Sometimes it will not be possible to park in a preferred location, and you will end up having to park deeper in the parking lot, where such natural surveillance doesn't exist. When parking, it is worth taking a moment—with the central locking on, using your mirrors, etc.—to observe your environment. Check who is either acting out of place within the environment (nobody should just be standing around in a parking lot; they should be going to or from a car), or, more importantly, observing or expressing an interest in you.

The aim of the following technique is to control and choke out your assailant rather than disarming them, etc. This is an especially good technique to use against someone armed with a revolver, where grabbing the gun could get your hand badly burned (if your attacker pulls the trigger), causing you to possibly release your grip on the gun and lose control of the situation.

Most people are aware that they shouldn't leave bags and valuables on display in their car. Unfortunately, many people will move their bags/valuables to the trunk of the car after they've parked in the parking lot. This activity could be observed by any criminals/predatory individuals who may be in the environment.

A criminal may not be aware of what is in the bag that you are putting in the trunk, but it is safe for them to assume that it is something of worth. This means that they can wait for you to return to your car and force you to open the trunk for them.

If they are by your car and you use your remote key fob to unlock the car from a distance, they can also open the door (turn off the central locking, etc.) and pop the trunk themselves, gaining access to your valuables.

It is always good to question a person's reasons for being in a particular location, especially when their movement (or lack of movement) doesn't fit into the normal behavior of someone in that environment. For example why is a person just standing in the parking lot, rather than going to or from a car? Why have they chosen to stand by an entrance/exit—is it so that they can monitor who enters and leaves the lot?

If someone is still in the same spot when you return to your car after a period of time, or they are still in the parking lot, you should be suspicious. Parking lots are not places where people tend to spend a prolonged period of time unless they are engaged in criminal activities.

As you return to your car, the predator may follow you, timing their movement so that they arrive at your vehicle at roughly the same time as you.

As you pop the trunk to retrieve your bag, your assailant could pull a gun and hold it to your head, demanding that you hand the bag over to them.

Your safest option in this scenario is to hand the bag over to them. In the majority of muggings or robberies, once the criminal has what they want, they will leave. Most muggers have no desire to increase criminal charges against them by using violence.

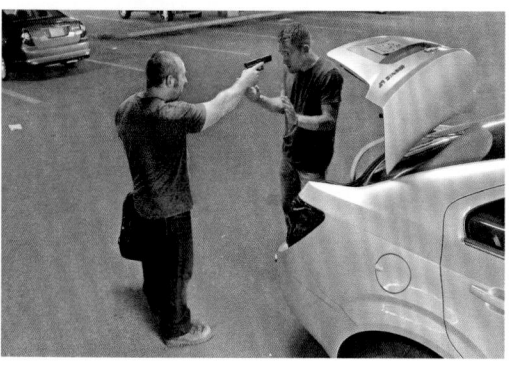

If, after you hand over the bag, the mugger does not leave, then they have gone "off script." A mugger's script would dictate that after acquiring what they want, they should leave. If they stay, they are working from a different script, which probably means they want to do something to you (shoot you, abduct you, sexually assault you, etc.). This is now not about your possessions, but about you and your survival.

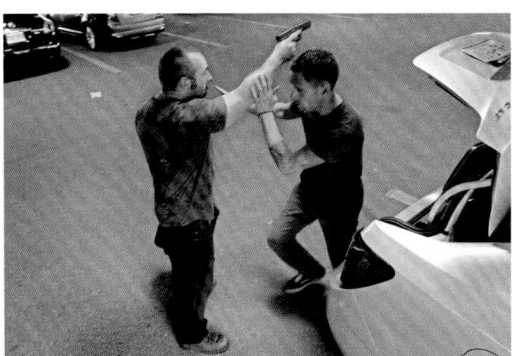

Once you realize that this is no longer a mugging and your assailant intends to cause you harm, you must act decisively.

Strongly "slap" your assailant's weapon hand away (hand defense), and move slightly to the side (body defense). At the same time, move rapidly forward in order to get behind the weapon.

The idea with this technique is to burst into your assailant and take away all movement of the weapon.

Your right arm should come up under your attacker's weapon arm and to the opposite side of their neck. Your shoulder should slam into their throat to help disrupt their balance.

Your head should be lowered against their shoulder.

Once you are close to them, start to wrap your right arm around their neck, pushing your right biceps and forearm against their carotid artery. At the same time, push your chin against their shoulder, so their own arm/shoulder blocks the other carotid artery.

For a blood choke to be effective, both arteries must be put under pressure.

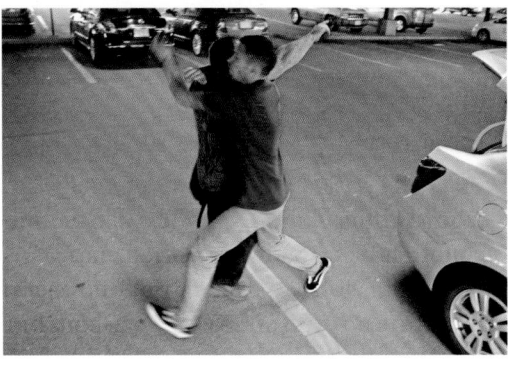

Join your right hand to your left forearm and upper arm. You should be pressing with your head into their shoulder and already be applying pressure with your right biceps even before you make contact with your upper arm (i.e., before you start applying the choke).

Grab your own head with your left hand and pull both of your arms in to take away all the space from around your attacker's neck. Your assailant should have started to experience the choke as soon as your arm made contact and your head pressed into their shoulder. Due to this, along with the way that they would need to first release the bag to do so, they will not be thinking about transferring the weapon to their other hand. Even if they immediately dropped the bag and thought about trying to do this, they would be unconscious before they were able to.

Lean back and lift your assailant off the floor, spinning them round to disorient them, as you complete the choke.

By turning as you choke your attacker, you will also be able to see what is going on in the environment, including any third parties who are coming toward you to assist your attacker. This will also allow you to plan your best escape route.

You don't have to apply the choke to completion. If you feel your assailant's body go limp, you can release them, pushing them away, and disengage from the situation. It will take them several moments to become fully conscious again, by which time you will have been able to exit the situation.

Don't try and get in your car. This will take too long. Rather, after disengaging to safety, inform law enforcement and ask that they return to your car with you.

If you are concerned about the length of time that it will take to choke your attacker and you want to cause them further distraction, rather than using your left hand to grab your own head you can use it to gouge and rip at your assailant's eyes.

Blood chokes, if applied correctly, are a very quick and effective way of shutting an assailant down. When applied at speed against an unsuspecting assailant, both the shock of the movement and the feeling of losing consciousness will override all thoughts about the weapon, as the assailant tries to stay on their feet and remain conscious.

The reason that blood chokes take effect so quickly is because they cause oxygenated blood in the brain to be flushed; without oxygen, the brain will shut down. When pressure is applied to the carotid arteries, blood ceases to flow to the carotid processes, which monitor blood pressure in the head/brain. Because they are not receiving new blood, they react as if there is too much blood in the brain and that pressure needs to be relieved. To achieve this, they flush the existing blood in the brain and lower the heart rate so that less blood is being pumped. This happens extremely quickly; a person may take 3 to 5 seconds to become fully unconscious, but the process begins immediately, and starts to override all other mental and physical functions. This means an attacker has no time to pass the weapon to their other hand and think about aiming at you with the non-dominant hand (while making sure they don't put themselves in the line of fire).

Knife to Opposite Side of Neck

The same choke can be used against a knife threat where an assailant holds a knife against the side of your throat.

You will make exactly the same movements as you did against the gun, patting/slapping the knife away with your left hand and shooting your right hand up under the attacker's weapon arm and around the opposite side of their neck.

When you apply the choke, you should keep moving, spinning/turning your assailant around. If you can keep taking an attacker's balance, this will override any and every other thought process for them. Keeping them in a perpetually unbalanced state will allow you more time to apply the choke, if you find that you have not been able to sink it in perfectly in the first attempt.

Another way to control the assailant rather than the weapon is to perform a throw or takedown. These often cause the attacker to drop their weapon(s) as they put their hands out to break their fall. Some examples of these techniques are demonstrated in part V, "Throws and Pick-ups."

Combative Approaches as a Strategy Against Weapon Threats

If disengagement isn't an option, and you believe that striking and punching will be effective against an assailant—i.e., you are confident in your striking ability and can punch with real power—and that your assailant won't be able to withstand your strikes, you should work combatively against them. Combative solutions—controlling the weapon arm, and striking—are some of the most simple, direct, and effective solutions; however, they rely on your ability to overwhelm your assailant and deliver concussive strikes. Unfortunately, as good as this looks on paper, in reality, many assailants—especially those with prior experiences of violence—will be able to turn on their pain management systems and weather your storm of blows. This means that when you apply a combative solution, you should always be prepared to switch to another approach if you realize that your punches and strikes are having little or no effect. If you assume that your striking will always be effective, you are turning a simple solution into a simplistic one.

Combatives Against Knife to Side of Throat

Combative solutions do not have to end up in a disarm or control. They can simply be used as a means of incapacitating an assailant so you can exit a situation safely by overwhelming the attacker with strikes and disengaging before they have time to recover. This type of approach works very well when you are dealing with possible multiple assailants and you don't have the luxury of time to perform disarms and controls.

Many people get caught up in the performance of techniques, rather than the goal of survival, when they learn Krav Maga. It is not what you do to your assailant(s) that is important, but rather what happens to you. It may be satisfying to perform disarms in training, but in reality leaving the situation quickly and safely is often a better survival option, and can get you out of harm's way much sooner.

As soon as you realize your assailant is putting a knife to your throat, start to slowly raise your hands until they are level with your attacker's weapon arm and in line with their wrist. Make this movement natural by bringing your hands up in a submissive manner.

As you do this, drop your chin down so that it is resting close to your assailant's hands. This means that if they suddenly try to cut your throat, you will have a kind of barrier to restrict that movement.

Once your hands are in place and you realize that your assailant is planning to move/abduct you, or use the knife against you, make your defense.

Pivot on your toes, to push your left arm toward the knife, while at the same time pulling your neck away from the knife. As you pivot, pull your right hand back, ready to strike.

Continue pushing the knife toward your assailant's waist/hip, straightening your arm—if it is bent, the knife will be too close to you, or you will be too close to the knife.

Your body should be fully bladed now, with your striking/punching arm pulled all the way back and your fist (not fully clenched) against your chest.

Start to drive forward into your assailant, pressing the knife against them to take away all its movement. Make sure you are continually pushing forward into them so that they can't step back and create space in which to maneuver the knife.

As you move forward, start your punching action. Most of your power, in this case, will come from your bodyweight driving forward, rather than from the hips (though these will turn slightly).

Keep driving into them and striking, pumping your punching arm like a piston. With your body lined up like this (bladed, or side on), your punches will lack some of the power that they normally have. Your goal is to overwhelm your attacker with a multitude of strikes, rather than relying on a few solid ones.

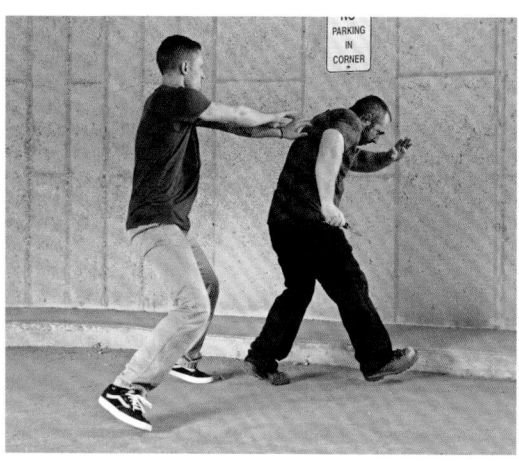

Once you have taken the fight out of your assailant, and they start to try and pull away from you to avoid being hit further, push them away and disengage.

Be aware that if you continue to punch them when they don't have an option to back away—pressing them up against the wall, for example—they may realize that their only survival option is to rally themselves and fight back. It is often a good strategy to leave an assailant with an escape route of their own, to avoid this.

Combatives Against Gun to Front of Head (with Assailant Retaining)

When disarming firearms, your goal should be to get the weapon out of your attacker's hand(s) as quickly as possible. This will generally involve getting two hands on the weapon and ripping it from your assailant's grasp (as demonstrated in *Krav Maga: Real World Solutions to Real World Violence*, pp. 97–102).

Sometimes, though, when you go to grab the gun, you can trigger an assailant's grab reflex, causing them to automatically pull back in response to your pulling action. This may happen if you hesitate or are too slow in executing the disarm, giving your attacker time to respond to what you are doing. If this happens, you will have to respond to what your assailant is doing and work with their pulling movement, rather than continue with your disarm.

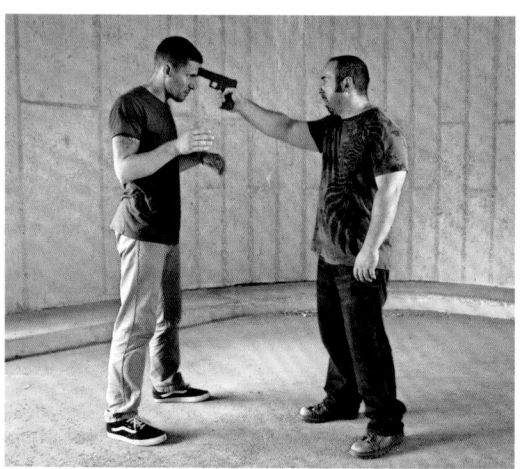

When someone points a gun at you, if you don't have the opportunity/distance to disengage, you should try to get as close to the gun as possible.

If you are dealing with a semi-automatic, pressing your head against the barrel can disrupt the movement of the slide on the rails, interfering with the weapon's ability to function. Never rely on this, though—this method is referred to as "Russian suicide" for obvious reasons.

As you go to make your standard disarm, grabbing the barrel as close to the trigger guard as possible, and pushing back on the slide slightly, your attacker may respond to your grabbing action by pulling the gun back, before you are able to get your second hand to it.

Immediately turn the barrel of the gun away from you, pointing it to the side and upward (working against your attacker's wrist), and start to move yourself offline, away from the gun.

It is important, when you attempt any disarm, not to extend/straighten your arm, but to keep it bent. Straightening your arm may push the gun further away from you, but locking it out will mean you won't have the ability to redirect the weapon.

As your attacker pulls their weapon back, work with their movement, redirecting the weapon toward their waist/hip. Your body should be bladed and off to the side, with the firearm pointed away from you.

As you step in and off to the side, use your momentum to power a disrupting strike to your attacker in order to start taking their focus away from retaining their weapon.

Keep delivering strikes and driving into your attacker. It is important to keep moving with them as you strike, as your punches could end up moving them back and away from you, giving them space and compromising your control of the weapon. At all times, you should be restricting the movement of the weapon.

In addition to controlling the weapon, it's important to keep your attacker moving so that they are concentrating on staying on their feet, rather than focusing on using their weapon against you.

Once you have disrupted your attacker, you can continue with the disarm. If your striking has delivered enough concussive force to render your assailant unconscious, you may want to disengage without disarming.

Pull your strike back along the same path that you made the punch. This will ensure that when you bring your hand to the gun, you are not muzzling yourself.

Bring your hand down and under the gun to grip around the area where the hammer and rear sight are. With this underhand grip, and the overhand grip you have on the barrel, you will be able to turn the gun sharply, training the muzzle on your assailant.

It is important that you are off to the side, and not in front of, or over the gun when you do this, otherwise you could end up muzzling yourself.

As you turn the gun toward your attacker by pulling with your right hand (the one on the back of the weapon), and pushing with your left (the one holding the barrel), pull your body back, away from your assailant, so that this ripping action has more power than you could create with your arms alone.

Continue moving back and away from your attacker. If you have the space and room to disengage safely without having to disrupt your attacker further, do so. If not, step back in and use the firearm as an impact weapon to deliver concussive strikes to your attacker.

Keep the gun close to your body so it is hidden as you back away, so that others in the environment do not become aware that you have a weapon, and potentially take you for an assailant.

Disarming a Knife to the Side of the Throat

Disarming should be considered when disengagement isn't an option; when you are unsure of your ability to control an assailant; when your combative solutions have not sufficiently disabled them; or when you need to use the weapon in order to increase your survival chances, as when there are multiple assailants.

You should really only disarm someone of a weapon if you are prepared to use it against them. If you take a knife from an assailant, you should be prepared to cut and stab them with it; if a gun, to shoot them and/or strike them with it; and have some understanding of how to do this effectively. If you don't have any training in weapons use, you are likely to hesitate. If your attacker decides to continue to fight, this hesitation could result in them disarming you and regaining their weapon. If you plan to use disarming as part of a solution, it is beneficial to learn how to use a knife and/or a gun (even if that simply involves you knowing how to make a firearm safe).

If you do carry a firearm for personal protection and end up disarming someone of a gun, you should secure your assailant's weapon under your armpit or elsewhere and draw your own weapon, rather than relying on your assailant's. Using their gun as an impact weapon to deliver concussive strikes will allow you the time to create the necessary space and distance to do this.

Don't assume that just because you have disarmed someone of a weapon, they will stop attacking you. In fact, they may decide that this is their only survival option, especially if they believe you are thinking about using their weapon against them. If you always train that the fight ends after you have disarmed your training partner, you are only training for one possible outcome, and may be surprised when your attacker responds differently.

It is rarely advisable to go straight to a disarm without first taking your attacker's attention away from their weapon. This is often best achieved by using a combative solution; i.e., repeatedly striking/punching your attacker.

After having employed a combative solution against a knife to the side of the neck (as described earlier), pull your punching arm straight back and open your hand.

It may be that as you were striking your assailant, you realized that your punches were having little to no effect, and you weren't going to be able to disengage safely.

Bring your hand to your assailant's weapon hand and start to wrap your own hand around theirs. This is very similar to the motion you made performing the gun disarm.

Gripping tightly with both hands, start to pull your attacker's weapon hand away from their waist/hip where you had initially positioned it when you were striking them.

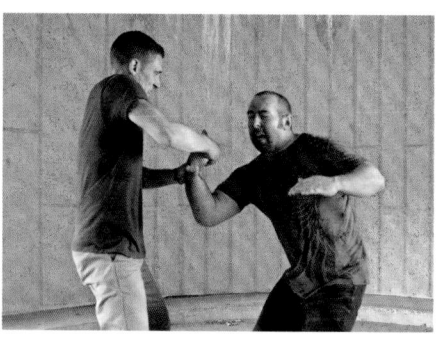

Abruptly move their arm in a counter-clockwise direction so that their hand is up and their forearm is vertical. From here, you should be able to press down on the back of their hand in order to open up their grip and take the knife.

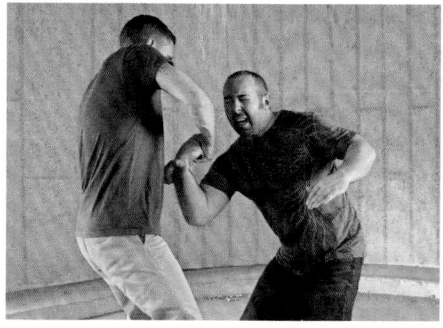

Keep pushing down, bringing your weight forward and over their weapon hand.

Your body motion should be like a wave, pulling their arm away from them and then coming back and crashing over it. As a result, you will be using your body, rather than your arms, to power the disarm.

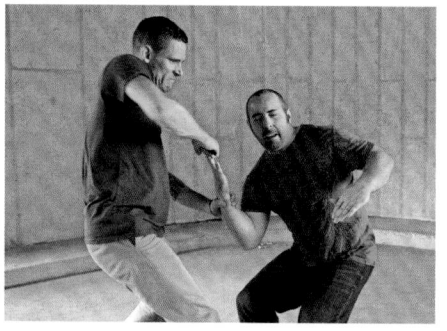

Once your attacker's hand has opened up and their grip has loosened on the knife, you can reach your fingers around and grab the handle.

Once you have a grip on it, pull back with both your hand and your body, ripping it from their grasp.

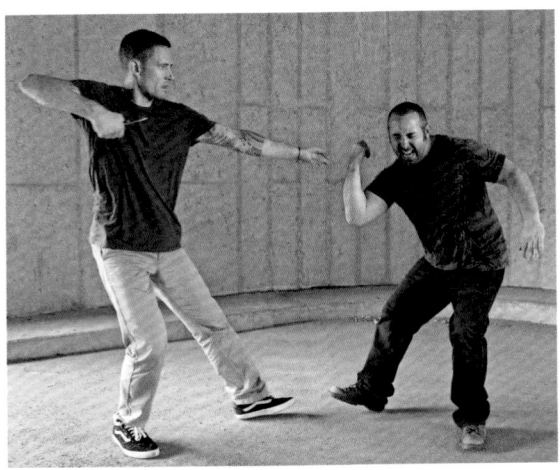

Keep backing away and making distance between yourself and your attacker.

If you stay close to them, they may believe that you are intending to use their weapon against them, and feel that their only survival option is to attack you and possibly try to disarm you. If this is the case, it is likely that you will end up using the knife against them as they move into you.

In order to open up your assailant's hand, you need to apply pressure to the back of their hand, rather than their fingers. You will need to be able to get their wrist to bend.

The easiest way to do this is to make sure that your own knuckles are over theirs. This will allow your palm to apply pressure to the back of their hand. If you find that their hand won't open when you apply pressure, pull your hand back and deliver a palm-heel strike to the back of their hand.

Disarming may well be a go-to option when you are dealing with multiple assailants. In such situations, you may want to disarm an attacker so that you have a weapon that can even the odds for you.

This is why it is important to have some training in how to use a knife offensively. You will want to know, for example, what the best targets are for disabling an attacker's movement.

Dealing with Clothing and Wrist Grabs During Knife Threats

It may be that an assailant grabs your wrist or clothing when they put the knife to your neck. These types of actions are normally performed either by highly emotional individuals who are consumed by anger and feel the need to get into your face (i.e., in spontaneously violent situations), or by predatory individuals who want to arrest your movement or move you to another location.

You may also find yourself being grabbed while a weapon is at your neck because your assailant's motive has shifted. What could start out as a mugging (the primary motive) could turn into an abduction or sexual assault (a secondary motive) if the assailant believes the situation/environment is conducive to such a crime. This may lead to your attacker grabbing you in order to control you as they move you to another location. It is worth noting that such incidents are rare, and that a mugger by default is not a sexual assailant, and will not suddenly turn into a sexual predator on the spur of the moment.

Unfortunately, in cases where weapons accompany a clothing or wrist grab, it will be necessary to break the assailant's grip in order to disengage, strike, or disarm.

In this situation, an assailant has grabbed your clothing with their left hand and placed a knife against the right side of your neck.

To get into position, you should raise your left hand up, with the palm up, facing their weapon arm, and your other hand between both of their arms.

Start to turn your body as you move your left hand toward the wrist of the assailant's hand that holds the knife, and grab it.

Use the turning movement of the body to bring your right hand up in a cutting motion in order to connect with your attacker's grip on your clothing.

Pull your right hand back so that your wrist makes contact against your assailant's hand that is holding onto your shirt. This movement needs to be extremely fast and explosive.

As your body is turning, it is actually pulling the material of the clothing away from your attacker's grip. The action of your right hand is to help pull the clothing out of your assailant's grasp.

Now that you have freed yourself, you can fully blade your body, and press your assailant's weapon hand to their body, restricting the movement of the knife.

The hand that you used to rip away your attacker's grip on your clothing should now be pulled back, and in position to strike.

You are now in a position to move forward and start raining down strikes/punches on your attacker, either in order to disengage or to set up a disarm.

The assailant may grab your wrist instead of grabbing your clothing. If someone holds on to you as they assault you, it is unlikely that they are trying to take something from you, as they wouldn't have a hand free to take what you gave them. The movement to break this grip is almost identical to the lapel grab break and disengagement, and you should think of them as being the same. Reusing movements is a fundamental concept behind Krav Maga techniques.

This scenario will look at what to do if your assailant has grabbed your wrist. This may be because they want to move you somewhere and will use your arm to direct you, or because they are concerned that you might try and do something with your arm.

As before, start by raising your free hand up in a submissive manner, getting it close to the wrist of the weapon hand/arm.

Start to blade/turn your body, pushing the knife away from your neck and pulling your neck away from the knife.

In the same movement, bend your elbow sharply, pulling your wrist upward and breaking your assailant's grip on it.

Drive the knife down and toward your assailant's body, and get set up to strike with the hand that is now free.

Your body should now be fully bladed, with your right arm pulled completely back, and ready to punch/strike.

Moving your weight forward, drive the knife toward your assailant and start punching, either to facilitate your disengagement or to set up a disarm.

Using an Assailant's Knife Against Them When It Is Against the Side of the Throat

It may be that, rather than attempting a disarm or taking the time to try a combative approach, you simply want to end the conflict then and there by using the attacker's knife against them while they are still holding on to it. This may seem an extreme response to a knife threat; however, if you analyze the situation, it is a morally appropriate one. If the threat is part of a premeditated assault, your assailant will either be trying to move you to another location (abduction)—in which case you are effectively fighting for your life, and should do anything and everything necessitated by that. Alternately, in the case of a mugging or robbery, they are after your possessions, which you should have handed over; if the assailant remains after that has happened, you should assume that they are going to use the weapon against you, and it is a case of you-or-them. If someone is prepared to use a weapon against you, you should be prepared to do the same.

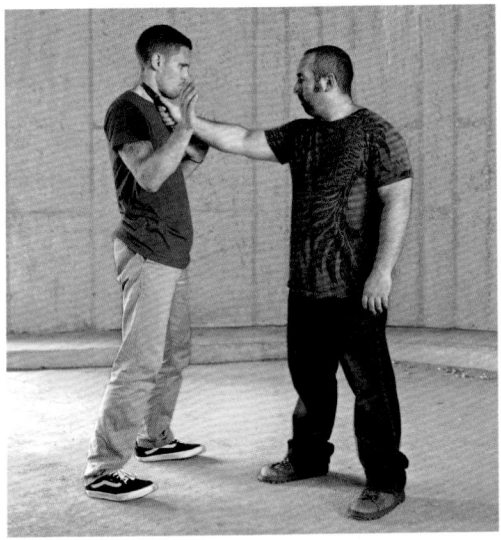

As the knife is put to your neck, raise your hands up in a submissive manner to demonstrate that you are not a threat, and that you are willing to comply with your attacker's demands—even though this may not be the case.

This will also allow your hands to be positioned close to your assailant's knife arm, so that you can quickly, and with a smaller and less discernible movement, gain control of it.

With your left hand, push/slap the knife away from your neck and smash your right forearm into your attacker's elbow. The opposing forces will cause the elbow to bend.

At the same time, start to move forward by taking a step with your right leg. When your assailant's arm is bent, the knife will be pulled away from you, so it is important to follow it in with your body in order to keep control of your attacker's arm.

As your assailant's arm bends, raise up your right elbow so that their forearm is vertical. This happens as part of the same movement that was detailed in the previous step.

The hand that slapped/pushed your attacker's knife arm should now be positioned over the back of their knife hand.

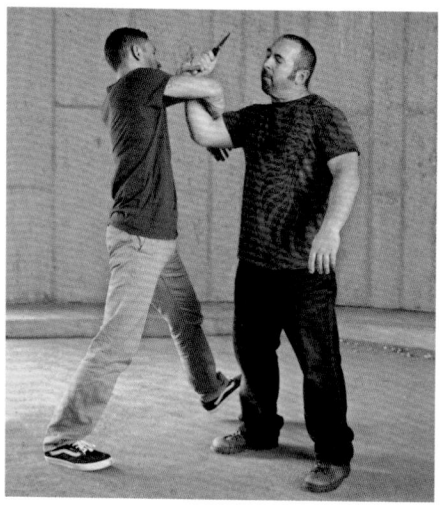

In this photo, you can see the arm movement(s) coupled with the body movement. Both should happen together, and as one single step.

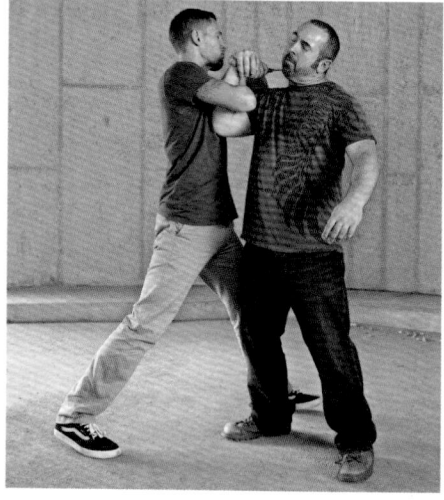

As you step in, move your chest into your assailant's vertical weapon arm, trapping it so that they are unable to move it, thus taking the movement of the weapon away.

Pushing forward with your chest/body like this will also push your attacker's knife toward their own neck, where you will be able to use it against them.

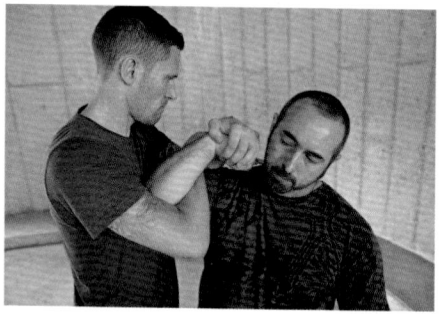

Once you have brought the knife toward your assailant's neck, use your left hand to control theirs, and position the blade against their neck. You are now prepared to cut them with it.

Your fingerprints should not be on the knife at all; this makes it very clear who the aggressor in the situation is. This might not be so clear if you perform a disarm and then end up having to use the knife against your attacker.

Rather than making a cutting/slashing movement with your arms, turn your body, with the arms fixed, to bring the blade across your assailant's neck.

Having disabled your assailant, you are now safe, to disengage from them, and make your way to safety. As with many of these scenarios, you may want to call law enforcement and the medical services to let them know there is an injured person—but only do this once you have gotten to safety.

You may also find yourself considering using the knife against your assailant after you have first tried another solution, such as combatively striking your attacker and/or attempting to disarm them. It may be that after repeatedly striking your attacker to little or no effect, you realize that another solution is necessary; or, when you try to bring their arm up to perform a disarm, they resist you. Being able to adapt and adjust to the changing nature of a fight is a necessary and essential survival skill. Otherwise all you will be able to do is persist with a technique that is failing.

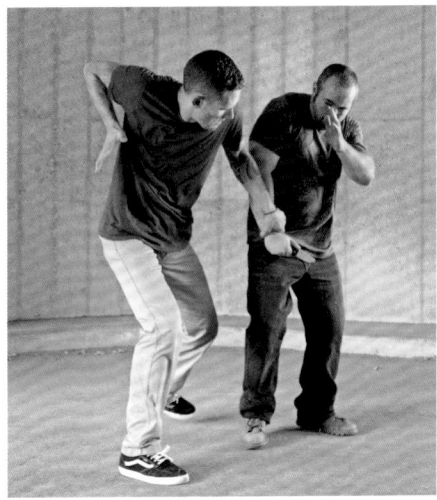

As you punch and strike your attacker, you may find that your punches aren't affecting them, either because you are not generating enough power, or because your assailant has a high pain tolerance due to adrenaline, drugs, alcohol, etc.

Although you are disrupting them, they may soon figure out how to respond to what you are doing, and so you will need to embark on another course of action.

After retracting one of your punches, roll your wrist over so that your hand is now positioned to make an underhand grip around your assailant's weapon hand.

Shoot the hand down to grab their hand, wrapping your fingers around theirs, so that you are now holding their hand as it holds the knife.

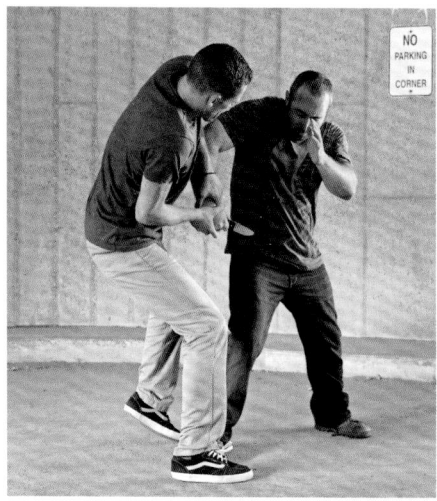

With both hands now on the assailant's weapon arm, step across and behind them, dragging their knife across the side of their torso.

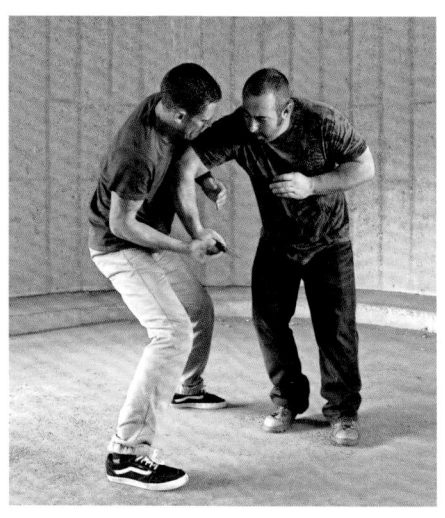

Once at their side, release your grip on their wrist and thread your arm through theirs, inside their elbow. Keep holding on to the hand that is gripping the knife.

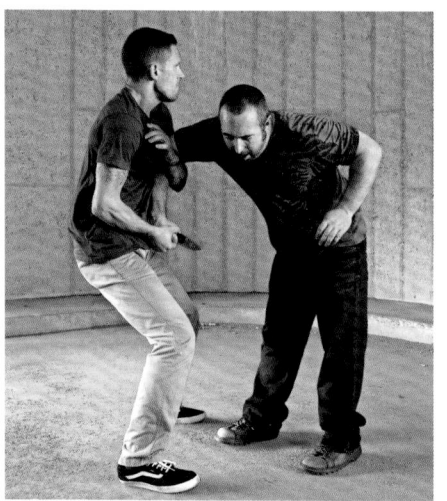

Pull their elbow to your chest, and the hand gripping the knife to your hips; their forearm should be vertical and flush to your body. You should have complete control of their arm, and their weapon should be pointed in their direction.

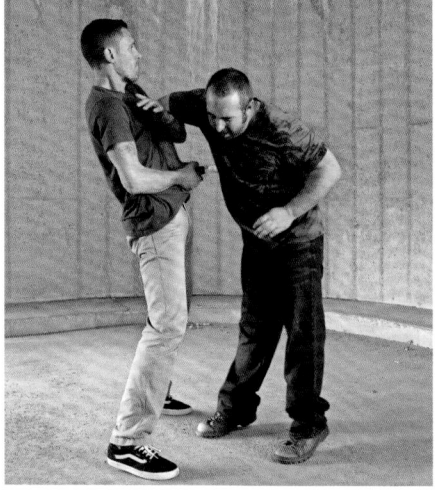

Drive your hips forward to bring the knife to their side, and lean back to pull them onto the blade. It may be necessary to reset the hips, and repeat this action several times, in order to fully incapacitate them.

It is not enough to only have one way of dealing with an armed assailant. It could be that your solution isn't appropriate or effective for the environment you are in. For example, if you have to deal with a knife threat in an elevator, it may be safer to use the knife against your assailant rather than acting combatively and/or disarming them; in such an enclosed space, you will not be able to disengage after disarming, and will have to use the knife against them. If acting combatively, you may find that you very quickly run out of space to strike effectively. You must be able to adapt and change your solutions based on the situations you find yourself in, as well as your assailant's responses to what you do. What if your strikes have no effect? What if their grip on the knife prevents you from disarming? Convincing yourself that these things won't happen is naïve and dangerous. Techniques can and do fail for these and a number of other reasons, and you will need to be able to respond when they do.

Some instructors will try to convince you that their techniques will work in every situation, against any and every assailant. Unfortunately, this is too simplistic an approach to take where your own survival is concerned. A technique that works nine times out of ten is an excellent technique, but you should be prepared for that one time when everything goes against you, and you have to adapt and change your solution.

Rear Hostage/Abduction Knife Threats—with Arms Pinned

In *Krav Maga: Real World Solutions to Real World Violence*, I detailed a solution to a situation where an assailant comes up behind you, puts a knife to your throat, and starts to pull you back (p. 104). In the scenario illustrated, the person being abducted had both hands free and was able to use them both in their defense and escape. However, an assailant may decide to control one of your hands by pinning it to your side, or even pinning it to your back. They may do this simply to feel they have better control of you, or because they are concerned that you might try to escape, and they want to limit your options.

One of the critical things to understand about an abduction is that generally your survival options diminish the further away you get from the location where the initial assault occurred; this means it is almost always better to act immediately, rather than later.

When you are abducted, you won't know how long your abductor intends to keep you, so escaping at the earliest opportunity is your best option. In most situations, the longer an abduction/hostage situation goes on, the more your survival chances are reduced. It is, in fact, very difficult to contain people, feeding them and providing bathroom facilities for them, while keeping their location secret. If the abduction has not been well planned and well executed, it is likely that as time goes on, the abductor(s) will have greater and greater difficulty containing and providing for their captive(s). All of this means that your actual value to your abductors will start to go down over time—especially if their initial demands are not met and they are forced to negotiate.

When someone puts their arm around your neck with a knife to your throat and takes hold of one of your arms, it is highly unlikely that you are dealing with a mugger. A mugger would not want to have their movement restricted by tying up with you in this way, and would require a free hand to take whatever they've demanded from you. As you are now dealing with someone who wants you, rather than your possessions, you will need to act quickly and decisively.

Rear Hostage/Abduction Knife Threat—with Wrist Held

Although you may not see yourself as a likely target for abduction or kidnapping, there are many different ways you can have value to someone (or a group). You may work in a venue such as a supermarket, restaurant, or bar, in which you have access to a lot of cash, especially if you are in charge of cashing out and locking up at the end of a shift. You may be the victim of an "express kidnapping", where an abductor kidnaps you in order to force you to withdraw money from an ATM (you may even be held overnight so the abductor(s) can make a second withdrawal, thereby getting around the bank's daily limit). Or you could be the victim of a "tiger kidnapping," in which you are kidnapped and taken hostage in order to get someone who knows you, such as a family member, to comply with an abductor's demands. This was a standard practice of the IRA in Northern Ireland: they would kidnap a person's family member(s) in order to get someone to plant a bomb for them or drive a truck of arms to a particular location. In the U.S., ex-partners and children involved in custodial disputes comprise the largest population that is abducted/kidnapped. It is always worth taking an honest look at your personal situation and making appropriate risk assessments based on the potential threats you may face, and the potential vulnerabilities that such threats could exploit.

One vulnerability that many of us have is a predictable schedule. If a person wants to commit a crime against you, knowing where you will be at a certain time makes it easy for them to synchronize their movement to yours and initiate an assault or crime. If you close up a business that deals in cash at the same time every day, and always go through the same routine, a criminal needs only a small amount of surveillance to plan to abduct you and force you to reopen the business so that they can gain access to the safe or other valuables.

In a similar scenario, someone might be aware that you have things of value in your house and get in at the same time every night. Rather than breaking in, they will wait for you to come home and then force you to open the house to them.

An abduction attempt could take place as you are leaving work, locking up for the day. It could be that an attacker armed with a knife comes up behind you, grabbing your wrist to control you, and places a knife at your throat, pulling you back. Their intent is to take you back into the building and force you to open up the safe.

This type of threat, where an assailant tries to restrict and control your movement, is more likely to signify an abduction than a mugging.

To set up your escape, hover your free hand over the attacker's knife hand. This can be made to look like a submissive/placating gesture. It is also unlikely that your attacker will even see your hand, as your head position relative to theirs will likely obscure it.

Explosively pull down on your attacker's knife arm. Your hand should be shaped like a hook, with your thumb open, ready to grab. The first thing your attacker should be aware of is their arm being plucked down. Don't first put your hand on the arm and then pull down, as this may give them time to react to what you are doing.

Start to rotate your wrist and bend your elbow to break your attacker's grip.

Continue to rotate your wrist and explosively pull up, keeping your elbow tight to your side. This makes the movement tighter and faster, preventing your attacker from reacting to the pull.

Once the knife is away from your throat, press your assailant's knife hand into your chest, securing it and preventing it from moving.

Once your hand is free from your assailant's grasp, bring it up and place it over your other hand, so you now have two hands securing your attacker's weapon arm. Continue to press it into your chest.

Start to bring your left leg—the one nearest to your assailant—back, and lift your right shoulder up.

Continue stepping back with your left leg and lifting your shoulder up. At the same time, begin to duck under your attacker's weapon arm.

As you do this, start to slide your top hand down so that it is over your attacker's hand, rather than over their wrist.

Continue stepping under the arm so that you are now behind and to the side of your attacker. Keep pressing their wrist into your chest and sliding your left hand down so that it is wrapped around their hand. The knife should now be pointing toward them, with your body behind it.

Straight away, drive the knife into your attacker's side, using the power of your body rather than just the arms. The knife should stay locked to your chest as you drive it into them. If necessary, pull back and repeat this action.

Once your assailant is no longer a threat to you, push them away and disengage. Don't try getting back into the building, as this will involve taking the time to unlock the door, etc. Under high stress and duress, fine motor skills—which would be needed to select a key and fit it into a lock—start to deteriorate, so it is safer just to run away, putting distance between yourself and your attacker. You can always return later with an armed police officer to finish locking up.

When performing any type of weapon control or disarm, you will be in a highly adrenalized state. You will likely be frightened, and your fear system will be telling you to comply with your assailant's demands, because while you comply, you are not getting hurt or experiencing any pain, and from an emotional perspective, this is a good thing. It doesn't matter if you know consciously that not acting in that moment will lead to pain later on; your emotional self simply knows that no pain now is a good thing, and you won't want to risk changing or upsetting this.

It is good to have systems in place that will force you to act even when you don't want to. When someone gets ready to do a bungee jump, they will normally count numbers and decide to jump on a particular count—for example, when they say "three." They therefore count out loud: "One, two, three," and then jump. You can do a similar thing by coming up with a sentence that you will say, and timing the initial movement of your technique to one of the words in it. Having a line such as, "I'll do whatever you want me to," and performing the first part of your disarm or control on the word "you" will not only help you be decisive, but will also force your abductor to start processing what you are saying, taking some of their attention away from the knife.

The Importance of Keeping Your Head In Contact with Your Attacker's Weapon Arm

 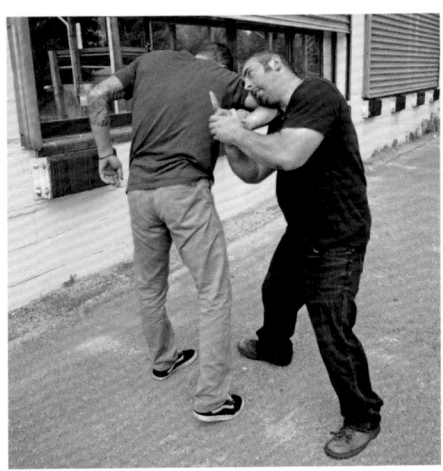

When you turn, ducking under your assailant's arm, you want to make sure that you keep your head pressed up against their elbow. Your head and neck are extremely strong and you can use them to put pressure on and help you control your aggressor's knife arm.

If, at any time, as you execute this technique, you feel that disengaging from your attacker is your most effective option (for example, if you see a third party coming to assist them), you should use your head to put forward/downward pressure on your attacker's elbow and push their wrist up behind their back.

This action should also start to make them bend at the waist and force them to take a step forward and away from you.

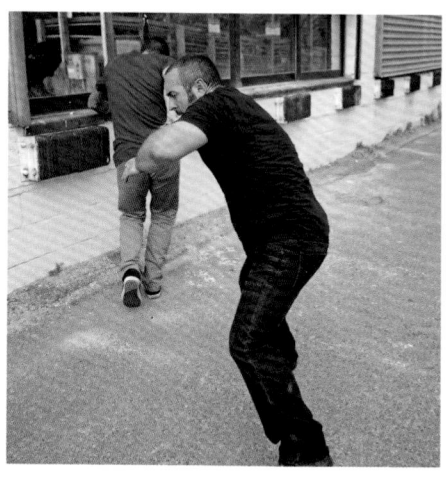

Keep forcing their arm up behind their back, pushing the knife toward their neck. At this point, you should no longer need to use your head to apply pressure, due to the inflexibility of your attacker's arm in this direction.

Once you have their weight moving forward, push them away by forcing their wrist up behind their back.

Now, put as much distance between yourself and your attacker as possible. If you aren't able to create distance, try to get an obstacle or barrier between them and you, such as a parked car—or find an improvised weapon.

Rear Hostage/Abduction Knife Threat—with Arm Held Behind Back

Your attacker, wanting greater control, may pull your arm up behind your back instead of grabbing your wrist. When they do this, they restrict your ability to duck under their armpit, forcing you to turn the other way in order to release your arm.

Now we will look at what to do if the attacker comes up behind you, pulling your arm down and behind your back, and places a knife to your throat. This would be someone who wants to control you and move you to another location.

A good rule of thumb/heuristic to work from is: if a person wants your possessions, acquiesce; if they want you, fight. An attacker may want to move you to another location because they're unable to do what they want to do to you in that location.

With your arm behind your back, it would be impossible to step back and under your assailant's weapon arm as you would if they were controlling your wrist. This means you will have to turn the other way.

You will still pluck your attacker's wrist down and pin it to your chest as you did before, so your first action should be to bring your hand up in a hook in order to do this.

Rotate your wrist and turn, pulling your arm out from behind you; turning will give you the space to do this. This movement should be explosive, and your palm should turn from facing your attacker to facing frontwards.

At the same time, pluck down on the wrist of your attacker's weapon arm, moving the knife from your throat to your chest. Once there, pin it tightly against you.

Using your hands, assisted by your body, bend your attacker's wrist so as to open up their hand and disarm them of their weapon. You can now take it and use it against them and any other assailants who may be in the environment, or simply disengage with it.

Keep turning so that you eventually face your assailant. Keep hold of their wrist with your right hand and bring your left hand to their weapon hand, grabbing it and placing your thumb against the back of their hand.

When you first turn, your right hand will be on the wrist of your attacker's weapon hand. This is the hand that plucked down and pressed the knife hand against your chest. As you turn, you should rotate their wrist so that their palm is not pressed to your chest, but is instead pointing upward.

The arm that was pinned behind your back (the left hand), should come around; you should aim to get that thumb to the back of their weapon hand.

Despite rotating the weapon hand as you turn, so that it is no longer pressed against your chest, you should not let your body lose contact with their knife hand. This allows you to lean your body forward against your own thumb on the back of their hand, so you can open their hand up and take the knife.

By bending forward, all of your weight will be pressed against your attacker's hand, causing their wrist to bend and their grip around the handle of the knife to be compromised. At the same time, this action will cause your assailant to bend at the waist, breaking their posture and forcing them to pull their hips back. In this position it would be very difficult for them to launch any type of counterattack while you take the knife from them.

What to Do If You Are Being Abducted by an Unarmed Assailant

Not everyone who may try to abduct you will be armed. Your attacker(s) may have to literally drag you away from wherever you are to a car, alley, doorway, or similar location where they can continue their assault unseen. In such situations, your primary goal should be to prevent yourself from being moved to their intended location. If your assailant doesn't feel the need to use a weapon to get you to comply with their demands, they have probably targeted you in the belief that they are stronger than you, and that they will be able to pull, lift, or carry you to wherever they want to take you. Your first tactic should be to start attacking them as they try to move you. If your attacks seem to have little effect, and you aren't able to escape from their control, your next step should be to start trying to hold on to objects in your environment, such as lampposts, the side mirrors of cars—anything that you can get your hands/arms around. This also includes people, if you are in a crowded location (abductions do happen in busy places as well). Grabbing on to someone else will make them part of your assailant's problem.

If your strategy is to grab on to objects and/or people, try to draw attention to yourself by shouting. There is a big difference between screaming/shrieking and shouting. If you simply scream, your assailant may become more emboldened, confirming your victim profile to themselves. Instead, issue commands to anyone who is around—instruct them as to how you would like them to act and behave. Don't simply ask them to help you, but tell them what to do—e.g., grab the assailant's arm and stop them from pulling you. If bystanders and those witnessing an abduction don't know what to do, they won't act.

An abductor might run up behind you and attempt to grab you as you leave a train station.

Transit stops are regularly chosen by criminals, as they have a high turnover of potential victims to choose from. If you are the last person off a train, and the platform quickly clears, you will now be isolated and on your own, despite having been in a crowd a few minutes before. It is always a good idea to exit a transit stop within a group for this reason.

This is a non-life-threatening attack, which would normally indicate that you should attack the attacker (in life-threatening attacks you attack the attack). If your balance is taken, however, you may not be in a position to attack your assailant, so you must do something to both regain your balance and disrupt their attack. At the same time, you must prevent them from moving you from this location to another.

As soon as you can, grab on to something so your assailant's attack is slowed down. It is not always necessary to inflict pain on your attacker. Sometimes all you have to do is stop them doing what they want to do to you—in this case, moving you from this location to another. The longer you can prevent someone from executing their plan, the more likely they are to give up on it.

If they manage to pull you away from what you are holding on to, don't feel that the situation is slipping away from you. Every second that you're able to delay your assailant puts them under more pressure.

It may seem that this would be a good opportunity to start attacking them. However, this may mean that you have to go forward in the direction that they are trying to pull you, which would take you closer to where they want to bring you.

If this is the case, keep grabbing on to things so that you are able to stay where you are. Your best survival strategy may be to simply delay your attacker and let the clock play out.

This may also be a more effective strategy than trying to engage with them physically if there is more than one abductor. It may be that you will be unable to overpower two assailants, but you could prevent them, or slow them down, from moving you.

Bystanders and other uninvolved parties are unlikely to intervene and help you. However, you may be able to directly involve them by grabbing on to them. This will both slow down your assailant's attack/abduction and complicate the situation for them by getting another person involved. Be sure to tell the person you grab onto what is happening and how they must stop you from being taken, etc.

Gun to Back of Head When Pushed Against Wall/Car/Door

Someone who has been planning to abduct you will have carried out some level of surveillance on you, and probably understands your movements and routine(s) better than you do. They will probably know when your car is in your driveway, when it is not, what time you leave and get home from work, etc. If you run your life like clockwork, it will give your assailant the ability to synchronize their movements to yours.

Home invasions are committed for a variety of reasons. For some criminals, it is an opportunity to enjoy power and control over a helpless victim and express their anger and frustration toward society. Others may need a homeowner present in order for them to reveal the whereabouts of any items of value or to give them access to a safe or similar. Others may look to enter your house to make a sexual assault. Rather than waiting until you are in your house to try and gain access, where you might have a security chain across your front door, decide not to answer the doorbell, etc., they may wait until you return home and force you inside as you open your front door.

It is easy to fall into the trap of thinking that once you reach your house you are safe, and that bad things will only happen to you in unfamiliar places. If a criminal believes you have something of value to them in your house, they may well wait for you to return home and then force you inside. Their intelligence could come from sources such as a girlfriend or partner who baby-sat your kids, or a friend who did some work on your house.

Many people feel safer when they are talking to or texting a friend, but there is a big difference between feeling safe and being safe. Whenever you are on a mobile device, your attention (situational awareness) is taken away from what is actually going on in your environment.

Part of your situational awareness is knowing entry and exit points within your environment, as well as points of concealment. This includes areas around your home.

Part of good situational awareness is recognizing when things in your environment change. If there were no cigarette butts by your door when you left your house in the morning, but when you return there are, something has changed.

A cluster of cigarette butts can be a clue that someone—a smoker—has been at that particular location for a prolonged period of time, either carrying out surveillance or waiting for someone.

If you have been talking on the phone (or texting), it is likely that you won't have picked up on these things and so will have missed some of the pre-violence indicators that could alert you to a potential threat or danger.

Many people, when they get to their front door, stop to look for their keys, rather than making sure that they have them in their hand and can look around before they unlock the door.

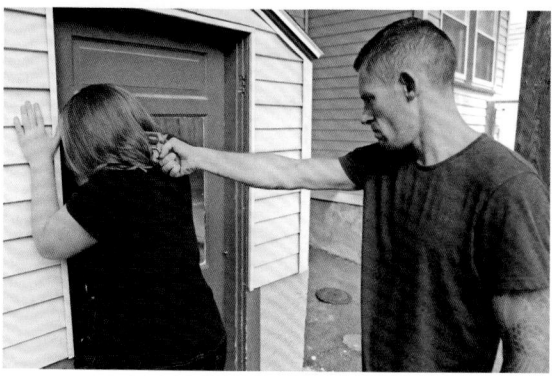

It may be that as you prepare to unlock your door you find yourself pushed up against it, with a gun at the back of your head, and an assailant demanding that you unlock it and let them in.

The first thing you should do is bring your hands close together so that you will be able to push yourself away from the door/wall. This will also mean that when you turn, your hands will be close to the gun.

You should push your head back into the gun so that your attacker pushes the gun harder into you; this will mean the gun will move forward when you turn (taking away the surface the gun is pressing into), helping you get behind the weapon more quickly.

Push off from the door/wall and start to turn toward your attacker.

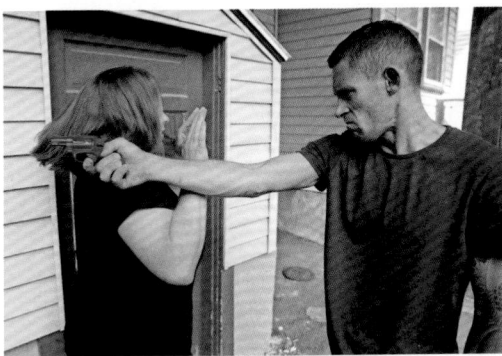

With your turning motion, your head should move out of the line of fire and your right wrist/hand should push the gun out of the way.

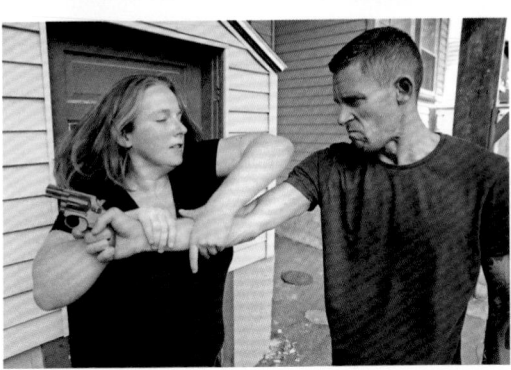

Grab your attacker's wrist with your right hand and start to bring your left arm over and inside their weapon arm, grabbing onto their forearm with your left hand.

In this position, you will be able to prevent your assailant from pulling back the weapon in order to try and retain it, which could put you back in the line of fire. If they try to pull the weapon back, they will end up with your elbow in their chest.

You should now be completely behind the weapon.

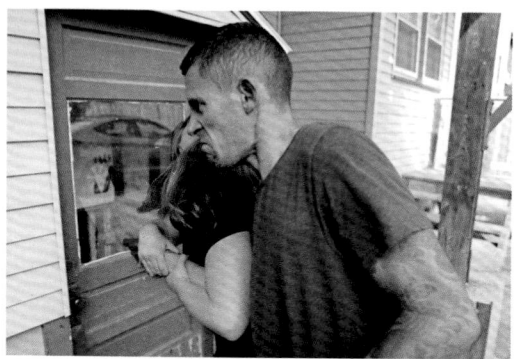

Keep turning so that you extend your attacker's weapon arm, locking their elbow and forcing them toward the wall.

Your largest and strongest striking surface is not your fist or any part of you, but the wall/door that you were pushed up against. Whenever you have the chance to use your environment as a weapon, you should.

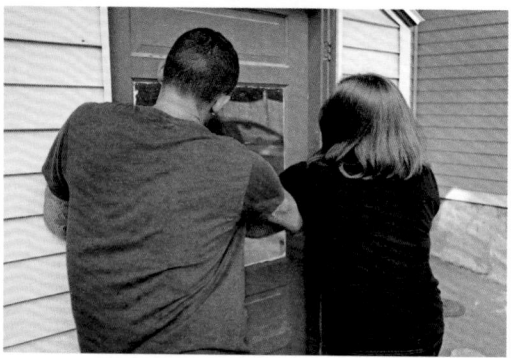

Turn your body so that your attacker is forced into the wall. You may want to pull back and keep slamming your attacker into the wall until you start feeling their grip on the gun weaken. You don't have to concuss your attacker, merely disrupt them.

As you do this, transfer your grip on your attacker's wrist to the gun so that when you are ready to disarm them, you already have a hold on the gun.

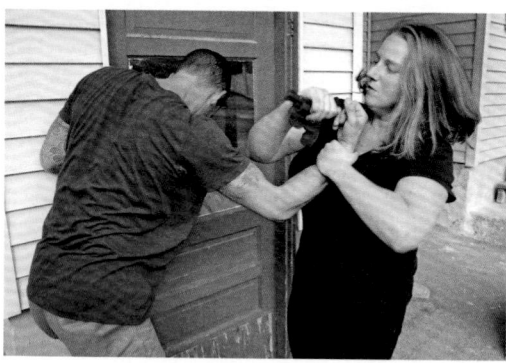

Once you feel that your assailant is stunned/disrupted, turn back out with your grip on the gun. Keep holding your assailant's arm with your left hand.

Your turning movement should be with your full body, rather than just your arm, to make sure that the gun is pulled clear of your attacker's grasp.

Once you have the gun in your hand, turn back into your attacker and use it as an impact weapon. You should have severely disrupted your assailant's ability to continue the assault, so it is probably safe to disengage.

Don't feel that you have to go inside your house. It is obvious that your immediate environment is a dangerous one, and you should get as far away from it as possible.

This technique will work if you are pushed up against any vertical surface, whether it's a wall, a door, a car, etc.

Gun Threat When Seated

When we think about the types of violent scenarios that we may find ourselves in, we often restrict ourselves to considering situations where we are on our own and standing. This may not always be the case, however. If you take public transport, you may be assaulted when seated; if you find yourself in the middle of a bar fight, you might have to start defending yourself from a seated position; if someone you know attempts to sexually assault you, you may be sitting next to them when they make their attack, etc. You should not always assume that you will be standing when you have to defend yourself, and you should train and prepare yourself for possible assaults at times when you may be seated.

Muggers and other predators follow a simple five-step process. This is:

1. Select a location
2. Select a victim
3. Watch/survey the victim
4. Synchronize movement with the victim
5. Interview the victim

A mugger wants to select a location with a plentiful supply of victims and a good number of potential escape routes. This means that shopping areas, transit stops, and the like are all places where you can expect a mugging to take place. It may seem strange that a mugger would choose a relatively crowded place to commit such a crime. Just because there are people around doesn't mean that they can see what is going on, though, and muggers are skilled at positioning themselves so that it is not obvious that they're committing a crime. One of the ironies of crowded places is that we feel safer in them, and drop our own awareness levels as we start to rely on other people to identify danger/threats for us. Unfortunately, the others we are relying on to identify danger on our behalf will also have lowered their awareness, and may not pick up on any dangers that are present. You should always aim to stay "actively" aware when you are in crowded situations.

When selecting a victim, predators will generally look for an individual who appears unaware, non-confrontational and, if possible, in a disadvantaged position, such as being seated, or on an escalator or stairway, etc. Your body language gives a predator a lot of clues about your physical and emotional state. Do you give off the impression of being tired, depressed, and lost in your thoughts? Is your head hanging down; are you looking at the ground; are you walking or sitting in a slumped manner? After selecting a victim, they will watch them for a period of time to confirm that they have made the right selection (you should be alert to individuals who seem to take an interest in you), and possibly, in this time, start to get themselves emotionally prepared to commit their crime. Their next step is to move toward their chosen victim in some way, synchronizing their movement with their target's (I have described the different methods of synchronization in *Krav Maga: Real World Solutions to Real World Violence*, pp. 61–62). Once they get to where their target is, they'll start their "interview process." This may be as simple as demanding the target's wallet, or it may involve some sort of "ambush" in which they first ask for directions, the time, etc. They may also attempt to "groom" their target, in order to get the person to trust them and hand over control of the situation to them, possibly even agreeing to move to another location.

Even if you don't normally take public transportation, there may be times that you are forced to do so; e.g., if your car is in the shop being repaired. Because you are unfamiliar with spending time at a transit stop, you may fail to identify when a person's movement, behavior, and manner is actually out of place; such as, if they move past a number of empty benches to one where you are sitting in an isolated part of the platform.

It could be that an assailant comes up to you while you are seated at a transit stop, pulls a gun, and demands your wallet. After you hand it to them, rather than leaving with it, they may stay. Not knowing if their secondary motive will involve shooting you, your safest option now would be to attempt a weapon disarm.

From your seated position, your hand defense must precede your body defense. From a "hands up" position, drop your right arm/hand down to move the gun so that you are not in the line of fire.

As you stand up, snake the hand that started to move the gun out of the way around your assailant's wrist. This technique is almost identical to how you would deal with a knife shank when seated (explained on pp. 140-143).

At the same time, take hold of the upper arm/triceps of your assailant's weapon arm with your right hand.

Your right hand should be rotating/pulling on your assailant's upper arm, while your left hand continues to snake around their wrist. Both actions should cause the attacker's arm to rotate.

One of the first actions you should make with your left hand as it wraps around your attacker's wrist is to hook it, so your assailant can't pull their weapon back.

As you come fully upright, pull your assailant's arm tight to your chest. It should be pulled/pressed flat against you, with your left arm controlling the gun at the wrist.

As you stand up, you can deliver a knee strike to your assailant's body in order to take their mind off the weapon and any thoughts they may have of fighting back. Against a tall aggressor, you can deliver this strike to their quads/upper legs.

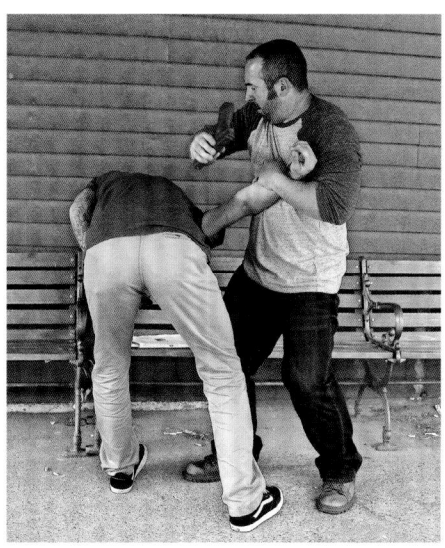

Keeping control of their wrist, reach over with the hand that was on the upper arm/triceps. Your thumb should connect with the gun around the area where the trigger is (the back end of the barrel). This will prevent you from taking a grip that would see you muzzle yourself.

Take the gun from your attacker's hand and immediately swing it into them, striking them with the barrel of the weapon.

Without releasing your assailant, rain down hammer-fist strikes on them, using the barrel to focus the force of your blows.

Once you have subdued your assailant, disengage, making your way to safety.

Improvised Weapon—Newspaper Mask

There is normally an abundance of free newspapers and magazines at transit stops and train stations. Even if you have no interest in their contents, it is worth picking one up, as it can be used as an easily deployable improvised weapon. With any improvised weapon, you need to make sure that it doesn't take much to alter or change the object's original form in order to use it as a weapon. Because violence usually happens very quickly, you may not have the time to spend fashioning a tool to use, and so must be able to use what is in your hand at the time. A newspaper may seem like it lacks any real structural integrity unless rolled up or folded, but depending how it is used, this isn't the case. Holding the newspaper in both hands as if reading it, you can quickly mask a person's face by wrapping their head in it. Hold the back of their head with your hands and start to deliver knee strikes into their groin and stomach. In response, they should double over with the strikes, presenting you with the opportunity to control their head and take them to ground.

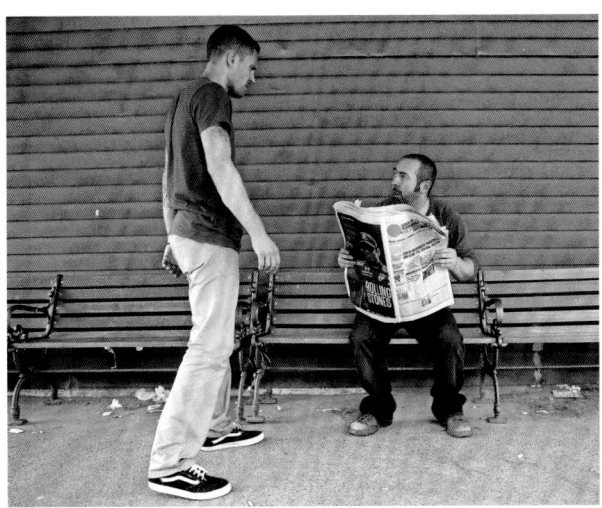

As you sit reading a newspaper, a person may approach you and begin posturing and acting in an intimidating manner. For whatever reason, they have decided that you are someone who looks like a potential victim/target.

Rather than staying in a disadvantaged position, (though you should still be intending to resolve the situation peacefully), stand up.

You may think that you need to put the paper down so that you are better able to deal with your assailant, but your newspaper can actually make a great improvised weapon and help you to gain an advantage over your aggressor.

If the situation cannot be de-escalated or resolved peacefully, you will need to make a pre-emptive assault against your aggressor.

Drive the newspaper into your assailant's face, wrapping it around their head so that their vision is obscured. Although it may seem like that the paper will simply rip, even the flimsiest of newspapers is strong enough to hold up to this treatment.

While holding the newspaper, grab the back of your attacker's head and pull it toward you, making sure that the newspaper is still obscuring their view/vision.

Deliver knee strikes to their body and legs while they are disoriented by their lack of vision. Don't spend too long doing this, but throw enough strikes that your assailant is left in a state of shock and surprise.

As soon as you recognize that it is safe to disengage, do so, throwing the newspaper back into your attacker's face. There is no reason to stay engaged with an attacker longer than necessary. Your job is to survive the situation, not to punish your attacker.

Knife Attacks

A knife attack differs from a threat in that your assailant has clearly demonstrated that they intend to cause you harm. Facing an attacker with a knife is a scary proposition; attacks are usually wild, frenzied, and committed, with the knife being recoiled sharply between attacks—something that is rarely replicated in the training environment. In reality, you may also be attacked within a confined space, such as in an elevator or a stairwell. For this reason, your first objective should be to try to take the movement of the weapon away by controlling your attacker's knife arm. This means that if you don't have an immediate disengagement opportunity, you will have to keep moving in toward your attacker in order to get control of their arm.

In my personal experience, trying to block and strike a committed assailant only really works as a distraction in order to disengage. Your chances of delivering enough concussive strikes to stop a highly adrenalized attacker before they have stabbed you enough times to incapacitate you are not great. If you can't block, strike and disengage, you should be looking to get control of the knife and restrict its movement.

It is always worth being aware that a knife can get pulled in the middle of a fight, not just at the beginning. Depending on how the fight started, your attacker may not have had the chance to draw their weapon at the outset; for example, if you attacked them preemptively. This may mean that the knife gets pulled later on in the fight.

Part of your training should involve training knife attacks when you are striking, grappling, and even on the ground.

In a real-life confrontation, be prepared that you may get cut, while at the same time understanding that, in general, a knife will have to penetrate to a depth of 2 inches to cause significant trauma. While there is always the risk of a major artery getting slashed or cut, such instances are not that common. Even if a block fails to stop the knife from reaching you, if it prevents the blade from penetrating too far, it has served a practical purpose—it will usually take multiple stab wounds in order for you to be physically unable to continue. Although you obviously want to avoid getting cut, if it does happen, you should never let it stop you from continuing to fight.

Adjusting Your Stance When Dealing with a Knife Attack

In most assaults involving a knife, you will be attacked before you realize what is actually happening, and you may end up getting stabbed. Be aware that a stab will often feel like a punch, and after a fight ends (in the post-conflict phase of violence) it is worth checking yourself to see if you were stabbed, even if you thought that your attacker(s) only hit you. On some occasions, however, an assailant may show you the knife in order to intimidate you. It may be that they are not yet emotionally ready to make their attack, and need to feed off your fear in order to work themselves up. In this moment, you should adjust your stance to be better prepared to deal with any attack.

If you are right-handed, your fighting stance and de-escalation stance should have you standing with your left foot forward and your right foot (and hand) back, where it can deliver the most power. However, if you are facing an attacker holding a knife in their right hand, blading or angling your body in this way would offer your attacker the shortest distance to be able to stab you.

If you change your stance over, the result is that you pull your body away from the knife hand, making it harder for them to reach you. This may seem like a lot of trouble to go to, but when you consider that the knife only has to penetrate by 2 inches to cause serious damage, this readjustment might provide the extra distance that prevents a stab from being fatal.

The key thing to understand about this is that your attacker is giving you the opportunity to do it. In most knife attacks, your assailant will deny you the time and distance to react, so this readjustment will not be possible.

Knife Shank to the Opposite Side

One of the key factors which differentiates real-world self-defense training from that of combat sports is that in combat sports such as MMA, Muay Thai, Boxing, Judo, etc., you are always aware of where your attacker is, and in all of these sports you start off directly facing them. Although most real-life violent situations start off with a face-to-face interaction and some form of verbal exchange, this is not always the case. You need to be able to defend yourself from attacks in all directions and have a 360-degree awareness of what is around you.

You may have had a dispute with someone in a bar that you thought was resolved—maybe they believed they were in front of you in line, that you were hitting on their girlfriend/boyfriend, etc. As far as you were concerned, the matter was ended and everybody had moved on. Unfortunately, you may have been dealing with an individual suffering from high but unstable self-esteem; someone who identifies themselves as occupying an "alpha" position but questions why others don't recognize them as such. This is the personality type of your typical bully. While they may have found themselves backing down over the original dispute, they may feel that it is necessary to reassert their authority and gain back the position/status that they feel they have lost. The human condition is such that people will work harder to regain lost status than they will to advance their original position. To this end, the person may wait for you to leave the bar with the intent of assaulting you. This is why it is sometimes better to leave a location at the first sign of trouble (i.e., after the initial dispute), rather than stay in an environment where someone may harbor harmful intent toward you.

If you are attacked on your left side by a right-handed attacker, your defense, control, and disarm will be almost identical to that performed from the front (see *Krav Maga: Real World Solutions To Real World Violence*, pp. 133–141, for a description of defending a front knife shank).

As you exit the bar, you may find that the individual you had the altercation with is waiting for you. Good situational awareness doesn't just involve identifying people who may mean you harm, but should also involve an understanding of your environment including, entrances, exits, concealment points, etc.

It is often worth leaving a location after a dispute even if you think an argument has been settled. That may be your interpretation of the incident; however, it may not be the other person's.

As your aggressor shanks the knife upward to your side, you will reflexively bring your nearest hand/arm out toward the attack, and pull your hips back from it.

At this point, you will still be side-on to your attacker.

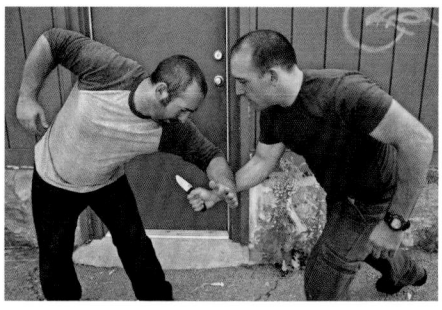

As you instinctively pull your hips back, start twisting your torso, so that you will eventually be able to face your attacker front to front.

Your blocking arm should be at a 90-degree angle so that it can stop, rather than deflect, the attack.

Your other arm should start to come up in preparation for grabbing your attacker's upper arm.

In this photo, you can see the 90-degree angle of the blocking arm (the right arm is pulled back for the photo so that this is clear; in a real-life dynamic situation, however, it would be reaching to grab their upper arm in order to help get control of the knife arm).

If the arm were at a greater angle (i.e., straighter), there would be the danger that the knife would be deflected and run up your arm toward your neck/head.

At this point, you should burst forward toward your attacker, with the goal of wrapping your arms around theirs, getting two arms on the weapon arm. Your left arm should "snake" under their arm and start to pull it to your chest as you burst in.

Your right hand should be on your attacker's arm, helping rotate it (so the blade points to the ground), and pulling it to your chest.

As you burst forward, pull your attacker's arm to you. Make sure it is flush with and pulled tightly to your chest. You want to have it securely locked onto you, allowing your assailant no space in which to move their arm.

If your movement allows it, you can deliver a knee strike to your attacker's torso. While this opportunity is "nice to have," often in dynamic situations it is not possible to make such an attack, as most of your effort will be on securing the arm and staying on your feet.

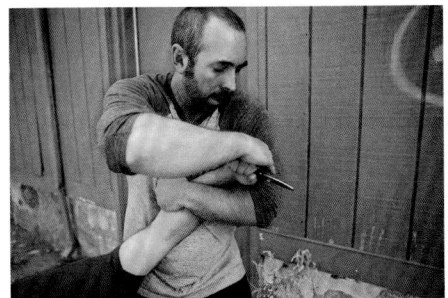

Keeping your assailant's arm locked to you (your left arm should be controlling their arm below the elbow—if you end up higher up, slide down the arm until you are in this position), bring your right hand over, placing your fingers and palm behind your attacker's knuckle line.

If you find you can't get deep enough to be over the knuckle line, it is likely that your left arm isn't close enough to the wrist, and you should slide down the arm toward it.

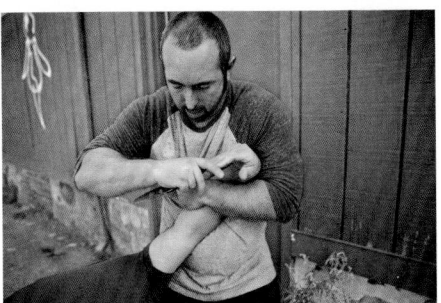

Pull strongly on their hand, folding it back toward the inside forearm, so that they are forced to release their grip on the knife. Use the three middle fingers to apply the pressure, and as the hand opens up, use your little finger to pull the knife out.

If you do this in one continuous motion, your little finger will pull the knife out and your middle fingers will be able to quickly wrap around the handle.

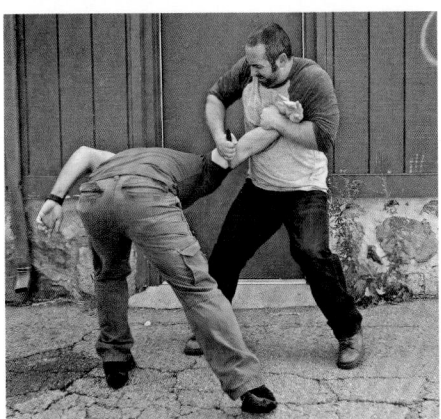

While still keeping hold of your assailant's arm, use their knife to make a deep cut around their upper arm/triceps. This is a necessary step to take, as you need to do something to disable/incapacitate your assailant so that they will be unable to continue the fight. Up to this point, you have done nothing to stop them from continuing to attack you.

Cutting their dominant arm (unless they are ambidextrous) will inhibit their ability to strike you or use another weapon they may be carrying.

Once you have disabled their arm, back away (the best way to cut them is to draw the knife through the muscle in one continuous motion, almost as if you were drawing a line around their arm with a pen).

As you back away, scan the environment and look for any other attackers and concealment points where someone could be waiting to assault you.

Blocks as Attacks

The first step in dealing with a knife attack is to protect yourself by making a solid block. You should think of your block as an offensive action, rather than a defensive one. Your blocking arm needs to attack the knife arm of your assailant with the aim of causing as much pain, damage, and trauma as possible. When an assailant attacks with a shanking action, they will do so repetitively, recoiling the knife to set up second and third attacks. Their attacks will have a rhythm to them, and part of your defense should be to break this rhythm so that you can prevent them from making multiple stabs/attacks. By striking into the knife arm and delivering a shot of pain to your attacker, you should cause them to hesitate as they react to your block/strike. This will give you a little extra time in which to execute your control.

The other reason for landing a solid strike on their knife arm is to prevent them from circling the knife and potentially cutting your forearm. Some assailants, when they stab, will bring the knife up and then pull it back in a circular fashion, so that their attack causes more trauma by opening up a larger wound. Even if your block manages to stop the knife from reaching your body (which should be judged as a success), as they cycle the knife back, they may end up dragging the blade across your inner forearm. If your block comes to meet their attack and strikes the knife arm before your assailant is in this recoil phase, you will prevent this from happening and have a better chance of controlling their weapon hand/arm.

If an attacker has any experience with a knife, they won't pull it directly back after shanking, but will rather aim to cause maximum damage by pulling it upward and back in a circular fashion.

The best way to prevent this movement from cutting your blocking arm is to make such a forceful block with your forearm that your assailant's attack, along with the recoil, is completely disrupted.

If your block isn't aggressive enough, your attacker will be able to drop their elbow and raise the blade in order to pull the knife back across the inside muscles of your blocking arm.

This is also one of the reasons you should start snaking your wrist around their arm in order to control it as soon as you've made the block.

If all this isn't done, your attacker will be able to pull the knife back, dragging the blade into your forearm and wrist. This will be an extremely forceful pull, and the cut will be a deep one, severing muscle and tendons.

Even if your attacker hasn't mechanically disabled your arm with the cut, they may well have caused you to become hesitant about using the arm to block with again.

It would be extremely difficult to force yourself to make the same block again, knowing the pain that could be involved in doing so. This is why it is so important that your first block is strong, and contains enough power and impact to interrupt the recoil motion of the knife.

If your attacker comes at you from your right side with a right-handed attack, you will not have the time to turn and block with your left arm, nor will you be able to move to the inside. Instead, you will have to block with your right arm, and move to their outside or "dead" side (the side away from their other arm). When blocking any strike, you should block with the nearest limb, rather than taking the time to position yourself so that you can block with your favored arm. This is one of the reasons it is good to practice defenses on both sides. While it can be harder to control an attacker from the outside, it is often easier to disengage from this position—which should always be your first option, especially where a knife is concerned.

In any situation, you must be flexible and able to adapt. Your initial thoughts may have been to control your attacker, disarm them of their weapon, and disengage; however, as the fight progresses/develops you may realize that you are dealing with a pain-resistant, highly motivated attacker who is intent on causing you extreme injury; i.e., you are fighting for survival. In such a situation, you will need a conclusive way of ending the conflict. It could be that disarming them will not deter them from continuing to fight, and that striking them is having little to no effect. One response in such a scenario is to use the attacker's knife against them while they are still holding it.

As you meet the attacker's arm with your block, avoid swiping or chopping it away. Your first job is to stop it dead, rather than redirect it, which would give it movement and a new direction from which to attack. You should now step to the side, circling your blocking arm around your attacker's elbow, making use of their recoil to pull you and your arm toward them. As you do this, keep your other hand up, covering your neck, so that if they try to redirect the knife toward you, you will be protected. This hand will also act to cover and control their knife hand and redirect the knife into their throat or neck.

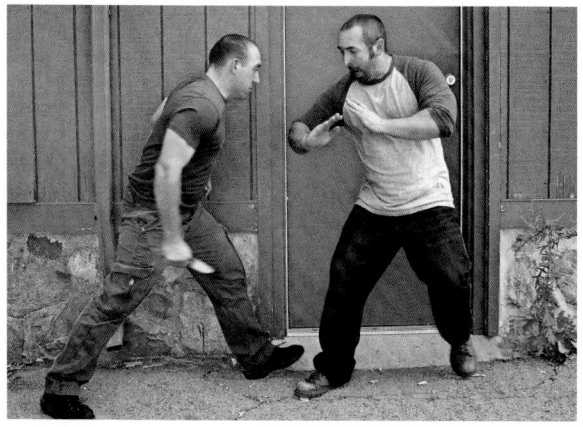

In this situation, your attacker shanks the knife toward your right side, which means you will have to block with your right arm; there won't be the time to turn and block with your left arm.

Your body will instinctively pull back from the attack, making your body defense. Your arm should drive out with the forearm horizontal, and forcefully impact your assailant's knife arm. Try to avoid making "chopping" motions from the elbow.

With your body pulled back away from the knife, make sure that your block has a 90-degree angle at the elbow. This will mean that you haven't chopped or deflected the attack, but have stopped it dead, taking away all the timing and recoil of the attack.

Your left arm should be up, guarding your neck, so that if the attacker were to suddenly move the knife around your elbow and toward your head, you will have a hand up, ready to block.

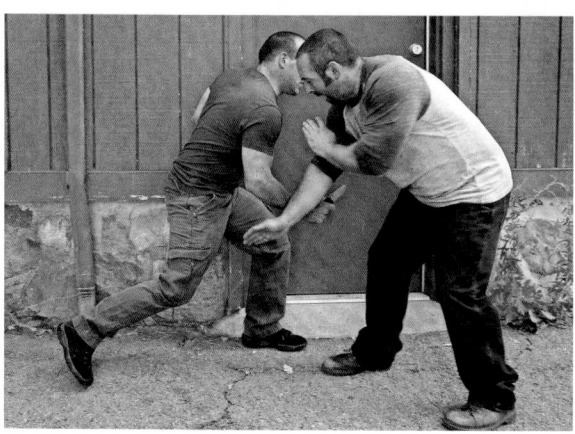

Start to snake your wrist around their arm in order to wrap/tie it to your body.

This is actually the same movement you made when the attack came from the other side, only on this occasion, you are going to clasp/wrap the inside of your attacker's arm, rather than the outside.

Continue to snake your hand under their arm, while keeping your other arm/hand up guarding your neck in case you lose control of their arm and they change their shank to a stab or slash to the throat.

Your arm should now start to wrap around your attacker's arm. You should be stepping/bursting forward as you make all of these movements so that your arm can get deep to the elbow. All the time, your other hand should stay up guarding your neck.

Start to wrap your arm over the crook of the elbow of your attacker's weapon arm. At the same time, continue to move your body toward your assailant. This will cause their arm to bend and bring the knife close to their own throat.

At the same time, bring up the hand that was guarding your throat and move it toward your assailant's knife hand.

Keep moving your body forward, toward your attacker, while at the same time pulling your assailant's forearm toward your chest and upper torso, taking away all movement from the knife.

Use your left hand to guide the knife to your attacker's throat/neck, using it to cut/slash him. Someone who is trying to shank/stab you is trying to kill you; therefore, for the sake of your own survival, you must be prepared to do what is necessary to incapacitate them.

Knife Shank When Seated

It may be that instead of following you outside, your assailant decides to attack you while you are still seated in the bar. The manner in which you are sitting can increase or decrease your survival chances greatly. Certain types of seating can restrict your movement more than others; for example, the type of molded and fixed tables/chairs that are used in many fast-food restaurants almost hold you in place, and need to be slid into and out of. Bench-type seating, such as that used on many types of public transport, is also restrictive, as the only way to stand up is to move the body forward. If sitting on a free-standing chair, on the other hand, it is possible to move the feet to the side of the chair so that they are under the body and stand directly up. If you believe that the situation around you is becoming dangerous, you should attempt to get to your feet at the earliest opportunity. If you are sitting on a chair, once up, you can also potentially use it as an improvised weapon.

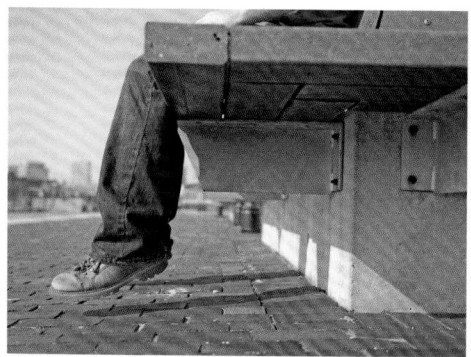

It would be naïve to assume that you will always be standing when you're assaulted. There are many situations in which we may find ourselves assaulted when sitting, such as when using public transport, when sitting in a pub or bar etc.

If you sit deep into a chair, seat, or bench, your center of gravity is a long way behind your feet, making it difficult to stand up quickly; in some instances, sitting this way could mean your feet won't even fully touch the floor.

By shifting your weight forward and possibly changing the way you sit, you can bring your center of gravity closer to your feet and assist yourself in getting up to standing much faster.

If you are seated and you detect that there may be harmful intent in your environment, you should adjust the way you sit so that you are able to get up quickly. This usually involves moving to the edge of the seat and straddling your legs to the side, rather than having them positioned to the front.

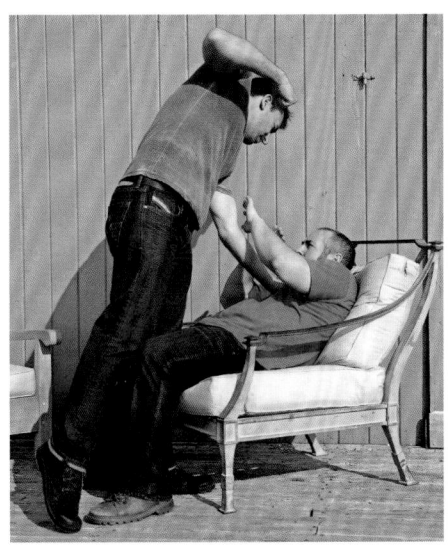

Many people, when they think about fighting from their back on the ground, forget that in real-life situations, the "ground" may involve seating. If your ground techniques require a lot of space and movement to work, you may find yourself having difficulty getting them to work in real-life settings/ environments.

Often "groundwork" in real-life incidents of violence involves fighting from your back in restricted spaces. It is often worth taking a training partner into the back seat of your car, positioning yourself on your back, and working out ways to adapt the techniques you would normally use so that they are effective in these restricted and confined spaces.

If you are attacked while seated, your first job is to get up and out of your seat. If you remain seated, you won't be able to utilize the power of your hips and legs or perform any type of body defense or disengagement.

When you are put in a disadvantaged position (something most assailants will try to do before they attack you), and are limited by time and position as to the responses that you can make, the essential components of a technique become evident, because these are all you will be able to do. In the case of dealing with knife shanks, the most important component of the defense is bursting into the attack as quickly and forcefully as you can.

There are certain body movements and positions that should immediately trigger a response. One of these is someone pulling their arm back sharply. As soon as you see this, you should start to move in toward whoever you are dealing with, whether you are seated or standing.

Start to stand up, bringing your hands into a position from which they can make a forceful block.

Dive/burst in toward your attacker. Your block should be coming out forcefully to meet the attack, rather than waiting for the knife to come to it.

With the speed of the attack, and the position you are in, all you should be thinking about is gaining control of the weapon arm before your attacker has time to recoil it and launch further attacks.

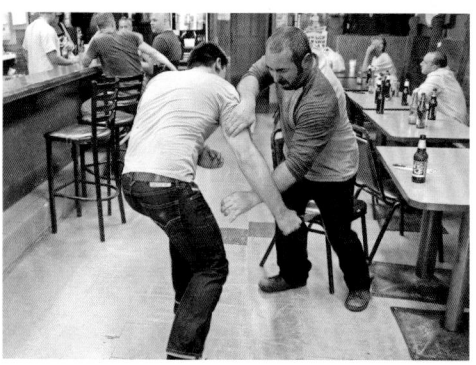

Once the block has been made—and not before you have stopped/interrupted the movement of the knife—start to snake/slide your blocking arm up under your attacker's weapon arm.

Your other hand should be placed on your attacker's upper arm/triceps, both rotating the arm so that the knife ends up pointing downward, and pulling you toward your attacker's arm. This should be coupled with your forward movement to get to your attacker's weapon arm as quickly as possible.

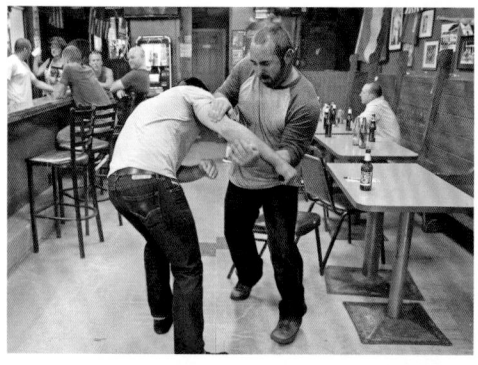

Start to wrap your arm under your assailant's weapon arm and pull it toward your chest; your body should still be traveling forward.

When you attempt to control the weapon arm, your number one priority is to take away the movement of the knife; if the knife can't move, it can't cut you. Blocking and striking should only be considered when you have the time to recognize an attack and where a quick disengagement from your attacker is possible.

Hugging the arm to your chest, making sure there is no space or room for movement, use your forward motion to deliver a knee strike. This is more to cause a distraction to your attacker and take their attention away from the knife (notice how it is instinctive for them to try and block the knee).

Make sure your control of the arm with your left arm is below the elbow on the forearm and wrist—this is where your assailant's leverage is weakest.

At this point you will have done little to disable your attacker—other than a knee strike, which may or may not have been particularly effective. One of the big myths that is often presented in self-defense classes is the reliability of striking. Often it is extremely difficult to deliver accurate, powerful, and concussive strikes in a dynamic confrontation, especially against a highly adrenalized attacker. This is why you will sometimes need other solutions.

Start to bring your right arm under the weapon arm, maintaining a strong grip on the attacker's wrist/forearm with your left.

Wrap and hug the arm to your body, making sure there is no room for it to move. Once you have the arm secure, slide your left hand to your attacker's weapon hand, clasping it firmly. You should now be holding the hand that is holding the knife.

If necessary, reposition your hand to your hips, so that the knife is low and pointed toward your attacker. At every opportunity, try to get behind the knife—in this position you won't be at risk of getting cut.

Keeping the weapon arm pressed against your body, start to drive your hips forward, pushing the knife toward your attacker.

You may want to grab your own clothing with the hand that is under your attacker's elbow. If you and your attacker are sweaty, this will prevent their arm from slipping out from your control.

As you drive your hips forward, pull/lean back with your upper body. This has the effect of upsetting your attacker's balance and pulling them toward you; that is, bringing them onto the knife. This, coupled with your hips driving forward, will allow you to deliver a powerful stab into your attacker's side.

Improvised Weapon—Ceramic Plate Knife

If you are seated in a restaurant or bar where there are ceramic plates, you can craft yourself a ceramic knife extremely easily. When considering the use of an improvised weapon, it is usually better to choose something that can deliver concussive force (such as an unbroken bottle), rather than something that can cut (like a broken bottle, or in this case a ceramic knife). With a solid object that can deliver solid blows, you are likely to render an attacker unconscious far more quickly than you would by cutting/slashing them. Improvised cutting tools are useful if you need to clear your way through a crowd. People will pull away and try to clear space to get away from someone who is slashing with a blade or other sharp object.

This will work with any ceramic plate; however, it works best with smaller side plates, as opposed to larger dinner plates. In a restaurant, these are usually the ones that the bread is brought on, so they are relatively clean and can be gripped well.

Put your four fingers on the back of the plate, with your thumb on the front. Spread your four fingers out as flat and wide as possible to cover as much of the back of the plate as possible, and then smash the face of it downward against the edge of the table.

The noise of you doing this will also alert and draw the attention of people in your environment, so they will be able to see you brandish your improvised knife, and hopefully stay away from you.

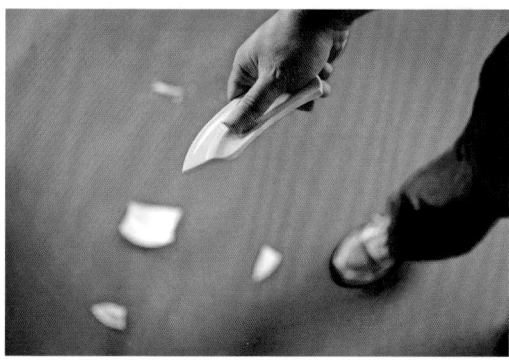

You will now be left with some pieces of ceramic that have sharp cutting edges and resemble something like a conventional knife.

Rather than using it as a stabbing tool, slash it at anyone who comes close to you, clearing a path to your nearest and safest exit point.

Troubleshooting the Knife Shank

No matter how much you practice and train, there is always the possibility that things will not go to plan, and you have to be able to adapt and change what you are doing accordingly. If you only ever train and practice techniques without considering what to do when an attacker reacts and responds to what you are doing, there is a huge and dangerous gap between your training and reality.

There are times when it isn't possible to get a good rotation on your assailant's knife arm, which means that the knife will end up pointed upward rather than with the blade down. There are several reasons why this could happen. Your assailant could have been fighting your control of their arm, attempting to slide the knife up toward your neck as you pulled it toward your chest. In this instance, you will need to be able to deal with the knife when it pointed upward. Because their palm is facing toward you, it is difficult to disarm from this position. You will need to get their arm to rotate before you attempt to take the knife.

As soon as you see the knife, burst forward to meet it. It doesn't matter if it is being pulled back to make the initial stab and isn't yet travelling forward. Your goal is to get both of your arms wrapped around the weapon arm as soon as possible.

As you dive/burst forward, you may fail to get the necessary rotation on the arm to get the knife pointed down, and/or your attacker may start to change their attack and try to bring the knife up toward your neck/throat. This means the knife will be pointing up when you have finished wrapping your arms around the weapon arm.

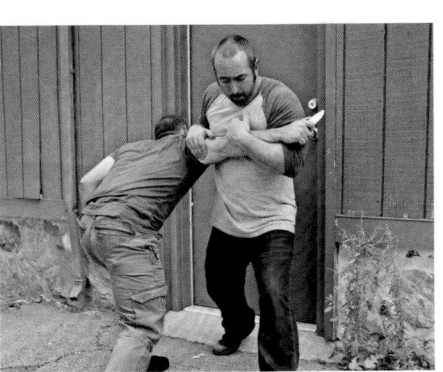

Although this is not ideal, you will have still accomplished the most important part, which was to trap the weapon arm and prevent any further movement of the blade. If from here you simply threw a series of knee strikes and moved back, dragging your assailant toward the ground before disengaging, you would have effectively solved the problem.

There could, however, be environmental factors preventing you from doing this, such as a wall behind you.

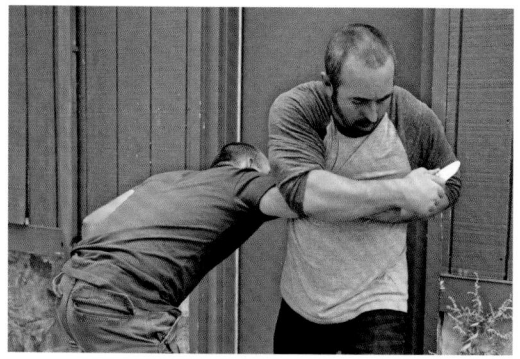

If this is the case, you will need to perform a disarm.

Keeping a secure grip on your attacker's weapon arm with your left arm, reach over with your right and take hold of your assailant's hand—the one that is holding the knife.

Once you have this secured, slide your left hand down and grab your attacker's wrist. Use your right arm to keep your assailant's arm pinned to your chest as you do this. Once again, your goal is to maintain control and deny the knife any space in which to move.

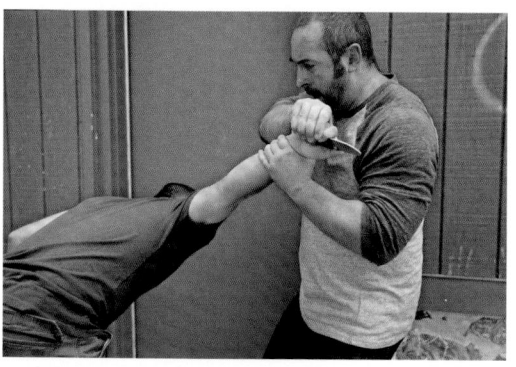

Now turn out with your body while stepping back. As you do this, start to rotate your assailant's arm.

It is important to take a step back as you do this; otherwise, you will be bringing the attacker's knife extremely close to your face. Although there is not a lot that your attacker could do from this position, it is always worth keeping the knife away from you when the blade is pointing in your direction.

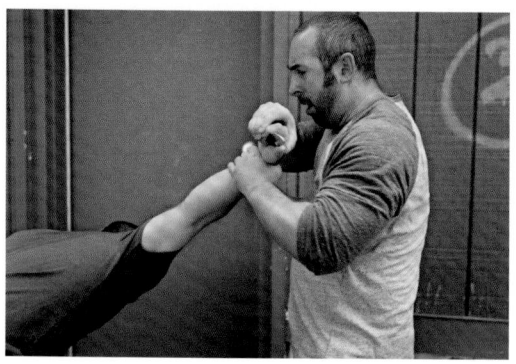

Once the arm has been completely turned over, push on the back of your assailant's knuckles with your right hand in order to force their grip on the knife to be released.

If they have a really strong grip on the knife, you can quickly release your right hand and slam it into their grip, as a palm-heel strike, to force their hand to open.

Keep pushing until their grip releases enough for you to scoop the knife out of their hand.

Once you have the knife, make a deep cut to their upper arm, cutting muscle and tendon. Your goal is to make sure it is mechanically unable to operate. This means that if they choose to continue the fight, they will be unable to use this limb to either strike or grab you, and/or to operate another weapon.

Ice-Pick Attack

"Ice-pick" attacks, in which the assailant holds the knife in an overhand grip and brings it downward toward your head and/or upper torso, are not the most common knife attacks you are likely to face. It is, however, important to know how to defend against them, as they signal an attacker's intent to kill you. Stabbing motions, as opposed to slashing ones (at least with untrained individuals), are intended to be fatal. A person who stabs rather than slashing has only one outcome in mind, and that is not to maim, wound, or incapacitate, but to kill. This may not have been their goal when they initiated the assault, but as they become more emotionally charged within it, their conscious control is reduced, and they enter an animalistic survival mode that makes them interpret the conflict as "kill or be killed." They could also start the assault in a state of extreme rage, with the goal of killing their intended target(s) from the outset.

Because these types of attack are emotionally charged, the attack is likely to be frenzied in nature, with the knife being moved rapidly, with fast recoils and repeated stabs. It is also probable that the angle of the attack will be altered if the stab is met with resistance (e.g., if the person defending themselves manages to get an arm up to block the attack). Dealing with someone in such an adrenalized state, who is probably going to be pain resistant or pain tolerant as a result, and who is committed to their goal, should be avoided at all costs.

Using Glisha Kick

If you have the time and space, your first response to someone making an ice-pick-style attack (after attempting to disengage, putting a barrier between you and them, obtaining a weapon, etc.) should be to try to move them away from you, using a strong kick (utilizing *glisha*/sliding) to the upper torso/ribcage. Kicking at this height will mean that they will be pushed back, whereas a lower kick might cause them to fold over and bend forward, bringing the knife closer to you. The kick should be delivered with maximum force, pushing your assailant backward and thus interrupting their attack. This is the time to put distance between yourself and your assailant.

Most fights happen at extremely close range. There are times, however, when you may be able to create distance between yourself and your assailant. There are also times where an attacker may run at you from distance in order to add momentum to their attack; this normally signals that they are in an extremely heightened emotional state. If this happens, rather than backing away, you should start to move toward your assailant, generating your own momentum.

As you step forward, start to lift up your opposite knee. With this action, you should start to lift your weight up off the supporting leg so that it will be able to slide.

The knee should be lifted high, and the angle between the upper and lower leg should be 90 degrees, so that you will be able to extend the leg forcefully toward your attacker.

It is at about this point that you should start your glisha/sliding step.

Propel your weight forward, sliding on your supporting leg. At the same time, thrust your kick out toward your attacker. Your kick should have your body's forward momentum adding to its power.

It is important that you slide, rather than hop/jump. If you hop, much of your forward momentum will be lost in the upward movement.

As you move into your attacker, extend the leg further to push them away.

By kicking your attacker's chest, you will propel them backward. If you hit their stomach or groin, they may well just bend forward at the waist, bringing the knife toward you.

In such a dynamic setting, a head kick would be extremely difficult to pull off, as the target is much smaller, and liable to be moving.

As your attacker is thrown back and their attack disrupted, recoil your leg (don't fall forward toward your attacker) and disengage from the situation. There is little to be gained by trying to engage with a highly emotional and committed assailant who has demonstrated their intent to kill you.

Disarming and Controlling

Most attacks will happen at close range, where there is neither the time nor the space to deliver such a kick. At this range you will have to use your hands/arms to block and control the weapon. Your most important task is to deal with the recoil action of the knife. With your assailant in such an emotional state, it is unlikely that any strikes you make will register with them—unless you manage to land a knockout blow, which is extremely unlikely. Any strikes you do make should have the goal of impeding and disrupting your assailant's movement in order to create a disengagement opportunity. This, however, becomes extremely difficult when an attack is at such close range.

When an ice-pick-style attack is made at close range, your goal should be to burst forward and wrap your assailant's arm under your armpit. There are times, however, when you won't get enough forward momentum to do this, and you will end up not being deep enough to make it happen. This will also be difficult to achieve if you are caught off guard (a distinct possibility), forcing you to make the most of your initial defense using just the arm.

If you are surprised and caught off guard, the movement of the knife will likely cause you to flinch, bringing your arm up in order to defend yourself. This is a natural, instinctive movement.

Because of the surprise element of the attack, you will not be ready to burst forward, and so will have to deal with the attack in a much more "defensive" manner.

You should start to wrap your hand over your attacker's weapon arm, with the eventual goal of continuing to wrap your entire arm around theirs, locking it under your elbow. If you are not deep enough to control the arm, you will need to control the wrist instead.

At this point, your blocking arm has a 90-degree angle at the elbow, and the hand has started to snake around the wrist.

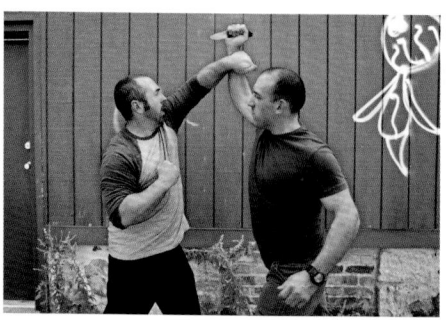

Your goal is to get your hand to form a hook around the attacker's wrist before they start the recoil motion of the attack (i.e., before they start to pull the knife back to stab again). If your block was forceful enough, it should have interrupted the rhythm of the attack and created enough of a pause for you to hook the wrist.

If they pull back forcibly while you have this hook, you should take advantage of this pulling action and move forward into them, punching them with your right hand.

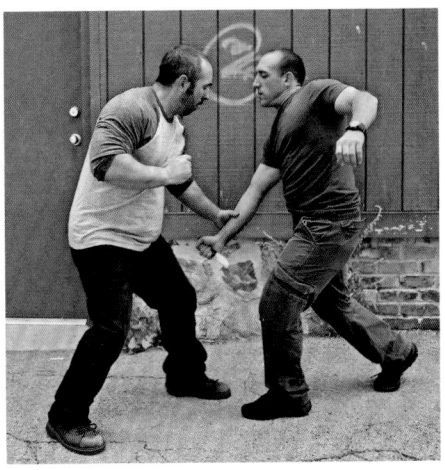

Move your arm outward in a circular motion, using your hand as a hook to scoop their weapon arm.

At this point, you are not gripping on to their arm; your thumb should be next to your fingers.

As the weapon arm is brought down, bring your thumb around their arm and start to slide your hand down toward their wrist.

As your hand moves down the arm, get ready to grab the wrist firmly (you will need to wait until you get to the wrist before you make your grip, as the forearm itself is often too big to get a solid grasp on).

Once you have hold of their wrist, pull your attacker's arm across your body diagonally; this will twist your attacker's body and unbalance them.

You should be pulling the arm until it is fully extended. When an arm is put at full extension, a person's grip will start to loosen. This is a good time to move your hand toward theirs in order to open their hand up.

Push on the back of the knuckles and start to move in toward your attacker. This should start to cause their arm to bend and allow you to get some bodyweight over the knife to assist you as you push on the back of the hand.

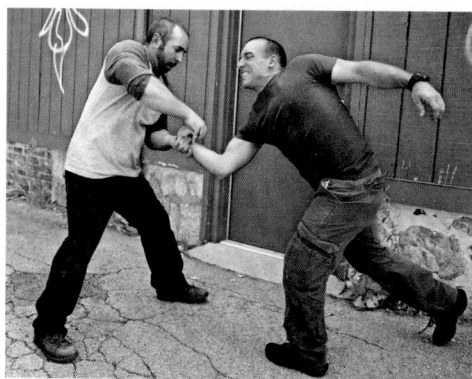

Step and lean your weight over your assailant's weapon arm, and push down, forcing the hand to open.

This downward motion should also break your attacker's frame, so that they are put in a biomechanically disadvantaged position.

The palm of your hand should push on the back of their hand, on the knuckle line or lower. This will cause the weapon hand to start to open up, allowing your fingers to reach over and under their grip and take the knife.

As you scoop the knife from their hand, step back and pull away. Disengage from the incident as quickly as possible, making your way to safety. You may have to put obstacles and barriers between yourself and your attacker first, if they choose to come after you. You may also want to look for an improvised weapon, such as a piece of scaffolding or pipe, that could be used to maintain range and deliver concussive force; i.e., a tool that will probably end the fight more rapidly than the knife would.

Do not assume that just because you have managed to disarm your attacker, the fight will be over. Your assailant may have another weapon; they may have friends/associates who have started to come to their assistance; or they may be so committed to their cause that they will continue the assault regardless of the fact that you are now armed. Whenever you disarm someone of a weapon, you need to be prepared and ready to use it against them. It is very dangerous to presume that disarming is where the fight ends.

Reverse Slash—Swaying

Krav Maga is a system based on natural responses and reactions. When a circular motion (such as a knife stab or slash) enters into a person's peripheral vision, they will instinctively flinch. Hopefully a successful block will be made; if they're trained, then a standard 360 block and response should be made. However, when the slashing movement is detected late, the natural response may not be to block, but to lean back instead, pulling your head out of the way. While this is a good initial defense, it does not put you in a good position to deal with a second or third attack, as it puts your body in a severely compromised position. Although you may be in a balanced position, you will not be in a stable one, and are therefore susceptible to further attack.

As soon as you can, you will need to get into a more stable and offensive position. If your attacker misses with a slash, it is natural for them to simply perform a reverse slash in the hope of connecting with the target they just missed. This means that as you move your body forward to get your head and shoulders over your hips, you must perform a 360 block to ensure that you aren't caught with this reverse slash. At the same time, you should use your other arm to help control the movement of the attacking arm, and, using both, position the knife so it can be used against your assailant.

In this scenario, the aggressor pulls a knife and starts to slash it toward your head. Ideally, you would burst in and control it, but being in an unprepared position like this means that you will not be able to do so.

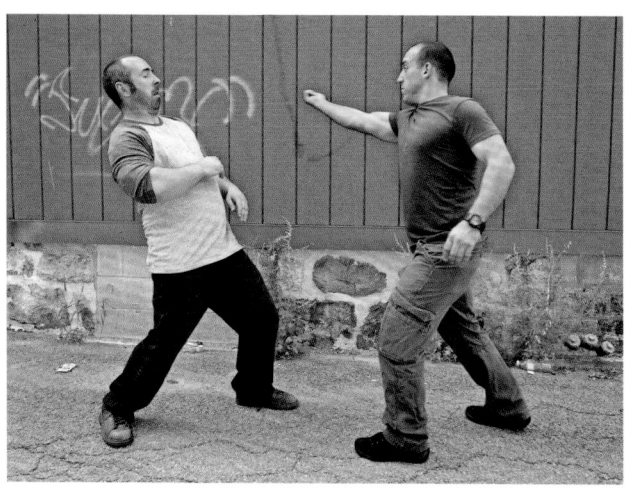

If the slash is very fast, your natural reflexes will pull you away from the attack, rather than causing you to flinch and bring your hands up.

Although this will initially make you safe, you won't be in a good position to deal with a follow-up attack, and unless you prevent the knife from moving, that is what your attacker will do.

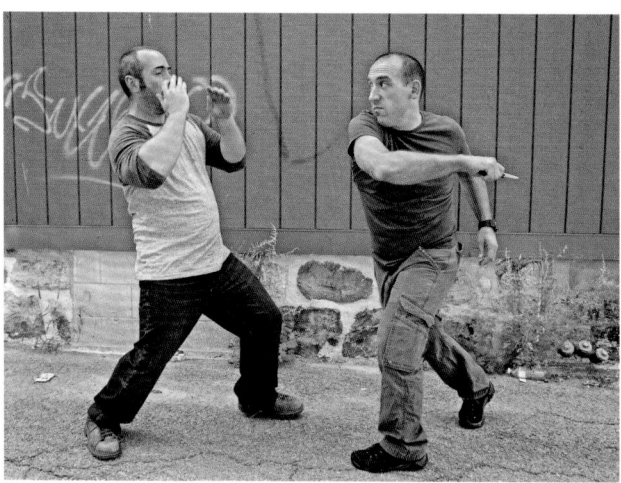

Bringing both hands up to defend, start to burst forward so that you can meet your assailant's reverse slash. This is the most likely attack that they will make, having failed to connect with their initial attack.

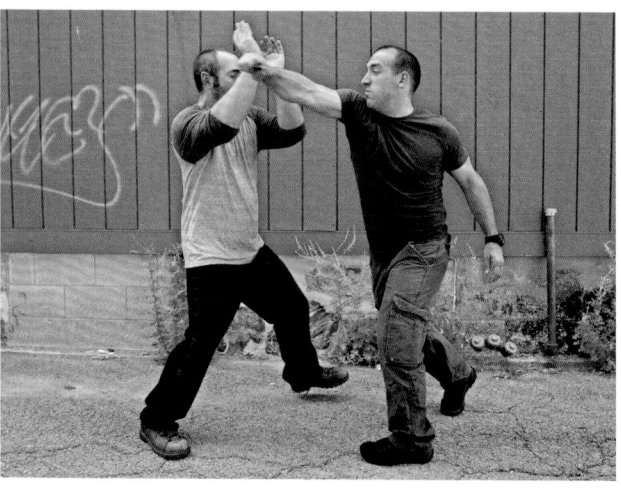

Both arms should come up: one is to take the impact of the slash—this is why you should be moving/bursting into the attack with momentum. The other is to reach behind your attacker's elbow.

Even if the slash is relatively wild and uncontrolled, your assailant may respond to the block by trying to draw their knife across your arms in order to cut them; this is a fairly effective way of getting you to pull back away from the knife, which will open you up to further attacks.

With your left arm behind your attacker's elbow, this movement will be prevented.

If your second arm is not there to restrict this drawing motion, you will end up with your arm being cut, and your attacker having the room to make another attack.

With the second arm up behind your assailant's elbow, the natural motion and movement of the knife will be restricted. Your assailant would have to pull the knife back toward them if they wanted to attack again.

As soon as you feel the impact of the block, start to hook your wrist over your assailant's arm in order to wrap your arm around it and pull it to your body. Once again, your goal is to take away all the movement of the weapon arm.

At the same time, start to move forward to your assailant's side so that you are behind the knife.

One way you can assist yourself in getting behind the blade is to use your left arm to put pressure on your attacker's upper arm. This will start to lock the arm out and bend them forward. This also has the benefit of breaking their base and their ability to counter what you are doing.

As you do this, pull your attacker's knife hand to your hips, so that it is locked onto your body. You should still be applying pressure to your assailant's upper arm/triceps so that their stability is compromised.

This action upon their upper arm, coupled with your movement to their side, should take their balance and cause them to spin.

As they are still spinning and concentrating on their balance, take your arm off the back of their arm and bring it under their elbow. The hand holding the knife should remain pinned to your hips.

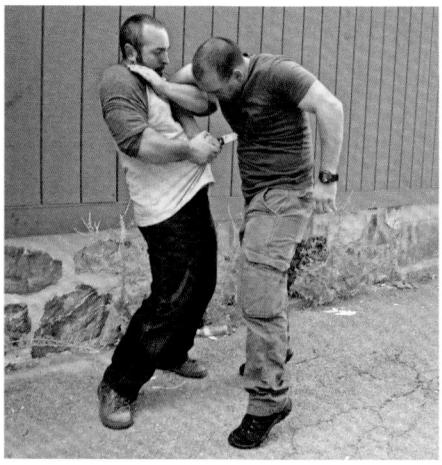

Bring your left hand up to your chest, pinning your attacker's forearm to your body, taking away all of the knife's movement and positioning yourself behind the blade.

Thread your arm all the way through so that the crook of your elbow is under the crook of your assailant's elbow. This means that your attacker would have to pull their arm across the entire length of your forearm to escape your control.

Once your assailant's arm is locked to your body, drive your hips forward, forcing their knife into their body. If necessary, you can pull your hips back and repeat this action until your attacker is no longer a threat.

Armed Assaults—Conclusion

If you can prevent a weapon from being drawn in the first place, you will solve a lot of problems for yourself, especially when dealing with a spontaneously violent situation where your aggressor has no predetermined outcome in mind. If it is a mugger, you will already know what they want, and what is likely to prevent them from using their weapon.

When someone threatens you with a weapon, they usually do so because they have an outcome in mind; a mugger, for example, wants your wallet. The easiest way to prevent such a predator from using their weapon is to hand the wallet over. If they go "off script" by staying after they have your valuables rather than walking away, you will then need to enact a physical solution.

When determining solutions to your situation, don't get caught up in considering variables that aren't relevant to your survival. A common variable that people consider when deciding whether to hand over their wallet is the amount of money that they are carrying; for example, if they are carrying less than $100, they'll hand the wallet over; if more, then they won't. This is an issue of ego rather than survival, as the amount of money you are carrying isn't directly proportional to your ability to physically deal with your assailant. That is, you don't become technically more proficient at knife controls and disarms based on the amount of money you are carrying. Understand that if you don't hand over what they are asking for, you will have to enact a physical solution, or risk getting cut/shot, etc. If you are carrying large amounts of cash, you may want to think about only carrying in your wallet the amount you'd be prepared to hand over, and carrying the rest in other places about your person. It may even be worth your while to carry two wallets—one with a slim profile, containing your drivers' license and most-used credit card, as well as some cash in larger bills; and a larger wallet containing expired cards and smaller bills, which you will hand over if mugged (most muggings are committed by drug addicts looking for enough money for their next fix).

In the picture are two "wallets". One is a traditional-looking wallet containing items such as loyalty, library, and business cards, along with a couple of expired credit cards. Muggings happen quickly, with little time for muggers to check these details, and in most instances muggers aren't interested in credit cards; they want cash. This wallet has about $20 in a number of denominations to make the amount look bigger. The other "wallet" has active credit cards, driver's license, and some cash.

The bigger wallet is the decoy. Everything in it has either a low monetary worth or can be easily replaced. It also has a much larger footprint. This is the one that you hand over if you are mugged.

The smaller wallet is slim fitting, and is unlikely to be detected even if your assailant pats you down as part of the robbery. It is also likely that once they find the larger wallet, they'll give up their search.

PART IV

Unarmed Assaults

Most violent incidents happen face to face, and involve some form of verbally aggressive exchange before any physical attack occurs. The initial attack is often very simple in nature, and not particularly dangerous; e.g., a push, a grab, etc. In many instances, people don't understand the significance or the danger of the attack, because there is no pain associated with it; however, these types of assault are normally a precursor to something more serious, such as a punch or a slash or stab. It is not the clothing grab or push that is the real danger—it is what will follow it.

It is also worth noting that these types of attacks often occur because the person is not yet emotionally ready to punch or hit you, and they are using the grab or push as a form of emotional escalation to get themselves ready to strike. If you can react to their grab or push straight away, you will actually have put them behind you on the curve and taken the initiative/advantage.

Clothing Grabs

It is easy to get caught up thinking about worst-case scenarios—being choked out, finding oneself on the ground, dealing with multiple assailants, etc.—and forget that the most common violent altercations usually involve simple, non-complex assaults such as pushing and grabbing. The vast majority of potential assailants haven't received any formal training, and so the types of attacks they are capable of making are usually relatively simple, such as pushing their victim and then punching them while they are off balance. If an attacker has a history of fighting, they will have learned that it is more important to out-match their intended target in terms of aggression rather than in technical ability. Most fights end when one party finds that they are emotionally, rather than physically, unable to continue, and so decides to take themselves out of the fight.

Some of the simplest forms of assault you may face will involve grabs to your clothing. These may be combined with punches and strikes, or act as precursors to such attacks, allowing your assailant to position you and restrict your movement to make their punches more effective. Someone may also grab you as a means of intimidation—perhaps grabbing both of your lapels as they verbally threaten you.

Clothing grabs are a simple and effective way of controlling and restricting someone's body movement. If someone manages to grab both of your lapels and has a good grip on your clothing, they will have a solid hold on you, and will be able to use this to move you around. Simply pulling away from them will be extremely difficult, as you will be unable to move your clothing in a way that affects their grip as you would be able to do if they were grabbing your wrist; i.e., you could turn and move the wrist in a variety of directions that can loosen their grip.

Lapel Grab—Combative Approach

Krav Maga is an approach to fighting that is based on concepts and principles, one of which is, "If an attack is life-threatening, attack the attack; if it is not, attack the attacker." When someone grabs your wrist or your clothing, the attack is not life-threatening—in itself it may not even be painful—and so the simplest and most straightforward option is to forget about the "grab" and start striking your attacker.

When striking, you should work from the premise that your "nearest weapon attacks the nearest target." If your hands are down, strike the groin; if your hands are up, the eyes or the throat—these are the targets on the body that don't require a great amount of force to have an effect. You should be aware that because you are being held (especially if it is a two handed lapel grab), you may not be able to generate a lot of power or force, and until your assailant releases you—in order to get away and protect themselves from your strikes—you may be restricted to attacking these areas or targets with "soft" strikes such as groin slaps, eye rakes, cradle-strikes to the throat, etc.

After accidentally knocking into someone, you may find yourself suddenly being grabbed and pushed into a wall before you have time to adopt your de-escalation stance or say anything. In such a situation, your aggressor will be too emotional to be talked down, and you will have no room to disengage. Therefore, you will need to be decisive and respond physically before they escalate the situation further. With your hands up, you should look for the nearest targets on the body that you can reach.

Solutions don't have to be complicated; they can be as simple and straightforward as getting fingers and thumbs into a person's eyes. Your hands are your nearest weapon to the target (their eyes) and so this should dictate how and what you attack. You might follow up your initial attack with hammer-fists and/or other strikes, or simply disengage.

If you find that your hands are low, don't waste time by bringing them up toward your attacker's eyes—a movement they may see and be able to react to—but instead strike the nearest target; i.e., the groin. For maximum effect, use either the palm or the back of the hand to slap upward. It may be that you don't make a solid and painful strike to the groin; however, just making contact should cause your attacker to pull their hips back, putting them in a disadvantaged position.

Lapel Grab—Thumb Lock

There is sometimes a difference between choosing the best solution and going with an effective one. If someone grabs your lapel (or your wrist), striking them and assaulting them could be an effective solution; but, depending on the situation, it may not be the best one. If you are in a bar and you get into a verbal altercation with someone, the chances are that they are not alone; they may well be out with friends. If, in the course of the dispute/argument, they grab your lapel and you respond by striking and punching them, it is likely that their friends, if in the bar, will come to their assistance, and you will find yourself having to deal with multiple assailants. In such situations, it may be more appropriate to try a more discreet solution.

If someone grabs you, pushes you, or even just stands in your way, blocking and restricting your movement, and you have reason to fear for your safety, it is an assault. Don't be under the illusion that someone has to punch you for it to be an assault (that would be assault and battery). If someone grabs your clothing, you are entitled to defend yourself. This may involve punching/striking them. However, this may not always be the best option for dealing with the situation.

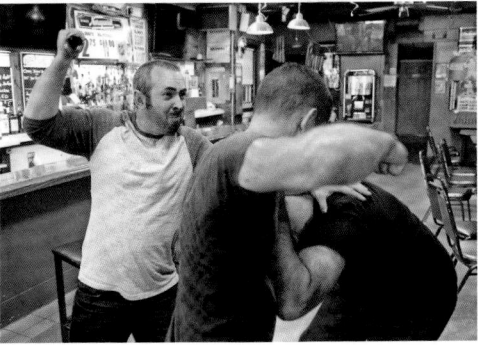

It is dangerous to assume that a fight will only involve you and the person in front of you who you are engaging with. In real life, a fight involves controlling the environment—not just the assailant you see. In fact, you may be enjoying a lot of success against your primary assailant, but because you are so narrowly focused on them, you will fail to see their friend who is coming to assist them, armed with a glass bottle. In this case, you would be failing to control your environment.

Despite having dealt successfully with the person who grabbed your clothing, you are now in a multiple-attacker scenario involving at least one armed assailant. In fact, there is nothing to say that the person who grabbed you (your primary assailant) isn't armed as well, and won't pull their weapon now that they have the time and space. In this situation, "attacking the attacker" has proved dangerous, and so using a more discreet technique would have been a better plan.

Principles are not solutions—they should guide us, but not blind us. Attacking the attacker, if it is a non-life-threatening attack, is a good rule of thumb to work from; however, it is the situation that should determine your solution. In the situation above, drawing the attention of others by attacking your assailant in this way would not be a good solution. Instead, a "softer" solution might be more effective. Rather than combatively assaulting your aggressor, it may be worth forcing them to release their hold on you. If you put extreme pressure on their thumb by locking the joint, you may be able to engage them in a simple pain-compliance process. Pain compliance works by putting a person in some form of lock or control where you have the ability to both increase and decrease their level of discomfort. For instance, if they struggle against the lock/hold, you can increase their pain and instruct them, "Calm down." If they comply, you can reduce the level of pain they are experiencing. In effect, you are educating them that when they comply, their pain decreases, and when they don't, it increases.

Pain compliance should be used wisely. At some point, you will have to release your lock, and if the person you were controlling has not calmed down, then you will have to engage with them in a physical confrontation. Also, if you are unable to immediately control the situation, after a while your assailant's friends may come looking for them, and you will find yourself having to deal with multiple assailants.

Perhaps the most important thing to take from the pain-compliance process is that one of the tools you have available to you is your voice, and there are times when it is appropriate and effective to use it—to talk to, inform, and control your assailant.

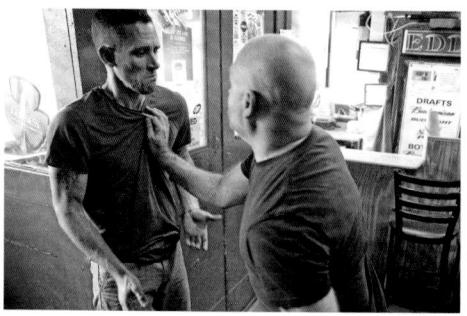

Although responding with punches and strikes would be an effective way to deal with this attack, in many situations (especially social ones), it would be dangerous to assume that you'll be dealing with only one assailant. Instead of striking, start to raise your left hand up, under your assailant's wrist. It is important to keep your palm facing up. If you try and grab overhand, your elbow will flare out, alerting your attacker to what you are doing.

Both of your hands should raise up at the same time. Your left hand should take hold of the attacker's wrist, while your right goes toward your assailant's thumb. If your attacker was to hold you with two hands rather than one, you would make exactly the same movement.

Once you have both of your hands on your attacker's wrist and hand, position your right thumb against their right thumb and push to compress it. Then start to push your attacker's hand down so that they start to release their grip.

Your thumb should be pushing on the nail of their thumb. Apply pressure both forward and upward (pushing upward helps if your attacker has flexible joints, and doesn't feel any pressure when the thumb is pushed back; they may have flexibility in one direction, but they are unlikely to have it in two).

You can push the attacking hand as far away from you as you need to. If you want to be discreet, keep your attacker more upright and talk to them, using pain compliance to control and de-escalate the situation. If you want to disengage, push your attacker as far away from you as you can, directing their elbow downward, so that their base and frame are broken.

You can also use this lock to take someone to ground if you feel the need to control and incapacitate them further.

If you need to completely control your assailant, either to create more time for you to disengage or to be in a more dominant position so that your pain compliance will be more effective, you may want to control/ take your attacker to ground. When you control and take an assailant to the ground, you should make sure they are positioned with their face to the floor, rather than their back. When they are face down, it is hard for them to use their second hand either to grab/attack you or to draw a weapon, etc.

To get your attacker to ground, keep rotating their wrist in a counterclockwise direction. As you pull your assailant forward, they will want to use their other hand to support themselves as they go to ground; this means they will not be able to use it to pull a weapon.

You can use your shin to help lock out their arm and direct them forward. You should still be applying pressure on their thumb as you do this.

Once you have them on the ground, you can either use pain/compliance to de-escalate the situation, and/or pull forcefully upward on their wrist, against your shin so that you hyper-extend and dislocate their elbow. Be aware that with many arm-bars of this nature that once you have dis-located the joint, the arm will snap back into place and may remain func-tional—if your attacker is highly adre-nalized, they may not register the pain of it, in that moment.

Double-Handed Lapel Grab

All of the defenses we are demonstrating against lapel grabs will work, whether it is a one-handed or two-handed grab. The problem that you may have against a double-handed lapel grab is that your assailant can use your clothing to push and pull you, throwing you around. This can make punching and striking very difficult to pull off, as you won't have a stable base from which to strike with any power. To try to reduce the movement of being thrown around, you will need to gain control of your attacker's wrist/hand, pulling it tightly to your chest so that they are locked on to you. Once that is done, they will have to push and pull your full bodyweight rather than just your clothing, meaning they are having to move a dead weight with each push/pull. The best time to try to grab their wrist is when they are in the push (rather than the pull) phase, as their hand will remain in contact with your body the longest during this phase of the attack. It's also when you can feel the attack rather than just seeing it.

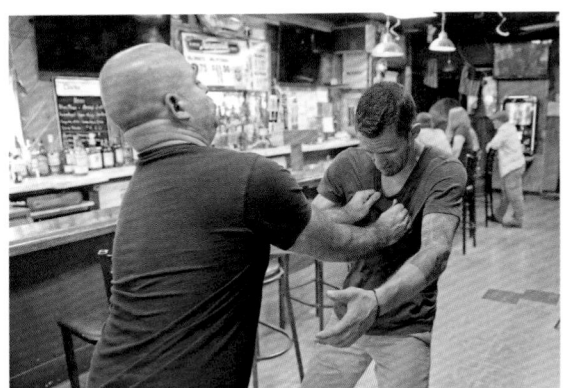

Real-life violence is dynamic, messy and frantic; something that is rarely captured or repli-cated in the training environment. Although a lapel/clothing grab can occur as a static threat, it is often used as a way of moving and throwing someone around.

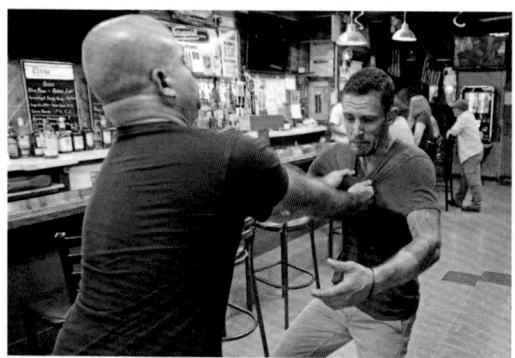

While you are being pushed and pulled around, with your assailant throwing you around like a ragdoll, you will not be in a position to strike and punch, whether this would be an effective solution or not.

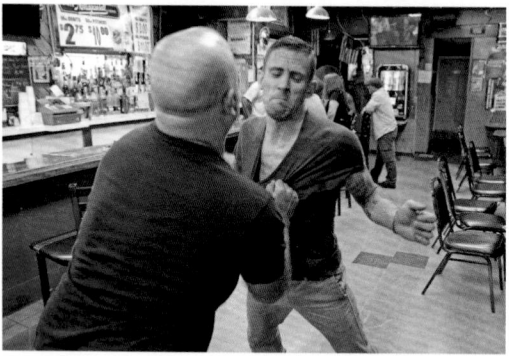

Before you can strike effectively, even with strikes to soft targets such as the eyes, which don't require any power behind them to be effective, you will need to at least be balanced. If you are being thrown around, all your thoughts and efforts will be directed at staying on your feet.

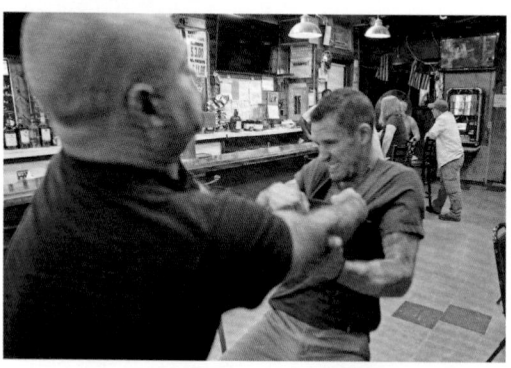

This means that your first concern should be to get based and stop being thrown around and disoriented. To do this, you must grab one or both of your assailant's arms and pull it/them toward your chest so that you can lock them onto you.

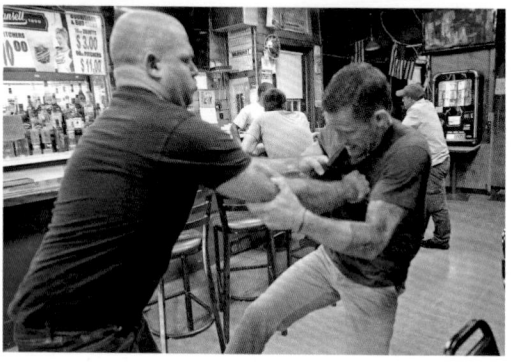

If you can pull their hand(s) to your chest, they will not be able to throw you around in your clothing, because they will now be pushing and pulling the "dead weight" of your body, rather than having your clothing amplify their pulls and pushes. Once they are locked to you, you can choose to strike them or use the thumb release/control explained previously.

When dealing with a two-handed grab, your first concern should be to tuck your chin to your chest so that your face isn't exposed to an assailant who is intent on head-butting you. If they do try to head-butt you, they will end up connecting with the thickest part of your skull, which, though painful for you, will hurt them just as much, or more.

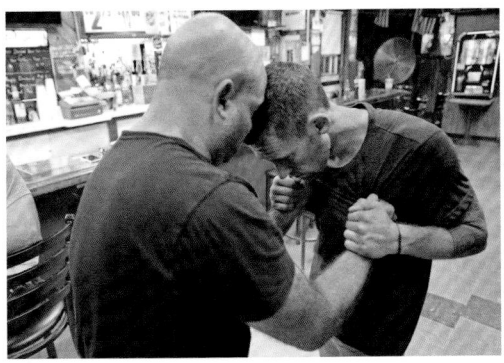

A common attack that follows a two-handed lapel/clothing grab is the head-butt. Head-butts are extremely effective and devastating strikes that are extremely difficult to recover from. If used correctly, they are likely to result in a serious concussion. If someone grabs your lapels, immediately drop your head, tucking your chin toward your chest. If your assailant delivers a head-butt when your head is in this position, they will end up smashing their face into the solid bone of your skull.

Lapel Grab—Wrist Lock

There are times when you might feel that you need a control hold that can be utilized while you protect/defend yourself. If you feel, when a person grabs you, that they are holding you in order to strike/punch you, then using both hands to deal with the lapel grab (such as with the thumb lock) isn't wise, as you will probably be hit before your attacker registers enough pain to disrupt their attack. It is possible to get your initial control on your assailant's hand/wrist while positioning the arm doing this in such a way that it shields your face/head.

Pushes and clothing grabs (and an initial push may turn into a grab) are used to set up a punch. In such an instance, your first job is to make yourself safe by covering your head. Sometimes a punch or strike will come when your balance is upset and you are disoriented. Trying to intercept a punch with a block when in this state is almost impossible, so your best way to deal with such an attack is to bring your hand up and cover your head. If you can do this as the person is pulling the arm back to make the punch, all the better.

You can use this blocking/covering movement to grab hold of your attacker's hand. Your left hand should come up at the same time to join the right, so that both hands are holding onto it. It is important to grab the hand that is holding your clothing, rather than the wrist. You want the wrist to be free to move for this technique.

Start to take a step back with your right leg, and use this body motion to help your hands rotate your attacker's arm. You should keep rotating it until the little (pinky) finger is pointing up. This equates to about a 180-degree rotation of the assailant's arm.

Once the arm has been rotated into this position, use your hands to push up and bend your assailant's wrist, taking all movement away from it; then lean in and over so that your bodyweight assists this movement. This is a painful lock and mechanical movement that will force your assailant to drop to the ground.

Keep pressing down with your body until you can go no further.

Once you have reached the point where you can press down no more, release your hands and raise your left foot high in the air...

...and then with full force, stomp down on the back of your attacker's ankle/heel to cause serious trauma to the tendons and ligaments of the ankle. Even if you don't cause a serious injury, your attacker will be reluctant to put weight on that leg, and will want to check what damage has been done before thinking about continuing the fight.

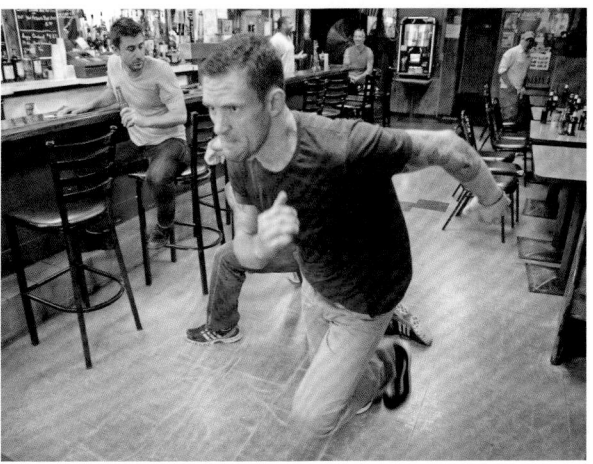

This will give you time to disengage to safety. After you have made an initial scan of your environment, exit the situation as quickly as possible.

It may make sense to go for a control hold, rather than taking a combative approach, if you believe that your attacker is attempting to draw a weapon. Although you may be able to beat them into unconsciousness with your strikes, it may be safer to try and get them into a position on the ground from which they will be unable to either access or use their weapon.

If someone grabs you and goes to draw a weapon, it will be extremely difficult to spoil their draw; in fact, this may be why they decided to grab you in the first place. Trying to get to the weapon hand may not be possible, so it is often more effective to work with the arm that is grabbing you. Once it is rotated, the elbow will lock, and it will be virtually impossible for your assailant to reach you with the knife.

Both solutions—either the thumb lock or the wrist lock—will work whether your assailant grabs you with one hand or two. This means you don't have to train different responses or spend unnecessary time trying to identify the specific nature of the threat.

If an attacker grabs you with both hands, you know that they will not be throwing a punch or reaching for a knife or other weapon; they will either be looking to head-butt you or throw you around like a ragdoll. It is still worth bringing your hand around your head in a protective manner, so that if they suddenly release one of their grips to strike you, your head will be protected.

With the elbow up, there is a good chance that if they try to punch or head-butt you, their head or fist will connect with your elbow. Once again, both hands should grab the hand of your attacker that is grabbing you. With a two-handed grip, you can work against either of your assailant's arms.

Don't worry about your attacker's other arm; simply rotate the arm you have hold of until their little finger is pointing up and their thumb is pointing down (this means rotating the arm about 180-degrees). Rotating and straightening this arm means that your attacker will be pushed away from you, and will therefore have to release or loosen the grip they have with their left hand.

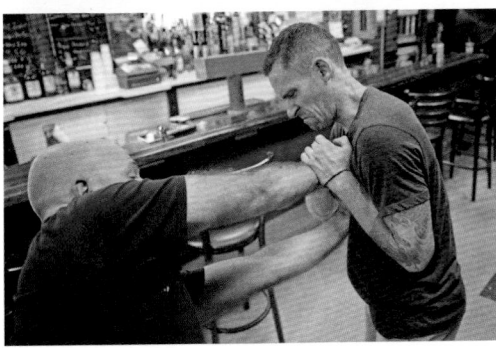

Bend your attacker's hand toward them and press in with your chest. It can be seen at this point that the assailant's left arm is virtually useless, even if they do continue to hold on to you.

Rear Naked Choke—Applying and Defending Against

The rear naked choke is an effective way of finishing a fight, whether it is applied by yourself against an aggressor, or by an aggressor against you. To fully understand how to escape and deal with an attack, it is important to learn how to make such an attack yourself. The first thing to understand about the rear naked choke is that it is a blood choke, as opposed to a strangle; that is, you are putting pressure on the carotid arteries rather than on the throat and windpipe—you are not preventing air from getting to the lungs. A common misconception with blood chokes is that you are preventing oxygenated blood from getting to the brain; in fact, by putting pressure on the two arteries, you are preventing blood from reaching the carotid processes, which measure and control blood pressure within the brain. When they stop receiving blood, they erroneously believe that there is too much blood (pressure) in the brain, and they respond by flushing the brain of blood (and hence oxygen), while at the same time reducing the heart rate so that no new blood is pumped to it. This results in unconsciousness.

One of the reasons it is so valuable to know how to choke someone out is that the application of a blood choke will quickly render even the pain-tolerant attacker unconscious—and take them out of the fight—where a combative solution may be unsuccessful. A choke will work equally well against an adrenalized, mentally ill, or conditioned person, where strikes and punches may fail. Knowing how to switch someone's lights off is an extremely useful skill to have.

Rear Naked Choke Application

To successfully apply a rear naked choke, you will need to be able to get behind your assailant—something that most combatants will not make easy for you. It is often easier to get behind someone before they believe the physical confrontation has begun—as a preemptive movement—while they are still engaged in the dialogue phase of the confrontation.

Whether from your de-escalation stance or in the middle of a confrontation, pushing and pulling on your assailant's shoulders is a fast method for getting behind your attacker. Once behind them, you can either disengage, or throw them, strike, choke, etc. One of your hands (in this case, the left), reaches behind your attacker's right shoulder, while the other (the right) gets ready to push their left.

Your right hand should push strongly against your attacker's left shoulder; at the same time, your left hand should start to pull the other shoulder toward you.

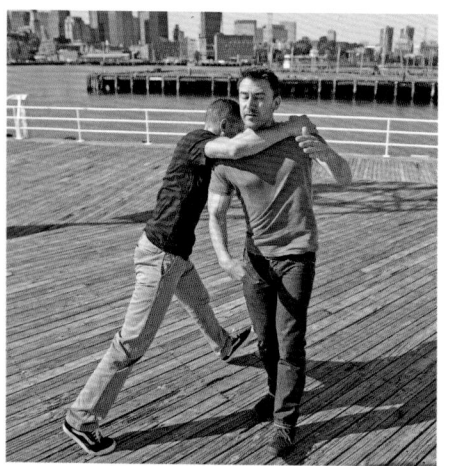

This will have the effect of turning your assailant's torso, creating room and space for you to step behind them. You are not trying to turn your attacker completely around; you just need to move their right shoulder enough to allow you to step behind them and take their back. Your right arm—the one that is on your assailant's left shoulder—should start to slide around their neck as you move behind them.

Step behind your attacker and turn, so that your chest is against their back. Your right biceps should be cutting/pressing into the carotid artery on the right side and the forearm should be doing the same against the other side. Your left arm should start to raise up so that your right hand can be placed on its biceps.

Place your right hand on your left biceps (upper arm) and bring your left arm behind your attacker's neck.

The trick to applying a fast choke is to take all space and movement away from the neck. To do this, you need to squeeze in a few directions at once. Pull your arms back toward you and hug the neck, bringing the elbows down. You can also take a deep breath in to expand your chest and take away space, which will push your attacker against your arms, increasing the pressure of your squeeze.

You can also lean back, pulling your attacker off their feet, to increase the pressure on their neck/throat, as well as take away any base they may have to try to counter what you are doing. Your attacker will have started feeling the effects of the choke the moment you started putting pressure on the sides of their neck; they may fully lose consciousness about five seconds into the application of the choke.

Rather than lifting their body up, you could kick their legs away by stomping on the back of their knee. You may want to do this if you intend to drag them to the ground in order to create more time to disengage safely.

This push and pull movement can also be used to set up other attacks, such as throws. One of these, the major outer reap, is demonstrated later in this book in the section on throwing.

To properly apply the choke, it is important to take away every bit of space in order to put full pressure on the carotid arteries while denying the aggressor any space to adjust their position and relieve this pressure. In order to accomplish this, you must squeeze the neck in more than just one direction. You can increase the pressure by bringing your elbows back and down, as well as by taking a deep breath in as you apply the choke—this will inflate your lungs and push your chest out, applying pressure from yet another direction. If you can combine all of these things, you will immediately stop the blood flow to the carotid processes and your aggressor will start to pass out in a matter of seconds. Even if the pressure you apply is more gradual, the body has no instinctual response to this type of attack, as it is replicating a safety mechanism that the body employs. This means that your assailant has to consciously identify the nature of the assault and then formulate a response against it—something which will be hard to do as they slip from consciousness.

Rear Naked Choke Prevention

In order for someone to apply a rear naked choke on you, they must first take your back. They may do this in the midst of the fight, either because they are a skilled grappler or because you have inadvertently presented your back to them. They could also manage it as an initial assault if they are able to come up behind you unseen. If you are too focused on what is in front of you, you may neglect to check the other directions from which an attack could come; this is why, from a personal safety perspective, it is good to adopt a 360-degree view of your environment. There are several reasons why your focus could be directed forward: you could be opening a door, or putting things in the trunk of your car; or you could be dealing with another assailant who is in front of you, either preceding or in the midst of a fight with them. In some instances, two individuals may work together, with one distracting you while the other launches their attack from behind.

When you are dealing with an individual in front of you (they may have made a request for directions, money, etc.), you should avoid focusing all of your attention on them. You should step back and scan so you can see anyone else who may be in the environment. Part of good situational awareness is understanding directions from which a person can enter the environment, as well as where they may be able to conceal themselves. You should try to position yourself in such a way as to be able to see such points, so that you can avoid having a third party attack you unawares.

As an individual engages you in conversation, you may become suspicious of their motives. For example, they may have asked you for the time, which is a strange request in an age where everybody carries a mobile phone. At this point, you should step back to control range and adopt your de-escalation stance. If you are too focused on what is in front of you, it could be that an accomplice who you had not seen comes up behind you to apply a choke. Good situational awareness would have allowed you to pick up on this individual.

As soon as you feel the arm come round your neck, bring your left hand up to protect it. This means that when your attacker's right arm comes around, your left will be there to meet it and prevent the choke from being applied. At the same time, you should raise your right leg up in order to kick the first attacker away.

Keeping your left hand on your attacker's forearm to prevent the choke, aim your kick at the first attacker.

Forcefully kick out, moving the first attacker back, in order to give yourself the time and space to finish dealing with the assailant trying to apply the choke—something that they will not be able to do with your left hand holding their forearm.

You should start to act before the choke has been fully applied; once your assailant manages to really start squeezing and denying you space to move, escaping will be much more difficult. Concentrate first on dealing with/preventing the choke, and then turn your attention to the attackers. In any multiple-assailant situation, you should accept that you are going to get hit and take some degree of punishment. This is one of the reasons it is worth spending some training time conditioning your body so that it is able to take shots and blows without being overwhelmed by pain. As soon as you have an escape option, you should take it and disengage. If you are unable to get a hand in to prevent the choke from being applied, you should try to create space around your neck as early as possible to avoid being choked out.

Once a rear naked choke has been sunk in, escape becomes extremely difficult. Solutions for dealing with such a situation will be described; however, it is preferable to deal with this attack as it's being made, rather than once it has been completed. If you miss the opportunity to get a hand between your attacker's arm and your throat, you should quickly bring up your left arm in order to shift your attacker's choke from your neck (where the carotid arteries are) to your jaw line.

Throw your left arm up and backward. Your goal here is to lift your assailant's upper arm up from around your neck, loosening the choke before they can fully sink it in.

Doing this will create the space for you to tuck your chin into the crook of your attacker's elbow. This will move your attacker's right arm up to your jawline, so that if they do try to apply the choke, they will be squeezing your jaw, not your neck. It is imperative in this life-threatening situation that you "attack the attack", before doing anything else. Once your neck is safe, you can start attacking your attacker by making a groin strike with your right hand.

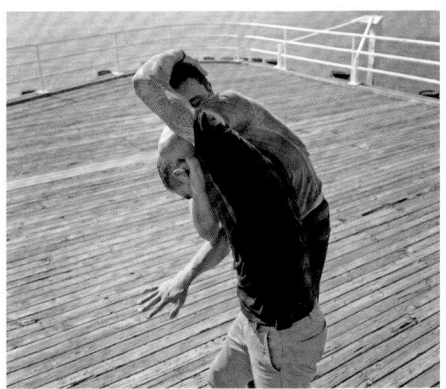

As you make the groin strike, use your left hand to push on your attacker's head, pushing them away from you, as you turn out to escape.

Keep pushing on the back of their head as you turn, and pull your head out from their grasp/hold.

As you pull your head out, push down on your attacker's head and take a step back. At the same time, raise your right hand up in preparation for making your own attack.

While pushing your attacker's head down and preventing them from standing, raise your right hand up and start to deliver hammer-fists down on the back of their neck.

Rear Naked Choke Escape

It may be that your attacker manages to sink the choke on and is able to apply pressure to your arteries immediately. If this is the case, you will only have a few seconds to make your escape. Fortunately, most people aren't skilled at applying such chokes, and will be trying to replicate something they saw in a televised MMA sporting contest or similar. However, if your initial movement to try and free yourself was not successful, then you will need to start altering your approach in order to escape. Using the hand that shot up to lift your assailant's choke, reach for their fingers and start to peel them off the top of your head, or the back of your neck, depending on where their second hand is positioned.

As you raise your arm up to prevent the choke, you may realize that your attacker has a good hold on you and there is little chance of creating enough space to turn your chin into the crook of their elbow to make yourself safe. To make the technique clearer and easier to follow, these photos show the attacker's left hand positioned on the top of the head. If they have buried it behind the neck, you would simply need to reach further behind in order to take control of their hand.

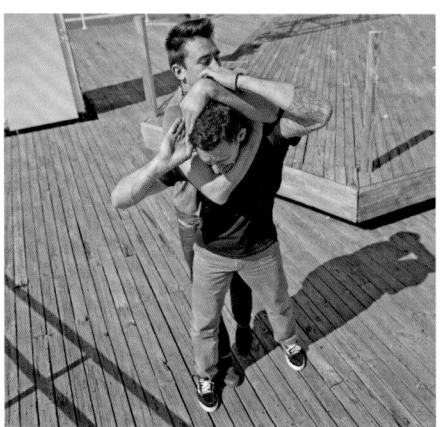

You should bring both hands up to their left hand (whether it is on the top of your head or behind your neck—you will be able to feel exactly where it is positioned). Immediately start to attack their fingers, peeling them away from your head.

As you bend their fingers or thumb backward, start to lift their arm up and away from your neck. Your first job is to create enough space to duck your chin into the crook of the elbow, thus making you safe from the choke.

Lift their arm high in the air...

...and then bring it violently down across your shoulder (you should still be bending their fingers back, causing pain and trauma to them). If you are the same height as your assailant or taller, you will cause damage to their arm by hyperextending it like this. If you are shorter than them, you will simply lift your attacker onto their toes, taking their balance and putting them in a position from which it will be difficult for them to make any other attack(s).

With your right hand, pull their arm away from your throat so that you can step under their armpit. As you do this, strike their groin with your right hand.

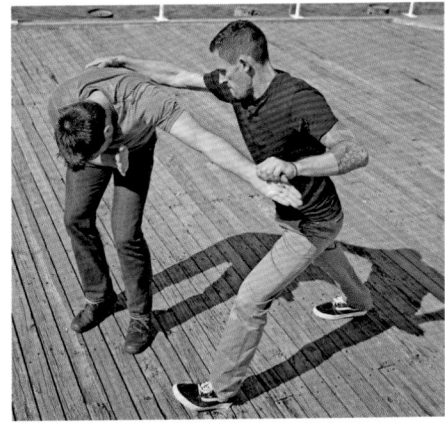

Step back, under their armpit. This will put you in a natural position to deliver a knee strike to their head.

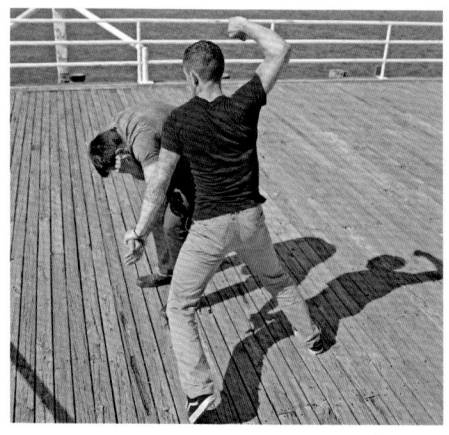

After making the knee strike, follow it up...

...with multiple hammer-fist strikes before disengaging to safety.

Once you have escaped from the choke, you will have various options. One (as illustrated above) is simply to work combatively against your assailant—delivering strikes, punches, knees and kicks, etc., before safely disengaging. Another option would be to throw/takedown your aggressor from here, using the control you have on their wrist/hand. When you throw someone, avoid the temptation to follow them to ground. Your goal is to create time and distance when you throw, so that you are able to disengage safely; you are not trying to win points in a sporting event. Often, when you throw someone, they will end up hitting themselves on something in the environment, such as a table or a car door, and this will increase the trauma that they experience. If you are dealing with multiple assailants, such as in this scenario, your goal is to cause enough pain, trauma, and disorientation that you will have effectively taken one of your assailants out of the picture. In such a scenario, you will not be able to devote the time to finishing them off, but instead must rely on your throw to have at least temporarily incapacitated them, allowing you room to escape or to decisively attack your other aggressor.

Once you have peeled your assailant's fingers away from your head and brought their arm down on your shoulder, you will have some options other than stepping under your attacker's armpit and finishing them combatively. One option would be to throw them from here. You will still need to pull their right arm away from your neck in order to do this.

After plucking the arm away, while still keeping tension on their right arm, start to turn away from your attacker.

As you do this, bring your right hand toward the edge of their left palm.

Take hold of their hand with both of yours and turn fully away from them.

You will now need to step back in, so as to bend their elbow. This entire movement should have a circular motion to it; i.e., your feet and body should be moving in a circular manner on a horizontal plane, and the movement of your arms should be circular in a vertical plane.

At this point, your attacker's elbow should be at a 90-degree angle, and their balance should be severely compromised.

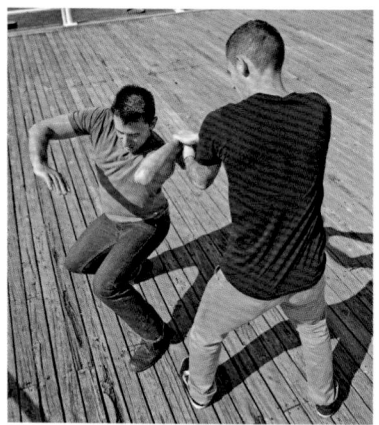

Keep turning from here, bringing your attacker's hand down toward the ground. With their arm and shoulder in this position, they will have no option but to follow this movement.

Pull their hand toward the ground, so that they land flat on their back and hit their head on the ground. As soon as this happens, disengage to safety.

Rear Tackle and Rear Bear Hugs

Rear Tackle

Sometimes the attacks that aggressors make aren't as sophisticated or technical as a choke, and are simply attempts to move you and/or put you on the ground. If you get into a verbal altercation with someone in a bar, you shouldn't assume that this is the only aggressor you will have to deal with. This is why you need to scan and check your environment any time you are involved in a verbal confrontation.

It may be that you have just dealt with the person you knocked into, who grabbed your lapel/clothing, by applying a thumb lock on them and breaking away. However, one of their friends witnessed what happened and has decided to get involved. Seeing that you are now separated, they may decide to tackle you to the ground before you can do anything further to their friend.

If you are in a bar where your assailant may have friends who can come to their assistance, you should break away from your attacker's lapel grab rather than trying to deal with them combatively. A combative solution could prove ineffective in this situation—you could find yourself with nowhere to disengage to, your back turned toward a wall, with your assailant between you and the door. You could also find yourself facing a second attacker.

Your attempt to disengage could also be misinterpreted by your attacker's friend(s) as a setup to launch a further assault on them.

To prevent you from reengaging with their friend, they may decide to try to rugby tackle you to the ground.

Their goal in tackling you like this is to take your balance and drive you into the ground face first. When you are attacked around the waist/upper body, you will be moved forward, causing your legs to fly out behind you.

To stop this from happening, drop your weight and throw your legs out in front of you. At the same time, lean back and wrap your arms around your assailant's head, hugging them to you. This is to prevent them from letting go of you, as you will need them for support.

Use your attacker's momentum to drive yourself forward as you lower your weight and direct them toward the ground.

You should have the feeling of walking forward on your heels as you drop your weight.

Once you have your attacker face down on the floor, start to turn your body over, while moving out to the side.

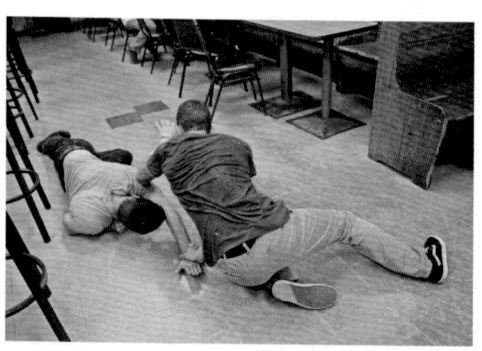

Keep turning, and get to your assailant's side, where you can pin them down with your hands, pushing them into the ground.

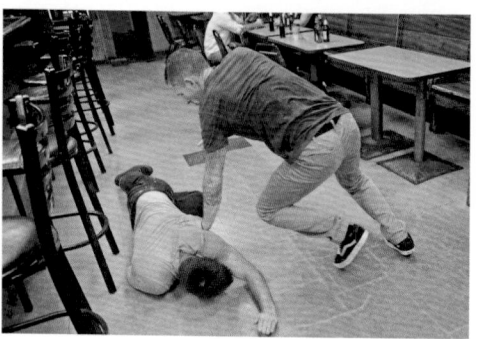

Push yourself to a standing position and then disengage. Be aware that you may still have to deal with your original/primary aggressor. This is why you should deal with the rear tackle as quickly as possible and get back to your feet.

Rear Bear Hug—Turning Away

A person will generally apply a rear bear hug for one of two reasons. They will either want to pick you up in order to move you, or to throw you down. It may also be that instead of tackling you to the ground, your primary assailant's friend wants to arrest your movement and hold you so that the other person is able to punch/strike you. When you are initially grabbed, you will not be fully aware of your assailant's motive. If they grab you high, around the chest, it is unlikely that they will try to pick you up, or be able to; in the heat of the moment, however, ascertaining the exact nature of the assault will be difficult.

As soon as you are grabbed, try to hook a leg around one of your attacker's legs (it doesn't matter which one). This will allow you to anchor yourself to your assailant, preventing them from moving or lifting you. If you are dealing with another potential attacker who is facing you, you can use this "anchor" as leverage to move yourself away from them, putting the person applying the bear hug between you and them. This will allow you to concentrate on releasing the hold without having to worry about being assaulted by another person as you do so.

As you are trying to de-escalate a situation with an aggressor who is facing you, a second assailant could come up behind you to put you in a rear bear hug. They may do this to move you, hold you, or pick you up. If they grab low, positioning their hips below yours, it is likely that they will attempt to lift you. Because your hands are up, they are not likely to get pinned to your body when the bear hug is applied.

As soon as you feel your assailant's arms wrap around your waist, pull your own arms back and squeeze them to your sides. If your attacker has their head low, you will catch it with one of your arms.

Your initial priority will be to turn away from the attacker who is facing you. There is little point trying to escape from the bear hug if the attacker facing you is able to deliver concussive strikes that could knock you out as you do so. To make the turn, reach behind one of your attacker's legs with one of your legs (it doesn't matter which one you use), and use it to turn your body away.

Use your attacker's leg to pull yourself around and away from your initial/primary aggressor.

You should now be lining up your attackers so that you have the assailant who was applying the bear hug between you and the first aggressor.

From this position, you can start to deal with the attacker applying the bear hug.

Rear Bear Hug—Arms Free

Once you have turned, you will need to release yourself so that you can deal with both assailants. One solution, if your arms happened to be free, would be to throw reverse elbow strikes at the person holding you; however, if they have pressed their head into your back, these are unlikely to be effective.

One solution for dealing with someone who has you in a rear bear hug is to try to throw elbow strikes at their head. This would be a good solution if they weren't pressing their head into your back. In reality, though, this is what most assailants will do.

If your assailant's head is pressed to you when you throw your rear elbow strikes, you will find that they won't connect. Rather than wasting time attempting a rear elbow strike only to find it doesn't work (and time will be of the essence if you are dealing with multiple assailants—which is a distinct possibility, given the nature of the attack), you may be better off attempting a solution that isn't dependent on your attacker's head position.

Because of this, it may be quicker and more effective to try to release the hold itself by attacking your assailant's grip and opening up their hands. This will also give you an opportunity to apply a finger lock on your attacker. When applying the lock, you may also want to consider breaking the finger so that their hand is put out of commission. In a multiple-assailant situation, anything you can do that will reduce one of your attackers' ability to fight will increase your survival chances.

As soon as an assailant puts a rear bear hug on you, slide your hands down their arms. You should do this as you are turning away from your primary attacker, if it is a multiple-assailant situation as described earlier. As you slide your hands down the arms, one hand will be stopped by the hand of your attacker that is gripping their other arm; your other hand will keep sliding. This will tell you, by feel, which of their hands is on top. Pull back the hand that kept sliding (off their top hand), and grab their wrist.

If this is the case, it is the left hand which slid off the assailant's top hand. With your left hand, get a solid grip on their left wrist. Place your right hand over your assailant's left fingers, toward the fingertips.

Start to pry off one of their fingers. Use all of your fingers/hand against one of theirs.

Once you have peeled off a finger and have it firmly gripped, start to turn away from your attacker in a counter-clockwise direction. Keep gripping their left wrist and start to bend their wrist back, using the finger as leverage.

Keep turning, making sure that your attacker's wrist stays close to your hip. You want to have a very tight turning circle around their wrist—this keeps maximum pressure on it, and prevents your assailant from turning away to reduce the pressure/pain.

Keep turning, keeping the pressure on the finger and continuing to bend it back, which in turn will force the wrist to bend back.

By bending the finger and the wrist while keeping them close to your body, you will force your assailant to stay crouched down in order to reduce the pressure. Once you start to turn fully out to their side, start to straighten their arm.

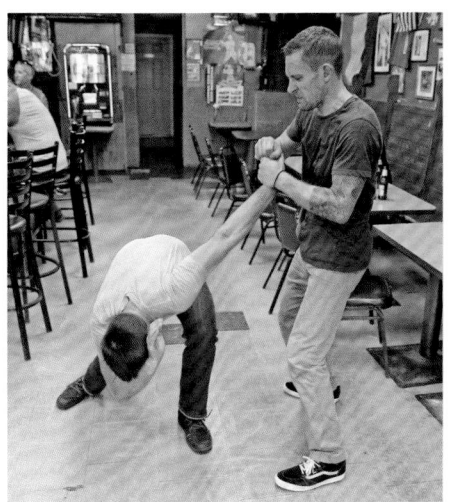

With their arm locked, drive them toward the ground by bending the finger back. Continue bending it until it breaks, and then either attack them combatively and/or disengage. With the pain of a broken finger, they may no longer want to continue the fight; even if they do, their left hand will be injured and severely compromised.

When you try to escape from the rear bear hug, you should keep your legs locked straight and lean forward, bending at your waist. By directing your head in this fashion, you are making it extremely difficult for your attacker to lift you up. The last thing you want in a multiple-assailant situation is to find yourself thrown to the floor. By keeping your legs locked, rather than bent, you will also prevent your attacker from pulling you to the ground from behind.

An attacker may change their attack based on your response(s) to their initial assault. This is something you have to be prepared for, regardless of whether you are dealing with an armed or unarmed attack. It is extremely dangerous to assume that your assailant will only respond in one way to what you do, or won't try to change what they are doing. The dynamic nature of violence often gets forgotten in the training environment. If you drop your weight too much and bend your legs, your assailant may alter their attack.

Their initial idea may have been to pick you up and throw you to the ground; however, they feel your resistance to this as you bend your legs and drop your weight. They can now change their attack and work with the dropping of your weight by pulling you to the ground.

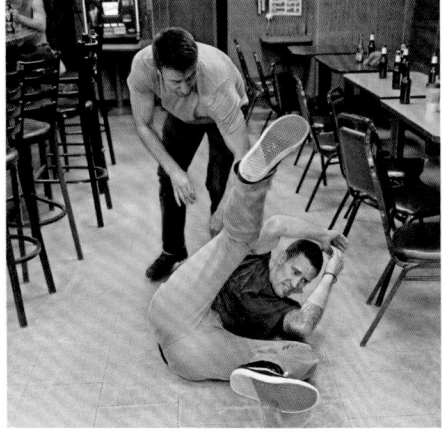

Because your weight is directed backward when you bend your legs (think about how you bend your legs to lower yourself into a chair) it wouldn't take any real effort on the part of your attacker to pull you to ground.

Once you have been dragged to ground, your attacker can stomp on you, "soccer kick" you, etc. It is very unlikely that they will follow you to ground, as remaining standing gives them a greater advantage. It is very difficult for you to attack them from the ground while they are standing; and they can easily pick up a chair or other improvised weapon and start hitting you with it and/or get others to join them in attacking you.

If you are concerned about being picked up or moved, drop your weight forward by bending at your waist while keeping your legs straight. With all your weight directed forward, it will be difficult for your attacker to either pull you back or lift you up. They can try to push you forward, but it will be difficult for them to keep hold of you if they do. From this position, you can work their fingers and wrist to release yourself from their hold.

Rear Bear Hug—Arms Trapped

If your arms are trapped, you will not be able to use them to break your attacker's grip. If your assailant's hold only traps your hands at the wrist/lower forearm, you may be able to pull them out and apply the finger lock/break. If their hold is anywhere higher than your mid-forearms, however, you are not likely to be able to get them free.

If an attacker pins your arms above the elbows, you will not be able to free your arms, so you will need to perform a defense/escape from this position. Someone who grabs/holds you like this is not trying to pick you up (they would need to get lower, bending their legs to do so), but rather to restrain and contain you—perhaps so another aggressor can assault you.

If your elbows are higher than your attacker's arms, it will usually be possible for you to pull your arms out and free them.

Simply pull your elbows up and out to free your arms.

Once free, start to escape from the bear hug by attacking your assailant's grip and prying their fingers away.

One of the principles we work to is "nearest weapon, nearest target." Although your body is in the way, the nearest, softest target to your hands is your attacker's groin. By moving your hips out of the way, your hands will be able to make strikes to the groin, which will help facilitate your release.

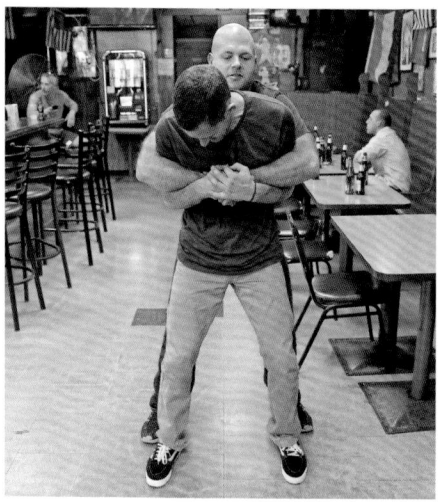

When the bear hug is high, it is advisable to keep at least one hand holding on to your attacker's arms. This prevents them from changing their attack to a strangulation or choke. Your attacker may be forced to give up a life-threatening attack for a non-life-threatening one, but you don't want them to go the other way—a bear hug, for example, is not as serious an attack as a strangulation.

Because your body is in the way of their groin, you should either step to the side or pivot so that the groin becomes available as a target. Keep hold of your assailant's arms with one hand as you slap their groin with the other.

Start to step and/or turn to the other side. Moving this way will start to loosen your attacker's hold on you. This is where your attacker might start thinking about changing their attack as they feel their hold on you slipping. The easiest attack for them to make from here would be to try and strangle you, so as you transition from one side to another, you will need to grip their arms with both hands to prevent this.

As you step to the right, deliver a groin strike with your left hand. The groin strikes are not just intended to cause pain; they are there to get your assailant to pull their hips back (an instinctive response to the groin being attacked). This will create more space in which for you to turn, and will aid your escape.

As you step/turn again, your attacker will be unable to maintain their grip, and their bear hug will open up. It is important to keep hold of their arms at this point, as they are at your neck level, making you vulnerable to a choke or strangulation.

As your attacker's grip loosens, prepare to step backward under their armpit. You should still be able to make a final groin strike with your left hand as you do this.

Step all the way under so that you can come out behind your attacker, away from their "weapons"—i.e., their hands, feet, head, etc.

Immediately start to strike them with concussive force before disengaging and/or having to deal with any other parties that may be in the environment.

Universal Rear Bear Hug Solution—Arms Trapped and Arms Free

In a real-life confrontation, it is often difficult to process everything that is going on; all of the information bombarding you will be overwhelming. It can be difficult to ascertain whether your arms are trapped or free, so having a solution that is independent of this fact can help you quickly escape and survive the situation. Rather than attacking the individual by using your elbows or slapping the groin, or looking to release the grip by attacking it, you can try to affect the assailant's balance by attacking their legs/ankles. When a person's balance is taken, they will usually release their grip on whatever it is they are holding in order to break their fall. (Picking someone up, lifting them, and throwing them to the ground is one of the quickest ways to get them to release any weapon they are holding.)

This technique is a good universal approach to dealing with a rear bear hug. It is worth knowing, as it doesn't rely on you determining whether your arms are trapped or free—something which might not be obvious to you when you are experiencing the stress and duress of real life violence. The one drawback of this solution is that your assailant could hold on to you as they fall. This isn't very common, but is of course feasible, and would see you end up on the ground.

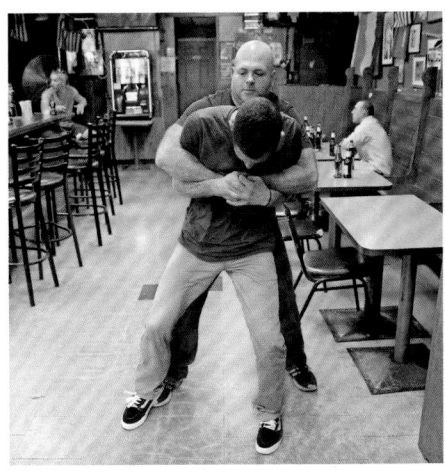

Bring your leg up and stomp down on your attacker's foot (toes/instep). Although it only takes around five pounds of pressure to break these bones, it is unlikely that such a degree of trauma will result, due to footwear, movement, and the difficulty of placing the strike. If you get the opportunity, however, it is worth getting a good stomp in.

When you strike, aim for their toes, and make impact with your heel. The primary reason you are stomping is to make contact with the foot, so that you can feel where it is.

Pull your foot back so that your toes are over your attacker's instep and your heel is where their ankle is—at this point, it is pointed at the ground.

Keeping pressure on the front of your assailant's foot, turn the heel of your foot toward your attacker's ankle. Keep holding their arms to your body so they can't change their attack.

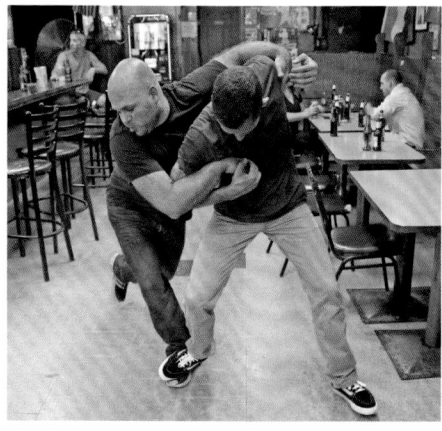

Start to drive your heel into their ankle, causing their foot to roll over. At this point, they will be biomechanically forced to fall/move to the side, and their balance will be compromised.

Keep pushing/driving your heel into the inside of their ankle. As your assailant realizes they are falling, they will likely release their grip on you so that they can use their arms and hands to break their fall. As you feel their grip on you loosen, release their arms—they will not, from here, be in a position to strangle or choke you, and you don't want to be tied to them as they go down.

Keep pushing and driving so that your attacker is forced to fall to the ground. This puts them in a disadvantageous position, and you in an advantageous one. Be aware that you are not likely to have caused them any serious pain or damage, so they will still be mechanically able to fight.

Back away from them, checking your environment before disengaging and/or dealing with any other assailants who may approach you.

Rear Bear Hug with Lift—Arms Trapped and Arms Free

Sometimes it is impossible to prevent someone from making an assault. If an attacker is determined to grab you and lift you up, it may not be possible to prevent them from doing so. If they do attempt it, you will need to be prepared to enact a solution straight away. If an attacker has been able to force/cause you to move, there is little point in trying to reverse what they have already accomplished. If you can prevent someone from doing something, that is one thing, but if they have started to do it—e.g., lift you—it is usually easier and more effective to work with their movement than to try to fight it. In the Krav Maga Yashir system we have the concept of "adding" to a movement, rather than trying to reverse it. If an assailant has managed to lift you, rather than working against the lift, you should go with it and try to take advantage of the movement of their attack.

If someone has started to get you airborne, you should add to this movement rather than fight it. It may be that you need to assault the person in front of you as well as the person lifting you. As you are elevated, kick your legs forward. This will pull your assailant forward, making it difficult for them to lift you, because they would need to push their hips forward and lean back to successfully lift your weight. Another effective way to get them to bend forward and drop you is to attack their groin. An easy way to do this is to use one leg or foot as a support against their thigh, using the other to make a mule kick to your attacker's groin. Striking their groin will cause them to pull their hips back, dropping you back to the ground. Once you are back standing on the ground, you can begin the necessary escape, whether your arms are free or trapped.

When someone has committed to picking you up, it is not always possible to prevent this attack. If they come up behind you quickly and decisively, you may find yourself being lifted before you can move to stop them.

Once you realize you are being lifted, don't try to fight your attacker's movement. You will need to work with it so that you can prevent the next stage of the attack, which may involve them throwing you on the ground, etc. As you are lifted, start to bring your left knee up.

Start to bring your foot back to push against your assailant's thigh/upper leg. At the same time, swing your right leg up and forward.

Push back with your left leg to create enough space to swing your right leg back...

...toward your attacker's groin. When you land a solid groin strike, the natural response of the person being hit will be to immediately bring their hips back to protect themselves. This will mean that the person lifting you will have to lower you—you can't lift someone with your hips pulled back. You may need to make several of these kicks to get this result; however, with your left foot placed where it is, your attacker will be hard pressed to continue what they are doing.

As you drop back to the ground, start working and prying your attacker's fingers away so that they are unable to maintain their hold on you.

You should be leaning forward as you hit the ground, and your attacker's grip should be broken.

As soon as you are free, disengage to safety. In this case, make for the door/exit.

If you were to recognize the threat quickly enough and are able to do so, you may be able to wrap/grapevine your shin and ankle around your assailant's leg, which would prevent them from picking you up. One of the indicators that someone is planning on lifting you is that they take a low grip on your body. A person who intends to pick you up with a bear hug will grab you around the waist/hips rather than around your upper torso.

As you hook your leg around your attacker's so as to pull yourself around them, you may realize that they are trying to lift you. If this is the case, wrap one of your legs around theirs.

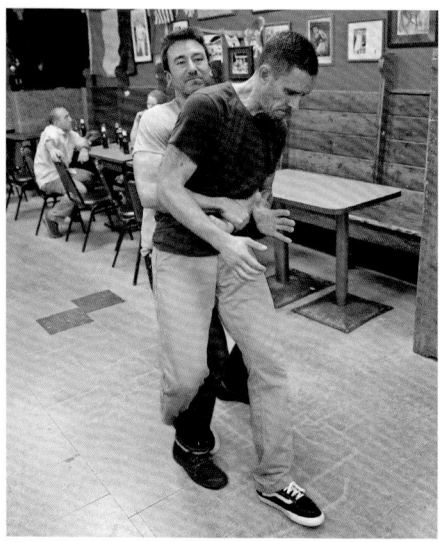

Position the instep of your foot against the inside of your attacker's ankle.

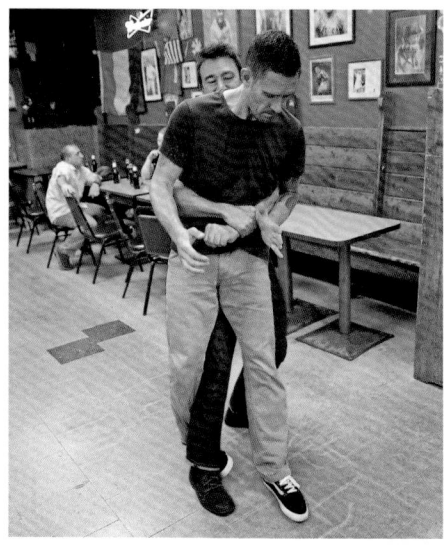

If your assailant tries to lift you now, they will find it difficult, as they will be pulling at their own leg, and you will be rooted to the ground. Now you can start to work your escape, prying your attacker's fingers away.

Unarmed Assaults—Conclusion

It is extremely tempting to present solutions to violence in a simplistic manner—as if, whenever you attempt to use a particular technique, the outcome will always be the same. In reality, this is not the case; attackers will often respond in ways that you weren't expecting and alter their attack(s) to counter what you are doing. If you try to blindly continue with your initial technique/solution and are unable to adapt to your changing situation, you will be found wanting. Solutions do not have to be complicated, but they do need to be flexible.

PART V
Throws and Pick-Ups

In some of the photo sequences, you will notice that the final execution of certain throws takes place inside on a matted surface, rather than outside, on concrete. This is due to the severe impact that these throws can cause, and the fact that even with a good break-fall, the risk of injury is high. Rather than demonstrate the entire throw in a studio setting, we felt that it would be better to demonstrate as much of the throw as possible in the context of the situation where it would be used. As with all of the photos in the book, everything has been shot at full speed.

Knowing how to throw someone is an extremely useful skill to have. While some throws take a great deal of skill and timing to pull off in real-life situations, others are relatively simple to learn, and can be applied in a number of situations.

There are many good reasons to learn how to throw. Throwing an assailant onto concrete or a similarly hard surface is one of the most unsettling, frightening, and painful things you can do to them. Not only is it extremely disorienting—one of the fears we are born with is the fear of falling—but it will also result in full-body trauma. When someone is thrown, their entire body is affected, whereas a punch or kick targets a specific body part/area. With a throw, not only will their head be hit, but if they are unable to break their fall (and most people don't possess this skill) their torso, arms and legs, etc. will be struck as well. Also, what will hit them (the ground) is a much harder and larger striking surface than any striking tool on your body, such as a fist, elbow or similar. As one of my old Judo instructors used to say, "Nothing hits harder than concrete."

When people are forcefully thrown, they do not get back up immediately, even if they have not sustained any major injuries or trauma. At the very least, most are shocked and winded, and will want to check themselves for injuries before trying to get back up. Another reason that many people stay down longer than they may physically need to after being thrown is that they recognize their position within the fight; there is no clearer position of superiority and dominance than that of someone who has put them on the ground with a technique that wasn't in any way a result of luck. You may get "lucky" punches, but there is no such thing as a "lucky" throw, and people understand this. The fact that people take several moments before getting back up, and receive a clear indication of their position in the fight, means that throwing provides you with more time to make distance between yourself and your assailant.

In the throws/pick-ups that I am going to describe, the goal will be for you to put your assailant on the ground, while you remain standing. There are times when it is expedient to follow your attacker to ground, but these are few and far between, and represent the exceptions rather than the norm. If you assume your assailant is armed, and has friends/acquaintances in the vicinity who can come to their assistance, it can be appreciated that fighting on the ground is largely inadvisable. To this end, the throws described will be done with the goal of leaving you in a relatively stable position with the option of disengaging.

Preemptive Throwing—Major Outer Reap

Just as you can use a strike as a preemptive attack, you can also use a throw or reap preemptively. One of the benefits of doing this is that you can effectively end the fight in one move. Any throw has three essential components:

1. The breaking of your assailant's balance
2. "Fitting in"/entering/positioning to make the throw
3. The execution of the throw

The first thing you need to do when throwing someone is to break their balance. This is where the true power of the throw comes from—your movements simply assist a person who is already falling and help to direct their movement so that they land heavily, with a serious impact. This is why a good throw should feel effortless for the thrower. You will also need to unbalance your attacker so that they are not able to do anything to you while you get into position (fit in) to execute the throw.

Sometimes you will not be able to properly control the distance between yourself and your aggressor—perhaps every time you try to put some distance between yourself and them, they fill the space. This puts you in a good position to execute a preemptive throw. If someone is shouting, posturing, and moving in to intimidate you, it is very clear what their intentions are, and you are morally and legally justified to respond to this assault (there doesn't have to be physical contact for an assault to occur).

Having brought your hands up in a placating, non-aggressive manner, you are in a good and close position to break your aggressor's balance.

With your right hand, push on their left shoulder and with your left hand pull on their right. This should be done quickly and with power.

As their torso/upper body starts to turn, step forward with your left leg. Your foot needs to be behind theirs for you to be able to properly upset their balance. You should step out to create just enough room to bring your other leg through with the knee up.

As you step, use the forward movement of your bodyweight to pull your aggressor backward, so that their head starts to move back past their hips and their feet and they are bent backward. Whatever direction the head moves in, the body will follow.

Keep pulling their head backward and raise your knee so that you are in a good position to execute the throw.

You should have pulled your attacker back so that all their weight is on their rear (right) foot. Reaps work by loading weight onto a leg and then taking that supporting leg out (sweeps work by taking a leg out as weight is starting to be transferred to it). This is a reap, so their rear leg needs to be supporting all of their weight.

While still pulling them backward, straighten your leg and then swing it into the back of your aggressor's leg. Ideally, the back of your knee will connect with the back of theirs. If this doesn't happen, you will still get a solid throw; you just won't get your aggressor as high into the air as you would otherwise.

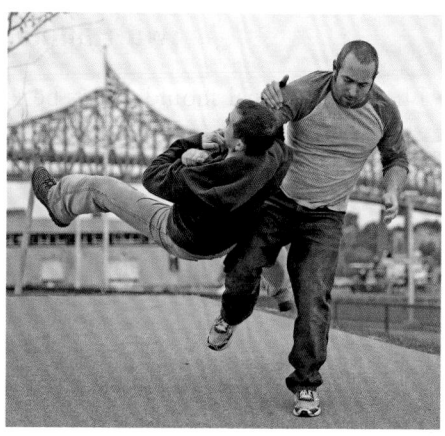

Don't put your foot on the ground, but swing it behind you. Bend slightly forward to allow it to swing as far behind and upward as possible, taking your attacker's leg with it. By bending forward, you will also help direct your attacker's head toward the ground.

Once your right foot has traveled as far as it can, you should get it back on the ground as quickly as possible. By this point, your attacker should be completely airborne, with both feet high in the air.

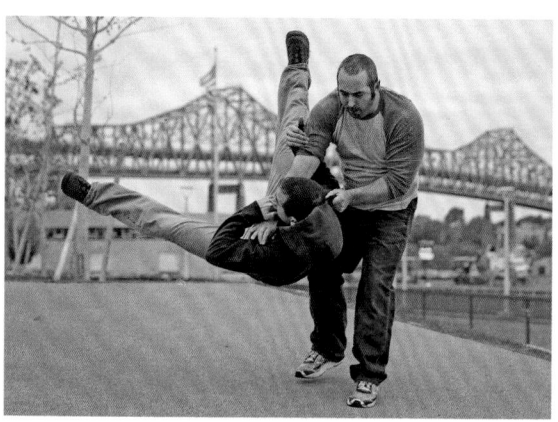

The swinging of your leg behind you, and the pulling of their head backward, should mean that their feet are above, or at least level with their head as they start to fall. An untrained person who doesn't know how to break-fall is going to land heavily on their head or neck. On concrete, this is likely to heavily concuss them.

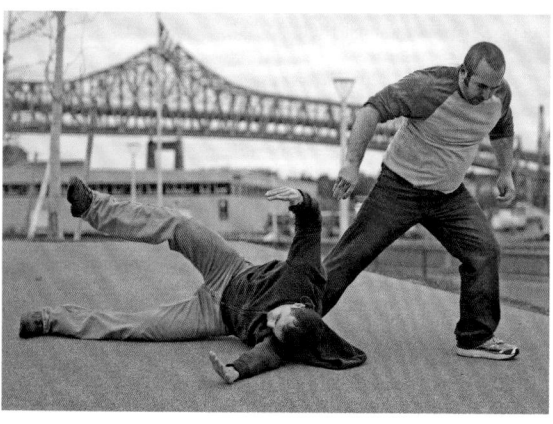

Don't wait to see exactly how they fall; instead, start to disengage as soon as you have completed the throw. Even if they are not concussed, they should be dazed, confused, and in a great deal of pain. If they put their hand out to try to break their fall, they will probably have a broken wrist and collar bone. The amount of potential damage and trauma that a throw can cause, compared to a strike/punch, makes throwing an essential skill to have.

Two-Handed Pick-Up/Reap

Although your goal should always be to try to control the range and prevent your attacker(s) from closing in on you, this will not always be possible. There may be times when you get caught in clinch/grappling situations. These can be bad positions in real-life conflicts: your assailant may be armed, and your visibility, understanding of the environment, and awareness of other potential assailants in it will be restricted. Making a quick throw that takes your attacker out of commission and frees you to deal with anyone else who may be looking to get involved can be an effective way of increasing your survival chances.

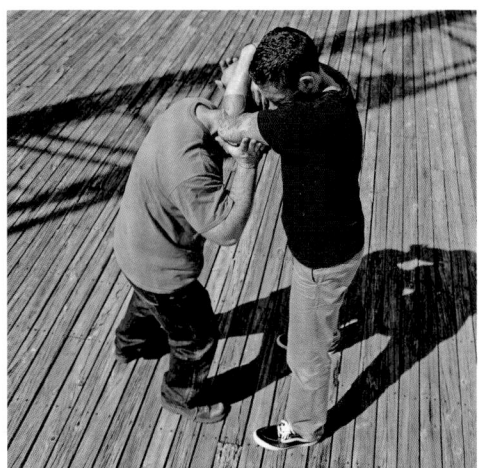

In real-life situations, getting tied up in a clinch is something that you want to avoid. If you assume that your attacker is "armed, assisted, and able," getting locked onto them is rarely a good idea. In such a situation, your objective should be to escape from your attacker's hold and finish them as quickly as possible, before they draw a knife or get assistance from friends. The first thing you should do is push up on your attacker's elbows.

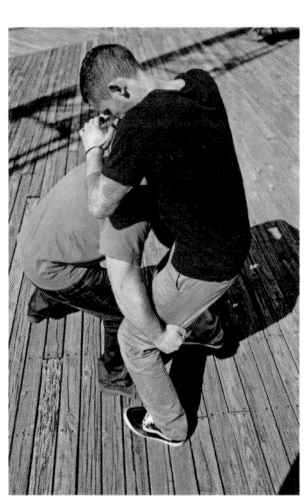

At the same time, drop down and then change your hand position so that you are now grabbing the back of their pants around their knees. This roots them to the spot and prevents them from throwing knee strikes.

Keep your head against their chest rather than moving it to their side, where it could be locked or guillotined.

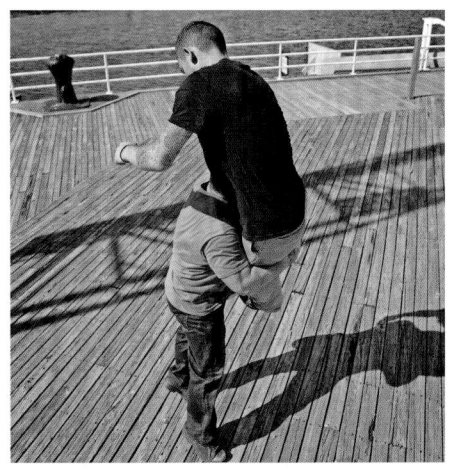

Change your grip so that your arms are wrapped tightly about their knees. They are now in an unstable position; when you go to lift them, they will be unbalanced and top-heavy, as your arms represent the pivot point.

Don't think about lifting your assailant. Simply keep your arms wrapped tightly about their legs, and hug them to you as you stand up.

Whenever you perform a throw, pick-up, or reap, you shouldn't think about the other person's size and weight, but simply perform the technique. If the person is heavy, you may not get their feet a good distance off the ground, but this doesn't matter; the throw works by tipping them, rather than lifting them.

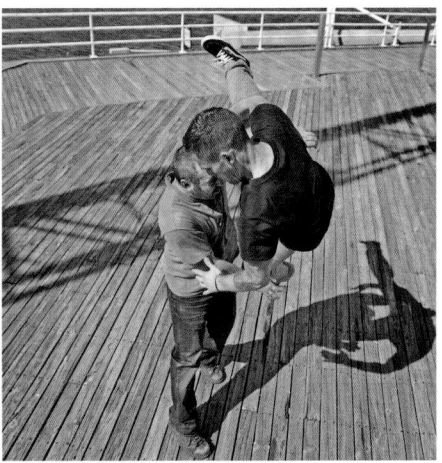

Once you have them as high as you can get them, start to tip them to one side. You can do this by leaning to one side and pulling their legs up to the other side. You can also use your head to direct their body.

If you have managed to stand straight up, they will be falling from height, and they will take a hard fall.

Once you have directed them onto their side, and their feet are higher than their head, release them. In this position, they will be landing on their head and neck, which is likely to cause serious trauma. It also means that they are likely to break their wrist and/or collarbone if they try to break their fall by putting their hands out.

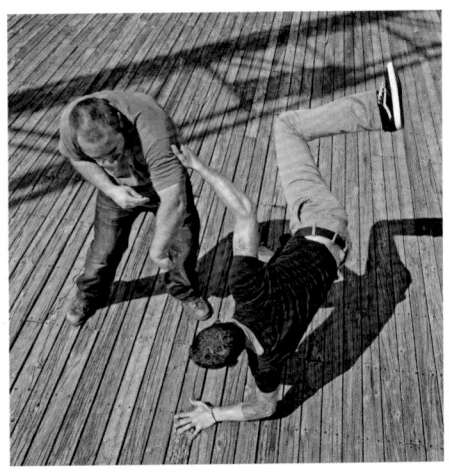

As they fall, they should continue to turn, so they land head first.

This is an extremely heavy fall to take, and even if your assailant is lucky enough to escape without injury, it will still take them some time to recover from the initial impact. This will allow you the time to exit the situation to safety.

With this throw/pick-up, it is essential to grab low around your assailant's knees. There are several reasons for this. One is so that when you lift your attacker, their center of gravity will be high, which means they will tip easily and can also be lifted high. This also makes it difficult for them to grab onto you, either to prevent the throw or to throw you, themselves (if they do hold onto you or try to prevent the throw, you will be low enough to simply throw them behind you). Another point of note is that when they are grabbed around the knees, they will not have the muscle strength to prevent you from pinning their legs together. This means that they will be unable to try to wrap their legs around you to take you to ground.

Throws Against Armed Assailants

Another, less obvious reason to throw someone is as part of a weapon disarm. One of the quickest ways to get a person to release their grip on something—be it a knife, stick, or short- or long-barreled weapon—is to throw them. For untrained individuals, the natural response when they find themselves being thrown toward the floor is to put their hands out to protect themselves. As they do so, whatever they were holding or carrying will be released. This isn't a method of disarming I would advocate for all situations; however, there are times when it is extremely useful, such as when you want to disengage quickly from a situation and need to create some time to do so without getting caught up in a fight for the weapon, etc.

Hand Wheel Throw

You may return to your car to find a person who believes you took their parking spot waiting for you. They want to confront you about this, and put a knife to the side of your neck. Their manner may suggest that they are too emotional to be able to resolve the conflict peacefully, in which case you should recognize that you will need to deal with them physically.

Immediately lower your chin so that the blade is on your jawbone rather than on your neck.

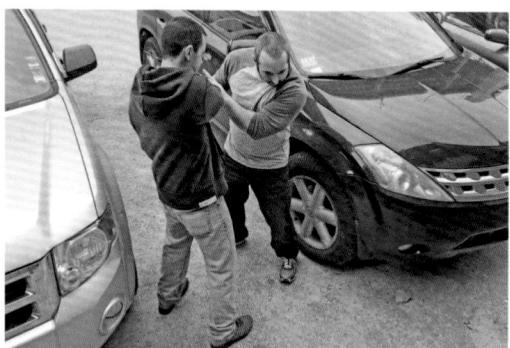

With a forceful strike, use your left hand to pat/push the knife away from your neck, while pulling your neck away from the knife (i.e., a hand defense coupled with a body defense). At the same time, start to move forward so that you can get behind the attacker's knife.

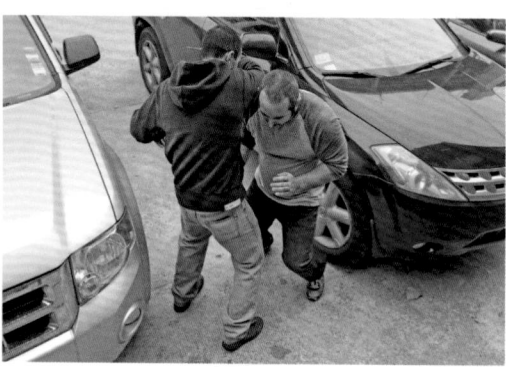

Stay close to your attacker's side so that if they try to make a reverse slash against your neck, you will be inside the arc of the slash. Also, because you will be looking to throw your assailant, you will want to be close to them.

With your right hand, make a strike to their groin and then thread your forearm between your assailant's legs. This is a distracting strike that will take their attention away from the weapon.

Step around to the side and slide your other arm between their legs. Each hand should grasp your opposite arm's wrist, creating a cradle that you can use to lift your attacker up.

While hugging your attacker's leg to your body, start to drive your hips forward and stand up. The goal here is not to lift them straight up, but to pivot them over your shoulder. You only need to lift them 5 or 8 inches off the ground to do this. Your hips should drive forward explosively. As soon as they are lifted/unbalanced, all thoughts about using the knife will go, as they will now have a new problem to deal with.

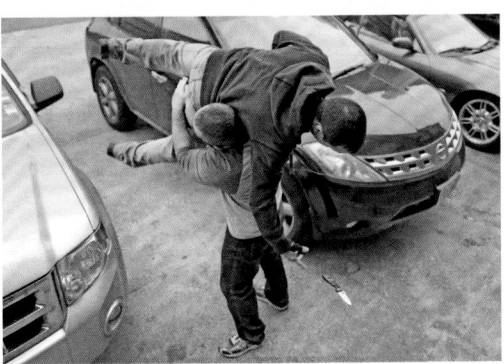

Once you have their ribcage at your shoulder height, start to pivot them onto and over your shoulder. At this point, all of their weight should be starting to shift forward, and they will begin to realize that there is only one direction in which they are heading—head first. This is probably when they will start to fully panic.

For many people, the natural response to finding themselves falling is to put their hands out in front of them, to help break their fall. This means they will instinctually let go of whatever it is they are holding, whether it is a knife, a stick, or a gun.

If you lean back slightly as you lift them, you will shift more of their weight forward and over your shoulder.

Continue to throw their legs up in the air as high as you can. This will add momentum to the throw and position their head toward the ground.

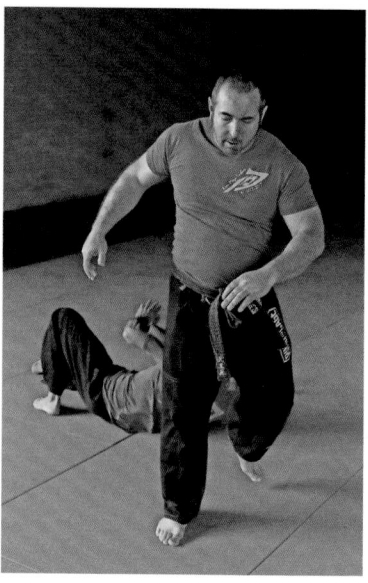

Even if they manage to make a break-fall, they will land heavily; on a hard surface such as concrete, their break-fall will merely reduce injury rather than preventing it.

As soon as there is no longer contact between you and your attacker, start to disengage. From start to finish, this throw should only take a few seconds, and is in fact a much faster solution than striking.

Don't look behind you to see what happens to your assailant. Simply trust that from the height they've been thrown, it will take them some time to recover—even if this merely consists of them taking a few moments to check themselves for injury.

This throw could also be used to deal with an assailant who is holding a firearm to your head (as in the next scenario), especially if it is a revolver, which, if you were to grab it as part of a "traditional disarm," could burn your hand if it went off.

Rear Throw

This is a heavy throw that gives your assailant little to no time in which to make a break-fall even if they have the knowledge and skill to do so. This throw is also extremely effective against larger and heavier people who you may feel are too big to be thrown with the "Hand Wheel Throw." With the rear throw, you don't need to actually lift your assailant into the air; you merely have to get them up onto their toes. The power of the throw comes not from the initial lift, but from your thigh sweeping into theirs and knocking them off their feet.

If you miss the opportunity to spoil the draw and find yourself with a gun pointed at your head, bring your hands up, level with the weapon. Your assailant will be expecting you to put your hands up, so this is not an unexpected movement. If the person had wanted to shoot you, they would have already done so; they are showing you the weapon for a reason—to get you to comply with their demand(s).

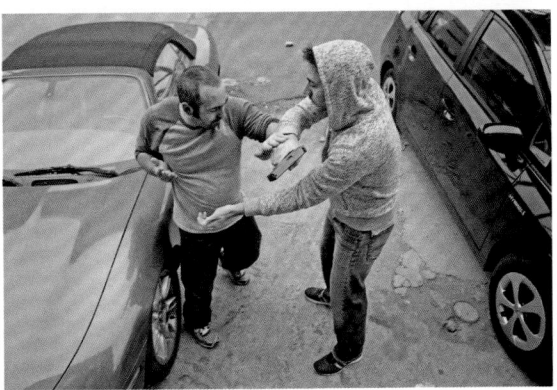

There are many reasons why you may choose not to try to control the gun, but rather knock it away, which is a much faster movement. This may be because you believe your assailant is trained/able to retain their weapon when they feel it being controlled. It may also be a firearm with a small frame, such as a snub-nosed revolver, which is difficult to get a good hold on, and which will burn your hand severely if your attacker pulls the trigger while you're holding it.

As you slap/strike your attacker's gun away, step forward so that you are behind the weapon, and deliver a groin strike with your other hand. In another situation/location it might be possible to simply disengage, getting distance, cover, and/or concealment; however, you may be in a situation where your escape routes don't allow this.

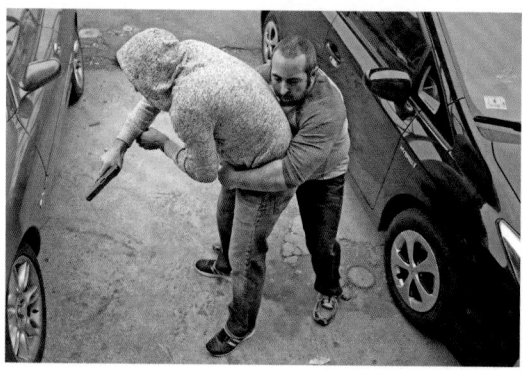

Spin around your attacker and bend your legs to get low—your hips need to be below your attacker's. Wrap your arms around your assailant, just below the waistline, and hug them to you. In this position, it would be extremely difficult for your attacker to turn the gun onto you.

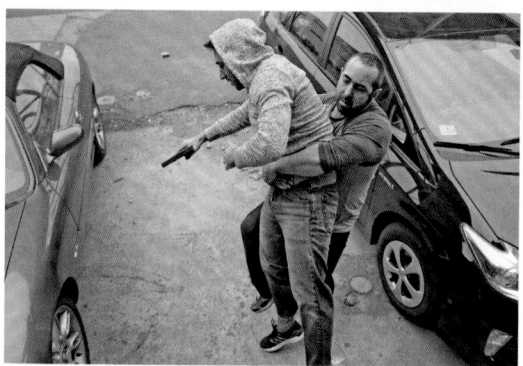

Drive forward with your hips and straighten up, while at the same time swinging your right leg into theirs. Your right thigh should connect with theirs, scooping the leg up.

With this throw, you don't even need to lift the person off the ground; you simply need to get them onto their toes so that your leg can sweep theirs away. This makes it a useful throw against much heavier assailants.

Keep scooping the leg until your attacker's body is parallel to the ground. It doesn't matter whether they release the gun or not, as they are likely to fall on to it if they don't. This is an extremely difficult throw from which to make an adequate break-fall, and most people will end up falling heavily on their shoulder and side, often with their arm under them.

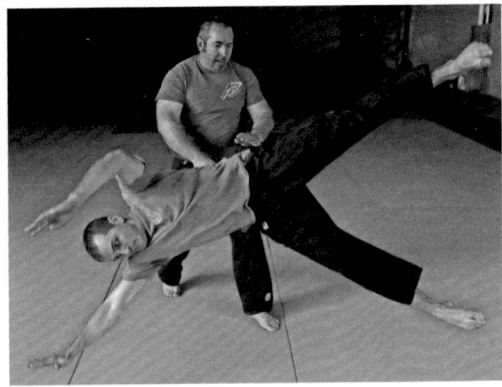

From this angle, you can get a better idea of what the throw looks like, and the level of contact between your leg and your assailant's. Your lifting and scooping actions are performed at exactly the same time. Don't lift the person up on their toes and then swing your leg; rather, do both simultaneously.

Due to the side-on nature of the fall and the speed at which you drop, the person being thrown will have little time and space to make an adequate break-fall, even if they have the training to do so.

The safest way to practice this technique is either to use a crash mat, or to return your partner back to their feet after you have scooped them up, rather than releasing them and allowing them to fall.

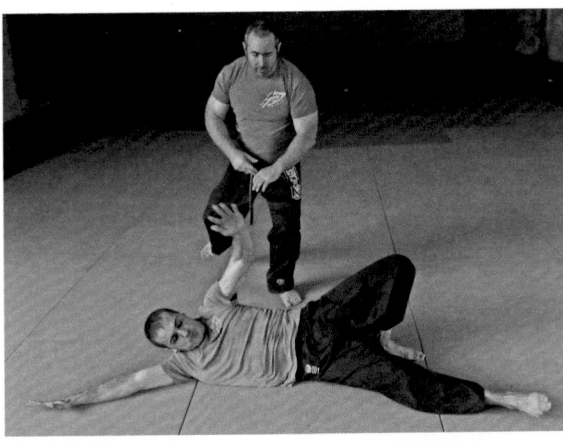

Once you have released your assailant, let them fall as you back away, scanning your environment. Don't waste time trying to access your vehicle. Leave the environment and return with law enforcement.

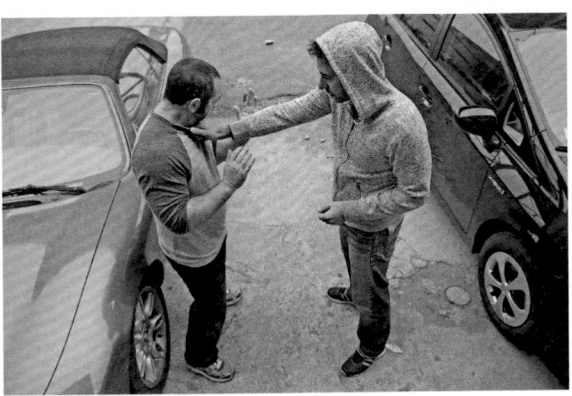

This same technique will work against an assailant who is holding a knife to the side of your throat. With your left hand, pat the knife arm away strongly (connecting at the wrist, where there is the most leverage) and make the groin strike with your right.

Many people put off throwing because they feel intimidated by having to face someone who is much bigger and heavier than them. This is something I can understand; however, I would point out that bigger people are usually less stable (due to being top-heavy) than shorter/smaller people, and once movement in one direction is created, they will have to shift more weight back in order to remain stable. This means that once you break a large person's balance, they have to work much harder, and put in more effort to ensure that they stay upright than a smaller, shorter person would. There is a lot to be said for the old adage, "The bigger they are, the harder they fall."

All of these throws result in very heavy falls, and for someone who doesn't know how to break their fall, they are as close as you can get to techniques which can conclusively finish a fight. If you throw someone, it is a clear indication of your superior fighting ability—both to the person being thrown as well as to anyone else who may be thinking of taking you on. While one might argue that you could make a "lucky" punch, there is no such thing as a lucky throw, and people understand this. In reality, it is likely that when you throw someone, they won't just land on the ground, but will fall onto tables, chairs, steps, and other objects, which will cause them more pain.

Sacrifice Throws

A sacrifice throw is one where you throw yourself to the ground as part of the execution of the throw. For real-life situations, this should not be your default option, as it is generally safer to stay on your feet. However, there are times when your attacker's movement and momentum don't allow you to remain standing, and you will find yourself being dragged or thrown to the ground. If this is the case, it is preferable to perform some kind of sacrifice throw so that you land safely and your attacker does not.

Rear Strangle to Ground

While your primary goal should be to stay on your feet, there are times when this is just not possible. When someone applies a rear strangle on you, it is best to perform the solution detailed in *Krav Maga: Real World Solutions to Real World Violence*. With this defense, you will remain on your feet and finish by disengaging from your attacker. However, attacks are dynamic, and it is not always possible to stay on your feet, especially if your assailant is dragging you backward—and potentially to the ground. When such assaults occur, you must be prepared to take the fight to the ground in a way that still leaves you in a dominant position.

Your first instinct when strangled will be to bring your hands up to your throat to pull your attacker's arm away so that you can clear your airway to breathe. One of the other problems you will likely have to contend with is the fact that your head will have been pulled backward so that it is now past your hips, putting you off-balance. If possible, you should try to take away your attacker's movement; to do this, lean your head on their shoulder and drive them backward. Sometimes, though, you won't be able to keep up with their movement and/or you may lose your footing. When this happens, you should be prepared to "sacrifice" yourself, and take them to ground with you.

As you are being pulled back and realize that you can't stay on your feet, your first move should be to step/move to the side. The last thing you want is to be dragged to the ground with your assailant directly behind you, where they can easily continue their attack and strangle you on the ground. Even if you have ended up on the ground, if you have moved to the side, your assailant will find it very difficult to make such an attack. Just as when you are fighting standing, when fighting on the ground, you don't want to give your attacker your back.

As you move to their side, slide the leg nearest to your assailant outward so that you can trip both of their legs with it. If you possess a bit more skill and timing, you can swing your leg into them so that it scythes/cuts them down and takes their legs from under them. If, at the same time, you can get hold of their clothing or pants legs and lift them upward as you do this, you will achieve a far more devastating throw.

If someone is strangling you, blocking your airway, your natural instinctive response will be to bring your hands up. This is also considered to be a "life-threatening attack"; if you don't clear it, your life will be in danger. Although your initial reaction may be to panic, strangling someone until they're unconscious in this way is a relatively long process. Because it is a life-threatening attack, Krav Maga principles dictate that you must "attack the attack."

Strongly and explosively tug your attacker's arm down as you drop down and step back under their armpit. You should be utilizing your large back muscles when you pull down on your attacker's arm. If you are successful, you will escape the strangle and end up behind your attacker. From here, you can either attack them or disengage. Sometimes, though, things can go wrong with this escape.

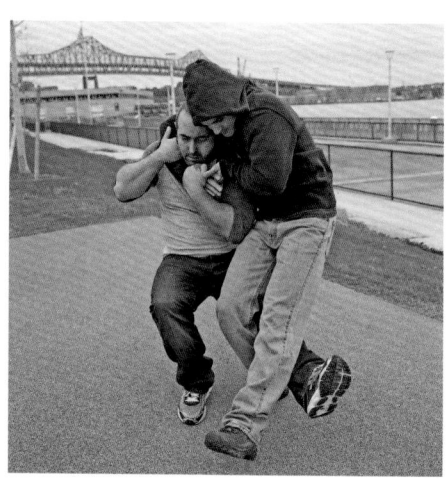

It could be that as you go to put your left foot down, your attacker starts to pull you in another direction, either to apply another hold or to try to prevent your escape. If this happens, you may find that you lose your balance before you can get your foot down. At this point, throw your left leg out behind both of your assailant's legs and start to sit down. If you have lost your balance, it is often easier to work with this movement rather than fight to regain stability.

Sit down and swing your leg into theirs, knocking their feet from under them. Continue to drop down as if you were going to sit on the floor. Rather than dropping straight back, fall at an angle (away from your attacker) so your attacker is pulled diagonally. This compromises their stability and makes the reaping action of your leg more effective.

Continue to drop, taking your assailant to the ground with you.

As you fall, your head will be protected by your assailant's arm, which will still be around the back of your neck. Once you've hit the ground, pin your attacker's upper arm to the ground with the back of your head. This will prevent your attacker from turning in to you and positioning themselves on top of you. As soon as you can, you should turn in to them.

As you turn, bring your left arm across their body to pin them, and strike their groin with your right hand. In all likelihood, the groin strike won't cause much actual pain due to the position you are in; however, it will focus your attacker's attention and momentarily take away any thoughts they may have of trying to control you.

Complete your turn so that you are now in a push-up position with your hands placed on your attacker's groin and torso. Your weight should be pinning them down. From here, extend your arms, explosively pushing off, until you are standing. Whenever you get up from the ground, if you are in contact with your attacker, you should use their body to support your weight and push off from.

Side Headlock to Ground

A common attack from the clinch position is the side headlock. Although it is a fairly unsophisticated attack, it is one that, if applied with sufficient force, can take you to ground. In *Krav Maga: Real World Solutions to Real World Violence*, I detailed how to prevent and escape from side headlocks when in a clinch situation. There are times, however, when your assailant will try to use a side headlock to take you to ground.

They may attempt this because they believe taking you to ground represents their best chance of dominating you, or because they know they have friends in the environment who will come and assist them. Although there are ways to prevent this from happening, sometimes the movement is so fast and hard that you are taken off-balance before you have the time to do anything to stabilize yourself. If you feel that you are already falling, and have little chance of staying on your feet, you will need to utilize your falling movement so that you can stay in control of the fight. Rather than fighting a losing battle to stay upright, you should instead go with your attacker's movement.

If you are going to be taken to ground, you should ensure that you go on your terms and end up in a dominant position that will allow you to get back to standing at the earliest, safest moment. While there are times that continuing to fight on the ground makes sense, in reality these are few and far between, and as a general rule you should try to get back to your feet as soon as possible. While you are on the ground, it will be difficult to deal with weapons or multiple assailants, and impossible to disengage to a place of safety—something that should always be your priority. While it is essential to know how to fight and survive on the ground, your goal should almost always be to get back to standing and disengage safely. How you end up on the ground will largely determine your ability to do this.

As your attacker tries to throw you to the ground, you should take advantage of the fact that, because they are tied up with you, they are also controlled by your movement. If you drop/roll close to them, they will end up being pulled directly down, which will unbalance them. If you combine this with a rolling movement, they will be pulled over you and find themselves being taken down to the ground, rather than taking you.

When someone attempts to put a side headlock on you, the simplest way to escape is to use one hand to strike the groin, using the other to "swim" over the shoulder to attack the eyes. Also, because with a side headlock you are pulled forward, you should take a step with your right leg to prevent yourself from being taken to ground.

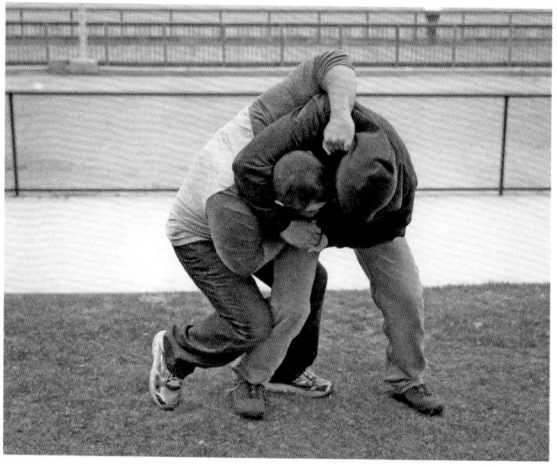

Unfortunately, sometimes the pull on your head is so strong that you either don't get the chance to make this step, or, as you make it, you are pulled down before your foot lands. Rather than resisting the pull, work with it, bending your forward knee as you start to turn your torso. If your assailant is committed to the headlock, they will be forced to come with you as you fall.

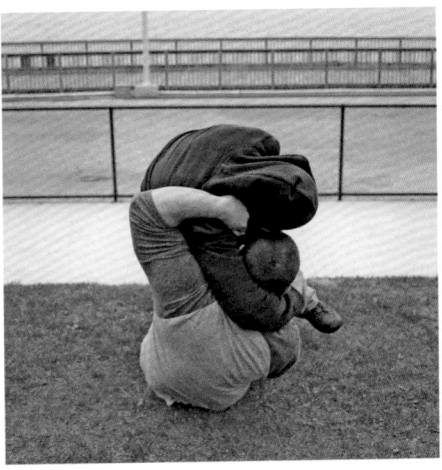

Keep turning and dropping. You are going to roll over your shoulders and upper back, with your attacker's arm protecting your head and ensuring that it doesn't come into contact with the ground.

The drop and roll will happen so fast that your attacker will be unable to let go, and will be forced to come with you. You are actually working with, and adding to, the initial force and movement that they were using to try to throw you to the ground.

Keep turning and rolling.

As you start to roll over your left shoulder and your attacker has moved past you, assist their movement by kicking and lifting their right leg with yours. This movement throws their leg over them and ensures that they keep rolling/moving.

Your attacker will now be in front of you. You should be thinking about starting to come up behind them so that you can take a dominant position and control them.

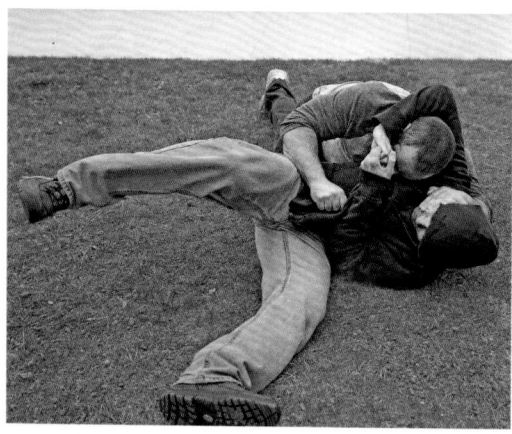

Keep your left hand on their face, pushing into their eyes, and move your right hand to the side of their body to keep them pinned down.

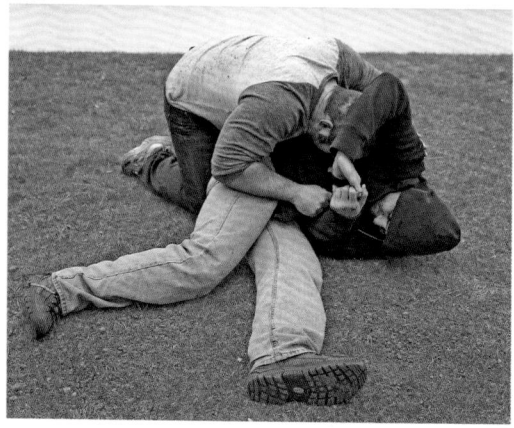

Bring your knees in and move your left hand to the back of your assailant's elbow/upper arm. Push the arm away from your head to free it from the lock.

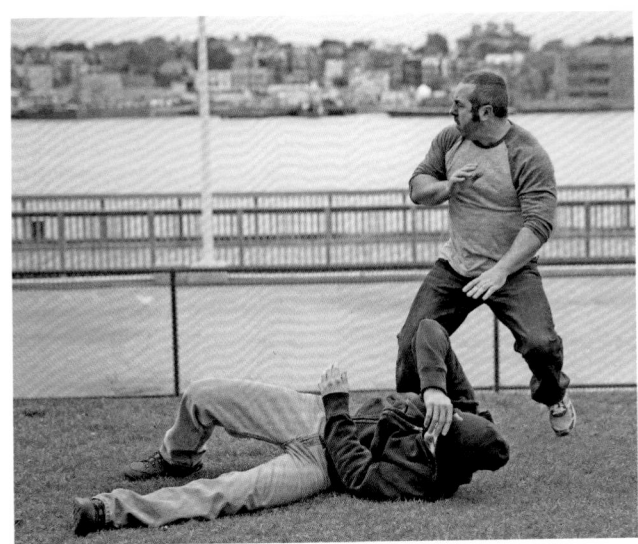

Immediately stand up and scan your environment as you back away.

How you go to ground is perhaps more important than what you do once you get there—though knowing how to fight and survive on the ground is an essential and important skillset to have. If someone can dominate and dictate the way you end up on the ground, it is likely that they will control the way the fight goes in this dimension. If they can't, it is likely that they will be the one who is controlled and dominated.

Conclusion

Real-world violence can be extremely simple to deal with—until it's not. A straight-forward solution to deal with an armed mugger is to control their weapon arm and punch them into unconsciousness, or strike them until you have the opportunity to disengage. This solution will work until you meet the pain-resistant assailant who is drunk, or on drugs, or who has been hit so many times before that your punches barely register with them. It will work until you're assaulted in a confined space where disengagement isn't an option, or in a location where you have little to no room to move (such as on an escalator, or in an elevator). These may be factors you've never experienced in a training environment, and so haven't had to consider them. However, they are regular occurrences in real-life situations and need to be thought about and rehearsed. It is all too easy to fall into the trap of believing reality will reflect your training environment. Unfortunately, this isn't often the case—if you train in an open, uncluttered mat space with plenty of room to move, it would be dangerous to assume that you will have the same amount of space in a real-life confrontation. It would be incorrect and dangerous to assume that an assailant won't continue to assault you after you've disarmed them of a weapon, and/or that every firearm you face will be real, loaded, and operable. You need to be prepared for these eventualities and realities. Rather than just practicing Krav Maga techniques, you need to rehearse real-life scenarios, developing your threat recognition and decision-making skills as well as your physical techniques, so that you understand the context of real-life assaults. This is how you will learn to get your Krav Maga to work for you, which should be your goal. Unfortunately, "knowing" Krav Maga is not enough.

If you train regularly, the assailants you are likely to face in real life will prob-ably not be as physically skillful as you are, or as fit/athletic as you are, yet they may have had a lifetime of being successful at what they do—not because of their phys-ical prowess, but because they know how to orchestrate situations to their advan-tage. The mugger who demands your wallet may well be in a state of withdrawal (most muggings are to support a drug habit), may not have slept for several days or eaten properly in weeks. Yet, even in this reduced physical state, they will have an advantage over you—they understand and know how to use violence; they are prepared to act without conscience; have little or no fear of the legal consequences of their actions; and they believe they are entitled to do whatever they want. They don't rely on physical prowess and abilities; they rely on their understanding of how to play every component in a confrontation to their advantage. They know how to limit any time and space that you may have so you can't respond, how to control and limit your movement, etc. They know how to reduce your ability to fight down to zero. Unless you know how to counter these things, it doesn't matter how much you train your physical techniques and solutions; you will never have the chance to employ them.

By understanding how violent situations occur and develop, you will be able to predict, identify, prevent, and avoid most violent situations; and if not, you will be able to set things up in the environment to be in your favor. This is the way you will get your Krav Maga techniques to work. To do this, though, you need to train yourself in the early identification of threats, how to position yourself relative to your aggressor(s), how to use the environment/geography to your advantage, etc. This means training your Krav Maga in context and in scenarios rather than just mechanically practicing techniques. Train not just to be the person that "knows" Krav Maga, but to be the person who knows how and when to use it. In the real world, you won't have the luxury not to.

Dedication

To Andy Rallings, a true martial artist—your friendship, input, contributions, and conversations over the years are truly valued.

Acknowledgments

Writing acknowledgements is always a difficult thing, as one always fears leaving out those who have played a part in the development of the book, even if their contribution was an indirect one. Probably the largest group of indirect contributors to the book have been the students at my schools, who, through their successes and challenges with techniques and solutions, have helped me evolve, refine, and develop the system that I teach, which is reflected in this book.

I would also like to take this opportunity to thank all of my instructors who have taken the time and the effort over the years to help develop me as a martial artist and a person. A special thanks goes to Miki Assulin (one of Imi Lichtenfeld's original black belts who was there from the beginning) for his training and teaching, and for giving me a window into the methods, instruction, intent, and original philosophy of Imi's Krav Maga. I'm indebted to Miki's honesty and integrity concerning his teaching of Krav Maga, and the fact that he has stayed true to the values of the method when many others have promoted themselves over the system. I would like to thank Miki for writing the foreword, and Oren Rippel for translating it from the Hebrew.

As always, special thanks goes to Andy Rallings, for both taking some heavy knocks and falls in the making of the book, and for always making himself available for these projects. His technical contribution over the years has been phenomenal and essential, and I am proud to be associated with him and the SEPS (Situation Effective Protection System) self-protection system that we developed together.

This book would not have been possible without the photography of Colin O'Reilly. His ability to capture the essence of the techniques when performed at full speed is truly remarkable, and I believe it is one of the major factors which distinguishes this book among self-defense instructional manuals. Colin has been a valued supporter of the system since he first came to train at Krav Maga Yashir Boston, and we are grateful for his efforts, both in the long days of shooting and the tireless editing of each photo afterwards. We could not have hoped to be in better hands.

I would like to thank Efe Atabay for taking some heavy falls (repeatedly) in the throwing section of the book (and for the conversations we have had over the technical aspects, the philosophy and ideas behind the martial arts, etc.); to Scott Campeau and Nick Zagami (who also provided the drawings in the section on de-escalation) for allowing me to kick them over and over again, without complaint; and to Carter Briggs for sustaining the longest bar fight of his life while playing the thankless role of antagonist. I would also like to thank Pat Gagnon for his enthusiastic support and willingness to do whatever is needed to help the school—in this case, managing to get a photo of a revolver expelling hot gases upon being fired.

A big thank you to Mike Merchant, who organized the shoot at Eddie C's bar in East Boston, and to Eddie Contilli, Jr., and the Contilli family for letting us use the bar to film in. The use of real locations to shoot the photographs in is one of the things which helps demonstrate the authenticity of the techniques shown.

Last but not least, this book would not be the book it is without the tireless editing provided by Liz Berrien, whose rewrites and revisions give the writing a flow that would otherwise not be present. Her contributions to this, the previous book, and other projects, and her ethic of the "good being the enemy of best," are truly appreciated.

ABOUT TUTTLE
"Books to Span the East and West"

Our core mission at Tuttle Publishing is to create books which bring people together one page at a time. Tuttle was founded in 1832 in the small New England town of Rutland, Vermont (USA). Our fundamental values remain as strong today as they were then—to publish best-in-class books informing the English-speaking world about the countries and peoples of Asia. The world has become a smaller place today and Asia's economic, cultural and political influence has expanded, yet the need for meaningful dialogue and information about this diverse region has never been greater. Since 1948, Tuttle has been a leader in publishing books on the cultures, arts, cuisines, languages and literatures of Asia. Our authors and photographers have won numerous awards and Tuttle has published thousands of books on subjects ranging from martial arts to paper crafts. We welcome you to explore the wealth of information available on Asia at **www.tuttlepublishing.com**.